Dear Colleagues:

This book, *Use and Interpretation of Tests in Clinical Immunology,* often referred to as the "SLI Green Book", is a succinct review of the latest information regarding the pathogenesis, diagnosis and normal or aberrant immune responses to infectious diseases.

Since Specialty Laboratories/Cytometrics' previous publication of this work in 1989, we have:

- incorporated significant developments in the field of immunology,

- added information on new techniques when they contribute to better understanding of the mechanisms of disease and immune response, and

- improved consistency of terminology and ease-of-use for all audiences referring to this booklet.

We welcome your comments and suggestions for improvements in our publications and resource materials. Please use the enclosed postage-paid card to request copies of SLI/Cytometrics' publications, including: the 1990-91 Fee Schedule, and educational booklets.

James B. Peter, M.D., Ph.D.

DEDICATION AND ACKNOWLEDGEMENTS

This book is dedicated to all those involved in the quest for greater understanding and control of the human immune system. Members of the research team at Specialty Laboratories, Inc. (SLI) are dedicated to keeping our Laboratories at the cutting edge of the rapidly changing field of clinical immunology. This booklet is our contribution to the challenging task of keeping up with the exciting advances in knowledge that are taking place every day. Dissemination of that knowledge is critical to the well-being of our ultimate clients--your patients.

The research and support staffs of SLI were instrumental in aiding the ongoing review of literature and synthesis of ideas that make updating a book of this nature possible. The author gratefully acknowledges the library support of Jui-lan Liu and Chris Ford, the excellent typing of Rose Yesowitch and Cassandra Brown and the publication design/coordination of Nancy Campman and Marion Logan, as well as the expert work of our publishers, Interstate Press, Omaha NE.

PREFACE

All those who participate in the care of patients know how explosively the field of clinical immunology is changing. This book is intended as a vade mecum to the incisive use and interpretation of the many assays now available for the detection of humoral and cell-mediated immune response to disease and for the evaluation of patients with immune disorders.

A **METHODOLOGIES and ABBREVIATIONS** Section which provides brief descriptions of diagnostic methods and a list of abbreviations is appended. The **INDEX** provides an alphabetical reference to the subjects and diseases mentioned in the text.

A tear-out card at the back of this text lists additional publications and resources available from Specialty Laboratories, Inc. Please fill out the card if you would like to be on the mailing list for the yearly updates of this booklet.

> *USE AND INTERPRETATION OF TESTS IN CLINICAL IMMUNOLOGY* is designed as an EDUCATIONAL and REFERENCE tool. For information on availability of specific tests, please contact the Specialty Laboratories Inc. Client Services Department: 2211 Michigan Avenue, Santa Monica, CA 90404-3900; (800) 421-7110, FAX (213) 828-6634.

ACETALDEHYDE ADDUCT ANTIBODIES

Present in approximately 73% of alcoholics and in 39% of nonalcoholic liver disease (e.g., primary biliary cirrhosis, chronic active hepatitis; acute viral and drug-induced hepatitis), the highest titers of acetaldehyde adduct antibodies are seen in the advanced stages of alcoholic and nonalcoholic liver disease.[1]

REFERENCES:
1. Hoerner M, Behrens UJ, Worner TM, et al. The role of alcoholism and liver disease in the appearance of serum antibodies against acetaldehyde adducts. Hepatology 1988;8:569-74.

ACETYLCHOLINE RECEPTOR ANTIBODIES

AChR *binding antibodies* (i.e., antibodies reactive with several epitopes other than the binding site for ACh or α-bungarotoxin) are present in approximately 88% of patients with generalized myasthenia gravis (MG),[1-3] possibly 63% of ocular myasthenia and in approximately 58% of MG in remission.[3] AChR *blocking antibodies* (i.e., antibodies reactive with the AChR binding site) are present in about 50% of patients with MG and are the only anti-AChR present in about 1% of MG.[3] AChR *modulating antibodies* (i.e., antibodies which crosslink AChRs and cause their removal from muscle membrane surfaces) are present in more than 90% of MG and occasionally are the only AChRA detectable.[1-3] AChRA of one or more types are reported to be found in at least 80% of ocular MG.[3] Approximately 1% of patients with rheumatoid arthritis being treated with D-penicillamine develop AChRA and MG, both of which disappear when the drug is discontinued.[4] Myasthenia gravis and antibodies to AChR are found occasionally in patients after bone marrow grafts for aplastic anemia and for acute nonlymphocytic leukemia.[5] One patient with motor neuron disease and AChRA was reported.[6] Antibodies to filamin were found in 100% of patients with ocular myasthenia[7], but confirmation of this work has not yet appeared. The characteristics of some AChRA-negative patients with MG have been described,[8] as having the characteristics of neonatal MG[9,10] and the characteristics of patients with thymoma and AChRA in the absence of MG.[11] Well-standardized methods for assay of AChRA are now available.[12] Epitopes of AChR that play a specific role in MG are being recognized.[13] Assays for AChR are useful for monitoring individual patients.[14]

REFERENCES:
1. Vincent A, Newsom-Davis J. Acetylcholine receptor antibody as a diagnostic test for myasthenia gravis: results in 153 validated cases and 2967 diagnostic assays. J Neurosurg Psychiatry 1985;48:1246-52.
2. Anonymous. The diagnosis of myasthenia gravis [Editorial]. Lancet 1986;1:658-60.
3. Lennon VA, Howard FM. Serologic diagnosis of myasthenia gravis. In: Nakamura RM, O'Sullivan MB, eds. Clinical laboratory molecular analyses. New York: Grune & Stratton, 1985;29-44.
4. Masters CL, Dawkins RL, Zilko PJ, et al. Penicillamine-associated myasthenia gravis, antiacetylcholine receptor and antistriational antibodies. Am J Med 1977;63:689-94.
5. Lefvert AK, Björkholm M. Antibodies against the acetylcholine receptor in hematologic disorders: implications for the development of myasthenia gravis after bone marrow grafting [Letter]. N Engl J Med 1987;317:170.
6. Abbott RJ, Holder D, Currie S. False positive anti-acetylcholine receptor antibodies in motorneuron disease [Letter]. Lancet 1986;1:906-7.
7. Yamamoto T, Sato T, Sugita H. Antifilamin, antivinculin, and antitropomyosin antibodies in myasthenia gravis. Neurology 1987;37:1329-33.
8. Soliven BC, Lange DJ, Penn AS, et al. Seronegative myasthenia gravis. Neurology 1988;38:514-7.
9. Morel E, Eymard B, Vernet-der Garabedian B, Pannier C, Dulac O, Bach JF. Neonatal myasthenia gravis: a new clinical and immunologic appraisal on 30 cases. Neurology 1988;38:138-42.
10. Melber D. Maternal-fetal transmission of myasthenia gravis with acetylcholine-receptor antibody [Letter]. Lancet 1988;1:996.
11. Cuénoud S, Feltkamp TEW, Fulpius BW, Oosterhuis HJGH. Antibodies to acetylcholine receptor in patients with thymoma but without myasthenia gravis. Neurology 1980;30:201-3.

12. Bonifacio E, Cobain TJ, Dawkins RL, et al. Comparison and standardization of measurement of anti-acetylcholine receptor antibody between laboratories. Autoimmunity 1988;1:59-66.
13. Brocke S, Brautbar C, Steinman L, et al. In vitro proliferative responses and antibody titers specific to human acetylcholine receptor synthetic peptides in patients with myasthenia gravis and relation to HLA class II genes. J Clin Invest 1988;82:1894-900.
14. Dawkins RL, Garlepp MJ. Autoimmune diseases of muscle: myasthenia gravis and myositis. In: Rose NR, Mackay IR, eds. The autoimmune diseases. Sydney: Academic Press, 1985:591-615.

ACUTE-PHASE PROTEINS

Which of these plasma proteins (in addition to fibrinogen) that increase 25% or more in response to inflammation and injury is under direct control of IL-6 (hepatocyte-stimulating factor) is not yet known. Other proteins which increase to varying degrees and at varying rates are ceruloplasmin, C3 and C4 (increase 50% or more); α-1 acid glycoprotein, α-1 antitrypsin, haptoglobin and fibrinogen (increase 2-4 fold); CRP and SS-A (increase several hundred fold). A recent detailed discussion of assays for CRP, SAA, ESR and viscosity was a disappointment, because data on clinical utility/predictive values of these assays in specific situations were not available.[1] Quantitation of serum CRP by rate nephelometry is expected to provide useful predictive values. See also **AMYLOID, C-REACTIVE PROTEIN, ERYTHROCYTE SEDIMENTATION RATE** and **VISCOSITY**.

REFERENCES:
1. Brahn E, Scoville CD. Biochemical markers of disease activity. Baillieres Clin Rheum 1988;2:153-83.

ADRENAL ANTIBODIES

Found in the majority of patients with idiopathic Addison disease[1-4] but only in a minority of patients with tuberculous adrenal insufficiency,[4] anti-adrenal antibodies (AAA) are detected by IFA or RIA (labeled adrenal microsomes). In females with normal adrenocortical function, AAA have very high sensitivity, specificity and predictive value for development of adrenocortical failure;[3] lower predictive values are found in non-Addisonian patients when tested for complement-fixing adrenal autoantibodies[4] and by IFA using ox adrenals[5] which are a less sensitive substrate. Some of the anti-adrenal antibodies in Addison disease react with the corticotrophin (ACTH) receptor and block the effect of ACTH on adrenal cortical cells.[6] Some AAA react with plasma membranes and others with microsomes.[7] See also **CORTICOTROPHIN RECEPTOR ANTIBODIES** and **STEROID CELL ANTIBODIES**.

REFERENCES:
1. Nerup J. Addison's disease—serological studies. Acta Endocrinologica 1974;76:142-58.
2. Kosowicz J, Gryczynska M, Bottazzo GF. A radioimmunoassay for the detection of adrenal autoantibodies. Clin Exp Immunol 1986;63:671-9.
3. Ahonen P, Miettinen A, Perheentupa J. Adrenal and steroidal cell antibodies in patients with autoimmune polyglandular disease type I and risk of adrenocortical and ovarian failure. J Clin Endocrinol Metab 1987;64:494-500.
4. Betterle C, Zanette F, Zanchetta R, et al. Complement-fixing adrenal autoantibodies as a marker for predicting onset of idiopathic Addison's disease. Lancet 1983;1:1238-40.
5. Eason RJ, Croxson MS, Perry MC, Somerfield SD. Addison's disease, adrenal autoantibodies and computerised adrenal tomography. N Z Med J 1982;95:569-73.
6. Kendall-Taylor P, Lambert A, Mitchell R, Robertson WR. Antibody that blocks stimulation of cortisol secretion by adrenocorticotrophic hormone in Addison's disease. Br Med J 1988;296:1489-91.
7. Bright GM, Singh I. Adrenal autoantibodies bind to adrenal subcellular fractions enriched in cytochrome-c reductase and 5 '-nucleotidase. J Clin Endocrinol Metab 1990;70:95-100.

AH50

Hemolytic activity of the alternate pathway (AP) is measured as AH50. This assay is useful as a screen for homozygous deficiencies of components of the AP, including C3, factor I (which causes a secondary deficiency of C3) and probably factor H. Deficiencies of factors I or H, which are regulatory proteins of the AP, cause secondary deficiency of other complement components (C3) in the same way that deficiency of C1 INH (a regulatory protein of the CP) causes secondary deficiency of C4. Absence of hemolysis in CH50 and normal AH50 suggests deficiency of an early component of the CP including C1, C2 or C4.[1,2] Plasma levels of factor Ba and SC5b-9 may be better indices of activity of SLE than are C3 or C4.[3] Activity of complement factor D of the alternative pathway resembles adipsia (the serine protease of adipocytes) in its cleavage of complement factor B complexed with activated complement component C3.[4] Activities of adipsia/complement factor D are decreased 58-80% in several experimental models of obesity.[4] Complement deficiency of factor D is associated with recurrent Neisseria infections.[5] Homozygous complete deficiency of complement factor H is associated with glomerulonephritis, recurrent meningococcal meningitis, hemolytic uremic syndrome, SLE or good health.[6] One or more components of the classical and alternate pathways are decreased in patients with multiple myeloma; elevations of the Bb fragment suggest that *in vivo* activation is a likely method for the occasional decreases seen in AH50.[7] See also **CH50, C3a, C4a & C5a and ANAPHYLATOXINS; COMPLEMENT SPLIT PRODUCTS (C4d, Ba and C3dg) and MEMBRANE ATTACK COMPLEX.**

REFERENCES:
1. Dalmasso AP. Complement in the pathophysiology and diagnosis of human diseases. CRC Crit Review Clin Lab Sci 1986;24:123-83.
2. Tucker ES III. Complement activation in autoimmune disease. J Clin Immunoassay 1984;7:310-20.
3. Petri M, Kolb W, Morrow P, Tamerius J. Association of complement activation tests with clinical measures of lupus activity [Abstract]. Clin Res 1989;37:510A.
4. Rosen BS, Cook KS, Yaglom J, et al. Adipsin and complement factor D activity: an immune-related defect in obesity. Science 1989;244:1483-7.
5. Hiemstra PS, Langeler E, Compier B, et al. Complete and partial deficiencies of complement factor D in a Dutch family. J Clin Invest 1989;84:1957-61.
6. Nielsen HE, Christensen KC, Koch C, Thomsen BS, Heegaard NHH, Tranum-Jensen J. Hereditary, complete deficiency of complement factor H associated with recurrent meningococcal disease. Scand J Immunol 1989;30:711-8.
7. Zurlo JJ, Schechter GP, Fries LF. Complement abnormalities in multiple myeloma. Am J Med 1989;87:411-20.

ALANYL-tRNA SYNTHETASE ANTIBODIES
Antibodies to alanyl-tRNA synthetase and alanine tRNA are quite rare but, as with other antisynthetase, are usually associated with myositis, arthritis and interstitial lung disease as seen in the Jo-1 syndrome.[1-3]

REFERENCES:
1. Bunn CC, Bernstein RM, Mathews MB. Autoantibodies against alanyl-tRNA synthetase and tRNA^{Ala} coexist and are associated with myositis. J Exp Med 1986;163:1281-91.
2. Bunn CC, Mathews MB. Autoreactive epitope defined as the anticodon region of alanine transfer RNA. Science 1987;238:1116-9.
3. Targoff IN, Arnett FC. Clinical manifestations in patients with antibody to PL-12 antigen (alanyl-tRNA synthetase). Am J Med 1990;88:241-51.

ALPHA₁-ANTITRYPSIN (α1AT)
α1AT is best referred to as α1 protease inhibitor (α1Pi) because it inhibits trypsin, elastin and several other proteases.[1-4] α1AT deficiency is an autosomal recessive disease characterized by reduced serum levels of α1AT (an inhibitor of neutrophil elastase which accounts for 90% of the anti-neutrophil elastase of the lower respiratory tract). This deficiency causes a smoking-accelerated panacinar emphysema in the third to fourth decades and accounts for approximately 2% of the 2 million patients with emphysema in the U.S.[1-4] α1AT-deficient patients typically have less than 50 mg α1AT/dL. Approximately 15% of neonates with the ZZ phenotype of α1AT (gene frequency of 0.03) develop hepatitis; 25% of these develop obstructive jaundice and cirrhosis and die before age 8.[5] About 9% of adults with nonalcoholic cirrhosis are MZ phenotype.[6]

REFERENCES:
1. Hubbard RC, Sellers S, Czerski D, et al. Biochemical efficacy and safety of monthly augmentation therapy for α1-antitrypsin deficiency. JAMA 1988;260:1259-64.
2. Anonymous. Proteases, antiproteases, and emphysema [Editorial]. Lancet 1987;2:832-3.
3. Pierce JA. Antitrypsin and emphysema: perspective and prospects [Editorial]. JAMA 1988;259:2890-5.
4. Crystal RG. The α1-antitrypsin gene and its deficiency states. Trends Gen 1989;5:411-7.
5. Dycaico MJ, Grant SGN, Felts K, et al. Neonatal hepatitis induced by α1-antitrypsin: a transgenic mouse model. Science 1988;242:1409-12.
6. Hodges JR, Millward-Sadler GH, Barbatis C, Wright R. Heterozygous MZ alpha1-antitrypsin deficiency in adults with chronic active hepatitis and cryptogenic cirrhosis. N Engl J Med 1981;304:557-60.

ALPHA$_1$-MICROGLOBULIN

α_1-M (also known as protein HC) is a 30 kd protein found in urine and serum, in which some α_1-M is present as monomeric IgA-α_1M complexes,[1] which can be elevated in IgA nephropathy.[2,3]

REFERENCES
1. Itoh Y, Kawai T. Human α_1-microglobulin: its measurement and clinical significance. J Clin Lab Analysis 1990;4:376-84.
2. Vincent C, Bouic P, Marceau M, et al. Alpha-1 microglobulin in IgA nephropathies. In: Revillard JP, Voisin C, Wierzbicki N, eds. Mucosal immunity. Fondation Franco-Allemande, Suresnes, 1985:188-90.
3. Murakami T, Kawakami H, Kobayashi K, Itoh Y. Glomerular alpha-1-microglobulin in IgA nephropathies. Am J Nephrol 1989;9:438-9.

ALPHA$_2$-PLASMIN INHIBITOR-PLASMIN COMPLEXES (α_2-PIPC)

α2-PIPC are rapidly formed when α2-PI (or α2-macroglobulin) combine with plasmin, the putative active component of the fibrinolytic process.[1] Although present in increased amounts in plasma of patients with vasculitis of SLE compared to SLE without vasculitis, the levels of α2-PIPC overlap greatly,[2] and the assay is not promising clinically.

REFERENCES:
1. Aoki N, Harpel PC. Inhibitors of the fibrinolytic enzyme system. Semin Thromb Hemost 1984;10:24-41.
2. Kawakami M, Kawagoe M, Harigai M, et al. Elevated plasma levels of α2-plasmin inhibitor-plasmin complex in patients with rheumatic diseases. Possible role of fibrinolytic mechanism in vasculitis. Arthritis Rheum 1989;32:1427-33.

ALVEOLAR BASEMENT MEMBRANE ANTIBODIES

Antibodies reactive with human alveolar basement membrane (ABM) are found in sera of patients with rapidly progressive glomerulonephritis and pulmonary hemorrhage (Goodpasture syndrome), and in sera from patients with anti-glomerular basement membrane (GBM) nephritis alone.[1] Different reactivities with ABM might explain why only some patients with anti-GBM nephritis have pulmonary involvement.

REFERENCES:
1. Yoshioka K, Iseki T, Okada M, et al. Identification of Goodpasture antigens in human alveolar basement membrane. Clin Exp Immunol 1988;74:419-26.

AMYLIN

Amylin (islet amyloid polypeptide), a 37-amino acid peptide found in the normal or the diabetic pancreas, is a major component of islet amyloid from patients with non-insulin-dependent diabetes mellitus (NIDDM), having been processed from proamylin by proteolysis at the N and C termini.[1] A potent inhibitor of glycogen synthesis in skeletal muscle,[2] amylin has an amino acid sequence which is 43-46% identical to the calcitonin gene-related peptides (CGRP1 and CGRP2). Serum amylin is said to be increased in NIDDM[3,4] and decreased in IDDM.[5]

REFERENCES:
1. Roberts AN, Leighton B, Todd JA, et al. Molecular and functional characterization of amylin, a peptide associated with type 2 diabetes mellitus. Proc Natl Acad Sci USA 1989;86:9662-6.
2. Cooper GJS, Willis AC, Clark A, et al. Purification and characterization of a peptide from amyloid-rich pancreases of type 2 diabetic patients. Proc Natl Acad Sci USA 1987;84:8628-32.
3. Leighton B, Cooper GJS. Pancreatic amylin and calcitonin gene-related peptide cause resistance to insulin in skeletal muscle in vitro. Nature 1988;335:632-5.
4. Cooper GJS, Leighton B, Dimitriadis GD, et al. Amylin found in amyloid deposits in human type 2 diabetes mellitus may be a hormone that regulates glycogen metabolism in skeletal muscle. Proc Natl Acad Sci USA 1988;85:7763-6.
5. Hartter E, Svoboda T, Lell B, et al. Reduced islet-amyloid polypeptide in insulin-dependent diabetes mellitus [Letter]. Lancet 1990;1:854.

AMYLOID

Amyloid, a group of proteinaceous materials with distinctive tinctorial features (birefringence with Congo red stain) ultrastructural characteristics (fibrillar structure by polarization microscopy and electron microscopy) and tertiary structure (β-pleats by x-ray crystallography), is associated with a variety of clinical syndromes in which it accumulates in different vessels and tissues. Amyloid A, the unique 76 amino acid amyloid protein which is the amino terminal two-thirds of a normal acute-phase serum protein (apoSSA), is associated with all types of amyloidosis previously referred to as secondary as well as with familial Mediterranean fever and the amyloid of renal cell carcinoma and Hodgkin disease. Amyloid L protein (AL), which is composed of NH_2-terminal portions of immunoglobulin light chains ($\varkappa$ or λ) found in patients with monoclonal plasma cell dyscrasia[1] and localized amyloidosis in bladder and lung.[1] AL is also distinct from amyloid F (AF), which is composed of transthyretin (TTR, prealbumin); mutated forms of TTR are found in the amyloid fibrils of the seven or eight types of familial amyloidosis (including familial amyloidotic polyneuropathy), whereas the primary structure of TTR is normal in senile systemic amyloidosis.[2] Other forms of amyloid include: amylin (islet amyloid polypeptide), a 37-amino acid peptide of which a decapeptide is important in amyloid fibril formation in NIDDM;[3] isolated atrial amyloid (IAA), composed of atrial natriuretic factor; β_2-microglobulin amyloid ($A\beta_2M$) which accumulates in joints and ligaments in dialysis patients; amyloid E (AE), which is composed of calcitonin in medullary thyroid cancer; cerebral angiopathy amyloid (CAA) or A4 or amyloid β-protein ($A\beta$ P), which is seen in blood vessels, neurofibrillary tangles[4] and plaques[5] of Alzheimer disease and Down syndrome. The subunit of cerebral amyloid called A4 or β is derived from protease nexin II/amyloid protein precursor (APP) found in platelet α-granules.[6] The ratios of different-sized fragments of $A\beta P$ change with aging and especially in Alzheimer disease.[7] A mutated form of $A\beta P$ is found in the Dutch type of hereditary cerebral hemorrhage with amyloidosis.[8] Normal processing of APP, which includes cleavage of APP in the interior of $A\beta P$, may prevent $A\beta P$ deposition.[9] The P-component amyloid (AP) is bound to most amyloid fibrils and is identical to a plasma protein (AP); the role of AP in amyloid formation is not known.[10]

At present, at least 12 different proteins are recognized components of different forms of amyloid,[11] including the recently described heavy-chain-related form of immunoglobulin-associated amyloidosis, tentatively designated AH amyloidosis.[12]

Immunoelectrophoresis (or immunofixation) of serum and urine is indicated in patients with unexplained cardiomyopathy, carpal tunnel syndrome, hepatomegaly, nephrotic syndrome, muscular pseudohypertrophy (shoulder pad sign or hip pad sign), peripheral or autonomic neuropathy, plasmacytosis and purpura. Biopsy of bone marrow, rectal mucosa or subcutaneous fat is often diagnostic.[1]

Thought to be a precursor of amyloid fibrils, serum amyloid A (SAA), the synthesis of which is stimulated by IL-1 and IL-6 as an acute-phase response, is of research interest,[13] but its assay[14] has no clinical utility at present. For additional information on **AMYLOID**, see **PRIONS** in reference 15. See also **AMYLIN** and **MONOCLONAL IMMUNOGLOBULIN DEPOSITION DISEASE (MIDD)**.

REFERENCES:
1. Gertz MA, Kyle RA. Primary systemic amyloidosis - a diagnostic primer. Mayo Clin Proc 1989;64:1505-19.
2. Westermark P, Sletten K, Johansson B, Cornwell GG III. Fibril in senile systemic amyloidosis is derived from normal transthyretin. Proc Natl Acad Sci USA 1990;87:2843-5.
3. Westermark P, Engström U, Johnson KH, et al. Islet amyloid polypeptide: pinpointing amino acid residues linked to amyloid fibril formation. Proc Natl Acad Sci USA 1990;87:5036-40.
4. Spillantini MG, Goedert M, Jakes R, Klug A. Different configurational states of β-amyloid and their distributions relative to plaques and tangles in Alzheimer disease. Proc Natl Acad Sci USA 1990;87:3947-51.
5. Spillantini MG, Goedert M, Jakes R, Klug A. Topographical relationship between β-amyloid and tau protein epitopes in tangle-bearing cells in Alzheimer disease. Proc Natl Acad Sci USA 1990;87:3952-6.
6. Van Nostrand WE, Schmaier AH, Farrow JS, Cunningham DD. Protease nexin-II (amyloid β-protein precursor): a platelet α-granule protein. Science 1990;248:745-48.
7. Palmert MR, Usiak M, Mayeux R, et al. Soluble derivatives of the β amyloid protein precursor in cerebrospinal fluid: alterations in normal aging and in Alzheimer's disease. Neurology 1990;40:1028-34.
8. Levy E, Carman MD, Fernandez-Madrid IJ, et al. Mutation of the Alzheimer's Disease amyloid gene in hereditary cerebral hemorrhage, Dutch type. Science 1990;248:1124-6.
9. Esch FS, Keim PS, Beattie EC, et al. Cleavage of amyloid β peptide during constitutive processing of its precursor. Science 1990;248:1122-4.
10. Hawkins PN. Amyloidosis. Blood Rev 1988;2:270-80.
11. Stone MJ. Amyloidosis: a final common pathway for protein deposition in tissues. Blood 1990;75:531-45.
12. Eulitz M, Weiss DT, Solomon A. Immunoglobulin heavy-chain-associated amyloidosis. Proc Natl Acad Sci USA 1990;87:6542- 6.
13. Kushner I, Mackiewicz A. Acute phase proteins as disease markers. Dis Markers 1987;5:1-11.
14. Sipe JD, Gonnerman WA, Loose LD, et al. Direct binding enzyme-linked immunosorbent assay (ELISA) for serum amyloid A (SAA). J Immunol Methods 1989;125:125-35.
15. Peter JB. The use and interpretation of tests in medical microbiology. 2nd ed. Nebraska: Interstate Press, 1990.

ANGIOTENSIN CONVERTING ENZYME

Serum levels of angiotensin converting enzyme (ACE) are less likely to be elevated in neurosarcoidosis than are CSF ACE levels.[1] CSF levels of ACE are increased in approximately 50% (11/20) of patients with neurosarcoidosis and in less than 10% (1/12) of systemic sarcoidosis without neurologic abnormality.[1-3] CSF ACE is typically normal in demyelinating diseases, cerebrovascular accidents and polyneuropathies (diabetic and alcoholic), but it can be increased in CSF in patients with CNS tumors and CNS infections, especially with widespread meningitis.[1] A sensitive method for detection is available.[4] Oligoclonal immunoglobulins and IBBB synthesis of IgG are also found in neurosarcoidosis.[5,6] Serum ACE is elevated in childhood and adult sarcoidosis; serum levels are age- and gender-related in children but not in adults.[7] Some work suggests that serum ACE might serve as an endothelial cell marker and might discriminate individuals at high risk of recurrent venous thrombosis.[8] Serum ACE can also be elevated in histiocytic medullary reticulosis, in Lennert's lymphoma (hematological malignancy characterized by the presence of a high content of epithelioid histiocytes, T cells and Reed-Sternberg-like cells) and occasionally in non-Hodgkin lymphoma (cf. 9 for review). The activity of ACE is increased about 15% after a single overnight storage at -20°C or -70°C.[10]

REFERENCES:
1. Oksanen V, Fyhrquist F, Somer H, Grönhagen-Riska C. Angiotensin converting enzyme in cerebrospinal fluid: a new assay. Neurology 1985;35:1220-3.

2. Schweisfurth H, Schiöberg-Schiegnitz S. Assay and biochemical characterization of angiotensin-I-converting enzyme in cerebrospinal fluid. Enzyme 1984;32:12-9.
3. Chan Seem CP, Norfolk G, Spokes EG. CSF angiotensin-converting enzyme in neurosarcoidosis. Lancet 1985;1:456-7.
4. Fyhrquist F, Tikkanen I, Grönhagen-Riska C, Hortling L, Hickens M. Inhibitor binding assay for angiotensin-converting enzyme. Clin Chem 1984;30:696-700.
5. Kinnman J, Link H. Intrathecal production of oligoclonal IgM and IgG in CNS sarcoidosis. Acta Neurol Scand 1984;69:97-106.
6. Mitchell JD, Yap PL, Milne LA, et al. Immunological studies on the cerebrospinal fluid in neurological sarcoidosis. J Neuroimmunol 1985;7:249-53.
7. Bénéteau-Burnat B, Baudin B, Morgant G, et al. Serum angiotensin-converting enzyme in healthy and sarcoidotic children: comparison with the reference interval for adults. Clin Chem 1990;36:344-6.
8. Drouet L, Baudin B, Baumann FCH, Caen JP. Serum angiotensin-converting enzyme: an endothelial cell marker. Application to thromboembolic pathology. J Lab Clin Med 1988;112:450-7.
9. Zachée P, Geboers M, Neels H, et al. Serum angiotensin converting enzyme: a possible marker in Lennert's lymphoma? J Clin Pathol 1989;42:1112.
10. Pietilä K, Koivula T. Increase of serum angiotensin-converting enzyme activity after freezing. Scand J Clin Lab Invest 1984;44:453-5.

ANTI-MYELIN BASIC PROTEIN ANTIBODIES

Antibodies to myelin associated proteins have been implicated as a possible factor in induction of demyelination characteristic of neurological diseases. These include multiple sclerosis (MS), Guillain-Barré syndrome, acute idiopathic optic neuritis, subacute sclerosing panencephalitis, chronic relapsing polyradiculoneuritis and carcinomatous polyneuropathy. Although anti-MBP antibodies are important in the pathogenesis of experimental allergic encephalomyelitis (EAE), which is an animal model for MS, such antibodies are detected with varied frequency in the CSF and sera of MS patients and other neurological diseases.[1-9] The use of a number of immunological techniques such as IFA, immunoblotting, RIA and ELISA offers a range of sensitivities which probably contributes to the varying reports on the incidence of anti-MBP antibodies in demyelinating diseases of man. In general, reports on the frequency of CSF anti-MBP antibodies in MS have been contradictory (cf. 9 for review). Assay for antibodies to myelin basic protein is of no clinical utility. The best evidence indicates that antibodies to peripheral nerve myelin are also of no pathological significance.[8] Careful studies have shown no major enhancement of cellular immune response to myelin basic protein in multiple sclerosis (cf. 10 for review). Immunization with modified peptides from MBP or with peptides from T cell receptors reactive with MBP protects rats against subsequent induction of EAE by immunization with MBP; EAE can be successfully treated with MAbs reactive with shared T cell receptor epitopes (cf. 11 for review). See also **MYELIN ANTIBODIES** and **MYELIN BASIC PROTEIN**.

REFERENCES:
1. Warren KG, Catz I, Bauer C. Cerebrospinal fluid antibodies to myelin basic protein in acute idiopathic optic neuritis. Ann Neurol 1988;23:297-9.
2. Sato S, Baba H, Inuzuka T, Miyatake T. Anti-myelin-associated glycoprotein antibody in sera from patients with demyelinating diseases. Acta Neurol Scand 1986;74:115-20.
3. Cruz M, Olsson T, Ernerudh J, Höjeberg B, Link H. Immunoblot detection of oligoclonal anti-myelin basic protein IgG antibodies in cerebrospinal fluid in multiple sclerosis. Neurology 1987;37:1515-9.
4. Edgington TS, Dalessio DJ. The assessment by immunofluorescence methods of humoral anti-myelin antibodies in man. J Immunol 1970;105:248-55.
5. Chou C-H J, Tourtellotte WW, Kibler RF. Failure to detect antibodies to myelin basic protein or peptic fragments of myelin basic protein in CSF of patients with MS. Neurology 1983;33:24-8.
6. Nobile-Orazio E, McIntosh C, Latov N. Anti-MAG antibody and antibody complexes: detection by radioimmunoassay. Neurology 1985;35:988-92.
7. Glynn P, Weedon D, Cuzner ML. Chronic experimental autoimmune encephalomyelitis: circulating autoantibodies bind predominantly determinants expressed by complexes of basic protein and lipids of myelin. J Neurol Sci 1986;73:111-23.

8. Cruz M, Ernerudh J, Olsson T, Höjeberg BO, Link H. Occurrence and isotype of antibodies against peripheral nerve myelin in serum from patients with peripheral neuropathy and healthy controls. J Neurol Neurosurg Psychiatry 1988;51:820-5.
9. Warren KG, Catz I. Neutralization of anti-myelin basic protein by cerebrospinal fluid of multiple sclerosis patients in clinical remission. J Neurol Sci 1988;88:185-94.
10. McFarland HF, Dhib-Jalbut S. Multiple sclerosis: possible immunological mechanisms. Clin Immunol Immunopathol 1989;50:S96-105.
11. Janeway CA. Immunotherapy by peptides? Nature 1989;341:482-3.

ANTINUCLEAR ANTIBODIES

The absence of ANAs is strong evidence against untreated systemic lupus erythematosus (SLE), because ANAs are positive in 95-99% of untreated SLE when tested on cryostat sections of liver, kidney and heart which are the substrates of choice because they are the only tissues on which standardization with 2800 healthy controls and 200 untreated SLE patients was done.[1-3] The amount of homogeneous pattern ANA should be reported in international units and can be used for monitoring the levels of homogeneous ANAs, but clinical utility of such monitoring has not been established. Standardization of the amount of homogeneous ANA is, however, useful; indeed, it is mandatory for comparison of results between laboratories. Recent, brief, analytical reviews are available regarding the wide variety of ANAs, their prevalence and clinical significance.[4-6] An international exchange of sera for quality control has resulted in remarkable improvements in agreement among expert laboratories.[7] Positive ANAs are found in approximately 3-4% of normal caucasoids.[1]

REFERENCES:
1. Hawkins BR, O'Connor KJ, Dawkins RL, Dawkins B, Rodger B. Autoantibodies in an Australian population: I. Prevalence and persistence. J Clin Lab Immunol 1979;2:211-5.
2. Peter JB, Dawkins RL. Evaluating autoimmune diseases. Diagnostic Medicine 1979;2:68-76.
3. Peter JB, Dawkins RL. The value of immunology tests. Diagn Med 1979;2:79-88.
4. Tan EM, Chan EKL, Sullivan KF, Rubin RL. Antinuclear antibodies (ANAs): diagnostically specific immune markers and clues toward the understanding of systemic autoimmunity. Clin Immunol Immunopathol 1988;47:121-41.
5. Tan EM. Antinuclear antibodies: diagnostic markers and clues to the basis of systemic autoimmunity. Pediatr Infect Dis J 1988;7:S3-9.
6. Wiik A. The value of specific ANA determination in rheumatology. Allergy 1987;42:241-61.
7. Hollingsworth PN, Bonifacio E, Dawkins RL. Use of a standard curve improves precision and concordance of antinuclear antibody measurement. J Clin Lab Immunol 1987;22:197-200.

AUTOIMMUNE HYPERLIPIDEMIA AND HYPOLIPIDEMIA

Autoantibodies to lipoprotein components, low-density lipoprotein receptor and to lipoprotein lipase and hepatic triglyceride lipase have been reported and are usually found in patients with other evidence of autoimmune disease (cf. 1 for review). These syndromes are usually accompanied by hyperlipidemia, but IgA anti-lipoprotein antibodies in multiple myeloma can be accompanied by hypolipidemia.[2] Whether immune complexes containing lipoproteins[3] and whether antibodies to oxidized LDL[4-6] or glycated LDL[7,8] contribute to human atherosclerosis is undetermined (cf. 9 for review), as is the relationship of infection to atherosclerosis (cf. 10 for review). Hypocholesterolemia in some malignancies (e.g., leukemia and prostate cancer) can be associated with increased LDL receptor activity in the tumor cells.[11,12]

REFERENCES:
1. Kihara S, Matsuzawa Y, Kubo M, et al. Autoimmune hyperchylomicronemia. N Engl J Med 1989;320:1255-9.
2. Noseda G, Riesen W, Schlumpf E, Morrell A. Hypo-β-lipoproteinaemia associated with auto-antibodies against β-lipoproteins. Eur J Clin Invest 1972;2:342-7.

3. Szondy E, Lengyel E, Mezey Z, et al. Occurrence of anti-low density lipoprotein antibodies and circulating immune complexes in aged subjects. Mech Ageing Dev 1985;29:117-23.
4. Palinski W, Rosenfeld ME, Ylä-Herttuala S, et al. Low density lipoprotein undergoes oxidative modification *in vivo*. Proc Natl Acad Sci USA 1989;86:1372-6.
5. Mitchinson MJ, Ball RY, Carpenter KLH, Parums DV. Macrophages and ceroid in atherosclerosis. In: Suckling KE, Groot PHE, eds. Hyperlipidaemia and atherosclerosis. London: Academic Press, 1988:117-34.
6. Parums D, Mitchinson MJ. Demonstration of immunoglobulin in the neighborhood of advanced atherosclerotic plaques. Atherosclerosis 1981;38:211-6.
7. Witztum JL, Steinbrecher UP, Kesaniemi A, Fisher M. Autoantibodies to glucosylated proteins in the plasma of patients with diabetes mellitus. Proc Natl Acad Sci USA 1984;81:3204-8.
8. Brownlee M, Cerami A, Vlassara H. Advanced glycosylation end products in tissue and the biochemical basis of diabetic complications. N Engl J Med 1988;318:1315-21.
9. Steinberg D, Parthasarathy S, Carew TE, et al. Beyond cholesterol. Modifications of low-density lipoprotein that increase its atherogenicity. N Engl J Med 1989;320:915-24.
10. Virella G, Lopes-Virella MF. Infections and atherosclerosis. Transplant Proc 1987;19;26-35.
11. Vitols S, Gahrton G, Björkholm M, Peterson C. Hypocholesterolaemia in malignancy due to elevated low-density-lipoprotein-receptor activity in tumour cells: evidence from studies in patients with leukaemia. Lancet 1985;2:1150-5.
12. Henriksson P, Eriksson M, Ericsson S, et al. Hypocholesterolaemia and increased elimination of low-density lipoproteins in metastatic cancer of the prostate. Lancet 1989;2:1178-80.

AUTOIMMUNITY

Recent annotated bibliographies on the origins of autoantibodies,[1] genetics of autoimmune diseases,[2] infection and autoimmunity[3] and autoimmunity in AIDS[4] are available.

REFERENCES:
1. Marshak-Rothstein A. Origins of autoantibodies. Curr Opin Immunol 1989;1:697-700.
2. Winchester R. Genetics of autoimmune diseases. Curr Opin Immunol 1989;1:701-7.
3. Vaughan JH. Infection and autoimmunity. Curr Opin Immunol 1989;1:708-17.
4. Wilkin TJ. Receptor autoimmunity in endocrine disorders. N Engl J Med 1990; 323:1318-24.
5. Via CS, Shearer GM. Autoimmunity and the acquired immune deficiency syndrome. Curr Opin Immunol 1989;1:753-6.

BETA$_2$-MICROGLOBULIN (β_2-m)

Levels of β_2-m (a 99-amino acid polypeptide) are sometimes increased in CSF (relative to serum) in CNS acute lymphoblastic leukemia (ALL),[1] lymphoma[2] and lymphoproliferative diseases,[3] but these increased levels are not helpful for early detection of CNS involvement in children with ALL.[4] CSF β_2-m is also increased in MS with severe neurological impairment.[5] Progressive decreases in β_2-m concentrations in CSF correlate with clinical improvement of neurological disease in myelo-lymphoproliferative disorders.[6] In HIV infection, there is a direct relationship between levels of β_2-m and neopterin in serum and CSF.[7] In man, β_2-m is typically associated with the heavy chains of MHC class I genes (which function to present antigen to T lymphocytes bearing $\alpha\beta$ antigen receptors and the CD8 coreceptor) and is also associated with the β_2-m-associated Fc receptor for IgG (at the epithelial brush border), the function of which is to transport maternal IgG across neonatal intestinal membranes. Mutations produced by homologous recombination in embryonic stem cells can be transmitted to the germ line by injection into blastocysts of mice which are thus rendered heterozygous for the disrupted β_2-m gene. Homozygotes for the disrupted β_2-m gene express no functional MHC class I antigens and are deficient in CD4$^-$8$^+$ T cell-mediated cytotoxicity[8-10] (cf. 11 for discussion). In mice, structural polymorphisms of β_2-m restrict the presentation of peptides by class I MHC to the immune system.[12] β_2-m determinations (cf. 13 for review) with CD4$^+$ counts may be useful for prognostication in HIV infection[14] but serum neopterin combined with CD4$^+$ counts is probably the combination of choice.[15] See also **BETA-GLUCURONIDASE** and **NEOPTERINS**.

REFERENCES:
1. Musto P, Tomasi P, Cascavilla N, et al. Significance and limits of cerebrospinal fluid beta-2-microglobulin measurement in course of acute lymphoblastic leukemia. Am J Hematol 1988;28:213-8.

2. Öberg G, Hällgren R, Venge P. β_2-microglobulin, lysozyme and lactoferrin in cerebrospinal fluid in patients with lymphoma or leukaemia: relationship to CNS involvement and the effect of prophylactic intrathecal treatment with methotrexate. Br J Haematol 1987;66:315-22.

3. Ernerudh J, Olsson T, Berlin G, von Schenck H. Cerebrospinal fluid immunoglobulins and β_2-microglobulin in lymphoproliferative and other neoplastic diseases of the central nervous system. Arch Neurol 1987;44:915-20.

4. Nagelkerke AF, van Kamp GJ, Veerman AJP, de Waal FC. Unreliability of β_2-microglobulin in early detection of central nervous system relapse in acute lymphoblastic leukemia. Eur J Cancer Clin Oncol 1985;21:659-63.

5. Bjerrum OW, Bach FW, Zeeberg I. Increased level of cerebrospinal fluid β_2-microglobulin is related to neurologic impairment in multiple sclerosis. Acta Neurol Scand 1988;78:72-5.

6. Storti S, Pagano L, Marra R, et al. Cerebrospinal fluid beta-$_2$-microglobulin: a reliable index of leukaemic infiltration of central nervous system. Scand J Haematol 1986;37:301-5.

7. Peter JB, McKeown KL, Barka NE, Tourtellotte WW, Singer EJ, Syndulko K. Neopterin and β_2-microglobulin and the assessment of IBBB synthesis of HIV-specific and total IgG. 1990; Submitted.

8. Koller BH, Smithies O. Inactivating the β_2-microglobulin locus in mouse embryonic stem cells by homologous recombination. Proc Natl Acad Sci USA 1989;86:8932-5.

9. Zijlstra M, Li E, Sajjadi F, et al. Germ-line transmission of a disrupted β_2-microglobulin gene produced by homologous recombination in embryonic stem cells. Nature 1989;342:435-8.

10. Zijlstra M, Bix M, Simister NE, et al. β_2-microglobulin deficient mice lack CD4$^-$8$^+$ cytolytic T cell. Nature 1990;344:742-6.

11. Parham P. Some savage cuts in defense. Nature 1990;344:709-11.

12. Pérarnau B, Siegrist C-A, Gillet A, et al. β_2-microglobulin restriction of antigen presentation. Nature 1990;346:751-4.

13. Bethea M, Forman DT. β_2-microglobulin: its significance and clinical usefulness. Ann Clin Lab Sci 1990;20:163-8.

14. Hofmann B, Wang Y, Cumberland WG, et al. Serum beta$_2$-microglobulin level increases in HIV infection: relation to seroconversion, CD4 T-cell fall and prognosis. AIDS 1990;4:207-14.

15. Fahey JL, Taylor JMG, Detels R, et al. The prognostic value of cellular and serologic markers in infection with human immunodeficiency virus type 1. N Engl J Med 1990;322:166-72.

BETA-ADRENERGIC RECEPTOR ANTIBODIES

Autoantibodies to β_2-receptors may play an important role in associated human diseases, including asthma, dilated cardiomyopathies and Chagas disease. Antibodies to β_2-receptors were reported in two patients with allergic asthma and one with allergic rhinitis.[1] Similar studies were reported[2,3] and reviewed[4] by the same group. Antibodies to β_2-receptors were subsequently reported in about 5% of asthmatics and in 8.8% of severely asthmatic children compared with 3.4% in the general population.[5] Antibodies to β-receptors were also found in diverse populations and did not correlate with a specific disease.[4] Antibodies to β_2-receptors from asthmatic and allergic rhinitis patients are associated with hyporesponsiveness of β_2-receptors. On the other hand, antibodies to the β_1-adrenergic receptor of heart muscle were demonstrated convincingly in human idiopathic cardiomyopathy,[6] as were antibodies to myocardial β_1-receptors and to spleen cell β_2-receptors in Chagas disease.[7] By contrast, anti-β_1 and β_2-receptor antibodies from dilated cardiomyopathy and Chagas patients are associated with an increased reactiveness of the receptors[6,7] (cf.8 for review).

REFERENCES:

1. Venter JC, Fraser CM, Harrison LC. Autoantibodies to β_2-adrenergic receptors: a possible cause of adrenergic hyporesponsiveness in allergic rhinitis and asthma. Science 1980;207:1361-3.

2. Harrison LC, Callaghan J, Venter JC, et al. Atopy, autonomic function and β-adrenergic receptor autoantibodies. In: Evered D, Whelan J, eds. Receptors, antibodies and disease. London: Pitman Ltd, 1982:248-62.

3. Fraser CM, Venter JC, Kaliner M. Autonomic abnormalities and autoantibodies to beta-adrenergic receptors. N Engl J Med 1981;305:1165-70.
4. Robinson DA, Fraser CM, Venter JC, The β-adrenergic receptor, autoantibodies, and allergy: how are they related? Clin Immunol Newsletter 1986;7:42-5.
5. Blecher M. Receptors, antibodies, and disease. Clin Chem 1984;30:1137-56.
6. Limas CJ, Goldenberg IF, Limas C. Autoantibodies against β-adrenoceptors in human idiopathic dilated cardiomyopathy. Circ Res 1989;64:97-103.
7. Sterin-Borda L, Leiros CP, Wald M, et al. Antibodies to β_1 and β_2 adrenoreceptors in Chagas' disease. Clin Exp Immunol 1988;74:349-54.
8. Collins S, Bolanowski MA, Caron MG, Lefkowitz RJ. Genetic regulation of β-adrenergic receptors. In: Hoffman JF, De Weer P, eds. Annual Review of Physiology. Palo Alto: Annual Review Inc., 1989;51:203-15.

BETA-GLUCURONIDASE (βG)

CSF βG is elevated in approximately 75% of patients with leptomeningeal adenocarcinoma and 25% of patients with myelogenous leukemia;[1] only slight elevations are seen with epidural or parenchymal metastases from solid tumors.[2] Elevations of CSF βG are 93% sensitive and specific for differentiating leptomeningeal metastases from other CNS metastases of breast adenocarcinoma.[3,4] Elevations of both CSF βG and beta$_2$-microglobulin are especially useful for prediction of leptomeningeal dissemination of solid tumors and non-Hodgkin lymphoma.[4] Elevations of CSF βG are also found in acute and subacute bacterial and fungal meningitis. CSF βG, as well as other lysosomal hydrolases including neutral proteinase (NP), are often elevated in MS but only CSF NP is associated with relapse.[5] See also **CSF CARCINOEMBRYONIC ANTIGEN** and **BETA$_2$-MICROGLOBULIN.**

REFERENCES:
1. Tallman RD, Kimbrough SM, O'Brien JF, Goellner JR, Yanagihara T. Assay for β-glucuronidase in cerebrospinal fluid: usefulness for the detection of neoplastic meningitis. Mayo Clin Proc 1985;60:293-8.
2. van Zanten AP, Twijnstra A, van Benthem V, Hart AAM, Ongerboer de Visser BW. Cerebrospinal fluid β-glucuronidase activities in patients with central nervous system metastases. Clin Chim Acta 1985;147:127-34.
3. Twijnstra A, van Zanten AP, Nooyen WJ, Ongerboer de Visser BW. Sensitivity and specificity of single and combined tumour markers in the diagnosis of leptomeningeal metastasis from breast cancer. J Neurol Neurosurg Psychiatry 1986;49:1246-50.
4. van Zanten AP, Twijnstra A, Ongerboer de Visser BW, Hart AA, Nooyen WJ. Tumour markers in the cerebrospinal fluid of patients with central nervous system metastases from extracranial malignancies. Clin Chim Acta 1988;175:157-66.
5. Halonen T, Kilpelainen H, Pitkanen A, Riekkinen PJ. Lysosomal hydrolases in cerebrospinal fluid of multiple sclerosis patients: a follow-up study. J Neurol Sci 1987;79:267-74.

BRUSH BORDER ANTIBODIES

Originally described in rats with Heymann nephritis, anti-brush border antibodies (ABBA) are also found in approximately 50% of patients with ulcerative proctocolitis and in approximately 20% of patients with antibodies to *Yersinia enterocolitica* 0:3.[1] The description of ABBA in patients with extensive burns[2] is another example of failure to recognize the pattern of reaction with various tissues of heterophile antibodies which are associated with blood transfusions and other forms of alloimmunization.[3]

REFERENCES:
1. Skogh T, Bodemar G, Kihlstrom E, Ljunghusen O. Anti-brush border antibodies (ABBA) in sera from patients with ulcerative proctocolitis and in sera with antibodies against *Yersinia enterocolitica* 0:3. J Clin Lab Immunol 1986;19:117-8.
2. Governa M, Benedetti E, Lorenzini M, Barisoni D. Autoantibodies in 16 patients with extensive burns and a review of the literature. Burns 1987;13:469-75.
3. Hawkins BR, McDonald BL, Dawkins RL. Characterization of immunofluorescent heterophile antibodies which may be confused with autoantibodies. J Clin Pathol 1977;30:299-307.

C-REACTIVE PROTEIN

Although likely to be greatly increased (greater than 6 mg/dL), elevated levels of serum CRP are only 39% sensitive and 93% specific for infection in systemic lupus erythematosus (SLE).[1] Nevertheless, very high levels suggest concomitant infection. Serum CRP levels are more likely to be elevated during bacterial rather than during viral meningitis, but the sensitivity, specificity and predictive value of CSF CRP for bacterial meningitis are too low to be routinely useful.[2] In patients with rheumatoid arthritis (RA), persistently elevated CRP concentrations (>4 mg/dL) are invariably present when the disease is active and usually fall to normal during periods of complete remission.[3] When very recent (less than 24 hours) changes in acute phase response are suspected, quantitation of serum CRP is the test of choice, because incremental increases (100-1000 fold) of CRP are greater than other acute phase reactants and hence provide the greatest sensitivity for detection of small, recent inflammatory stimuli. In later phases (greater than 24 hours), the ESR or plasma viscosity are complementary to quantitation of serum CRP.[4] Sera with very high CRP levels usually contain elevated TNF; the TNF/CRP ratio may have some disease specificity with elevations in renal allograft rejection and low ratios in bacterial infections and RA,[5] but more data are needed. About 60% of healthy newborns have a serum CRP concentration greater than 1 mg/dL at least once during the first twenty days of life;[6] hence adult levels may not be applicable to this group. Quantitative measurements of CRP are underutilized in infectious and rheumatic diseases (cf. 7). See also **ERYTHROCYTE SEDIMENTATION RATE** and **VISCOSITY**.

REFERENCES:
1. Mackiewicz A, Marcinkowska-Pieta R, Ballou S, Mackiewicz S, Kushner I. Microheterogeneity of alpha$_1$-acid glycoprotein in the detection of intercurrent infection in systemic lupus erythematosus. Arthritis Rheum 1987;30:513-8.
2. Lindquist L, Linné T, Hansson L-O, Kalin M, Axelsson G. Value of cerebrospinal fluid analysis in the differential diagnosis of meningitis: a study in 710 patients with suspected central nervous system infection. Eur J Clin Microbiol Infect Dis 1988;7:374-80.
3. Hind CRK, Savage CO, Winearls CG, Pepys MB. Objective monitoring of disease activity in polyarteritis by measurement of serum C reactive protein concentration. Br Med J 1984;288:1027-30.
4. Bull BS, Chien S, Dormandy JA, et al. Laboratory techniques: guidelines on selection of laboratory tests for monitoring the acute phase response. J Clin Pathol 1988;41:1203-12.
5. Maury CPJ. Monitoring the acute phase response: comparison of tumor necrosis factor (cachectin) and C-reactive protein responses in inflammatory and infectious diseases. J Clin Pathol 1989;43:1078-82.
6. Gussetti N, Ruga E, Giaquinto C, et al. Is C-reactive protein a reliable indicator of bacterial infection in the newborn? J Infect Dis 1989;160:909-10.
7. Okamura JM, Miyagi JM, Terada K, Hokama Y. Potential clinical applications of C-reactive protein. J Clin Lab Anal 1990;4:231-5.

C1 INH DEFICIENCY (HEREDITARY ANGIONEUROTIC EDEMA - HANE; ACQUIRED DEFICIENCY)

In type I HANE (∿85% of kindreds), which is characterized by low plasma levels of C1 INH protein and C1 INH function associated with partial deletions and/or duplications C1 INH gene, the remaining C1 INH is apparently normal, catalytically active C1 INH and present at 5-30% of reference range concentrations. In type II HANE (∿15% of kindreds), normal to elevated levels of C1 INH protein are consistent with structural gene defects manifest by the presence of both a dysfunctional mutant protein and less than 50% of the normal protein (cf. 1 for review). The decrease in synthesis of normal C1 INH (as expected in heterozygotes for types I and II HANE) is accompanied by elevated fractional catabolic rates for normal C1 INH so that serum concentrations of normal C1 INH are reduced to less than 50% of the usual reference range.[2,3] Increased levels of C1 INH complexes in plasma of both type I and type II correlate inversely with plasma C1 INH in type I. Although iC1 INH (a cleaved form of C1 INH) is normal in type I and normal in those type II patients with increased C1 INH antigen, it is greatly (∿20X) increased in some type II patients who have normal C1 INH antigen levels.[4] There is now ample evidence of genetic heterogeneity in both types of HANE.[5-7]

The most common variety of acquired deficiency of C1 INH (which is due to increased consumption as opposed to the decreased synthesis and increased consumption in HANE) is associated with benign or malignant B-cell lymphoproliferative disorders.[8,9] A less common form is associated with autoantibodies to C1 INH.[10,11] The decreases in serum C1q protein in the acquired forms of angioedema distinguish them from HANE.[12] All forms of HANE and acquired deficiency of C1 INH respond to attenuated androgens, but the individuals with acquired deficiency require higher doses.[9] In addition to angioedema due to deficiency of C1 INH, other diseases due to deficiencies of proteinase inhibitors (members of the serpin super family of serine protease inhibitors; cf. 13 for review) are emphysema and hepatitis (α_1-proteinase inhibitor), thromboembolism (antithrombin III) and bleeding (α_2-antiplasmin). Angiotensin converting enzyme inhibitors can precipitate angioedema in patients with a history of idiopathic angioedema.[14]

REFERENCES:
1. Davis AE III. C1 inhibitor and hereditary angioneurotic edema. Ann Rev Immunol 1988;6:595-628.
2. Lachmann PJ, Rosen FS. The catabolism of C1̄-inhibitor and the pathogenesis of hereditary angio-edema. Acta Pathol Microbiol Immunol Scand 1984;92(Suppl 284):35-9.
3. Quastel M, Harrison R, Cicardi M, Alper CA, Rosen FS. Behavior in vivo of normal and dysfunctional C1̄ inhibitor in normal subjects and patients with hereditary angioneurotic edema. J Clin Invest 1983;71:1041-6.
4. Cugno M, Nuijens J, Hack E, et al. Plasma levels of C1̄ inhibitor complexes and cleaved C1̄ inhibitor in patients with hereditary angioneurotic edema. J Clin Invest 1990;85:1215-20.
5. Cicardi M, Igarashi T, Kim MS, Frangi D, Agostoni A, Davis AE III. Restriction fragment length polymorphism of the C1 inhibitor gene in hereditary angioneurotic edema. J Clin Invest 1987;80:1640-3.
6. Stoppa-Lyonnet D, Tosi M, Laurent J, Sobel A, Lagrue G, Meo T. Altered C1 inhibitor genes in type I hereditary angioedema. N Engl J Med 1987;317:1-6.
7. Levy MJ, Ramesh N, Cicardi M, et al. Type II hereditary angioneurotic edema that may result from a single nucleotide change in the codon for alanine-436 in the C1 inhibitor gene. Proc Natl Acad Sci USA 1990;87:265-8.
8. Melamed J, Alper CA, Cicardi M, Rosen FS. The metabolism of C1 inhibitor and C1q in patients with acquired C1-inhibitor deficiency. J Allergy Clin Immunol 1986;77:322-6.
9. Sheffer AL, Austen KF, Rosen FS, Fearon DT. Acquired deficiency of the inhibitor of the first component of complement: report of five additional cases with commentary on the syndrome. J Allergy Clin Immunol 1985;75:640-6.
10. Alsenz J, Bork K, Loos M. Autoantibody-mediated acquired deficiency of C1 inhibitor. N Engl J Med 1987;316:1360-6.
11. Jackson J, Feighery C. Autoantibody-mediated acquired deficiency of C1 inhibitor [Letters]. N Engl J Med 1988;318:122-3.
12. Caldwell JR, Ruddy S, Schur RS, Austen KF. Acquired C1̄ inhibitor deficiency in lymphosarcoma. Clin Immunol Immunopathol 1972;1:39-52.
13. Carrell RW, Boswell DR. Serpins: the superfamily of plasma serine proteinase inhibitors. In: Barrett A, Salvesen G, eds. Proteinase inhibitors. Amsterdam: Elsevier, 1986:403-20.
14. Orfan N, Patterson R, Dykewicz MS. Severe angioedema related to ACE inhibitors in patients with a history of idiopathic angioedema. JAMA 1990;264:1287-9.

C1q ANTIBODIES

Antibodies to C1q are found in most, if not all, patients with the hypocomplementemic urticarial vasculitis syndrome (HUVS)[1] and in 30-60% of SLE.[2-4] In HUVS serum levels of C1q are profoundly depressed, but C1r and C1s are relatively normal and there is only slight activation of C5-C9.[5]

REFERENCES:
1. Wisnieski JJ, Naff GB. Serum IgG antibodies to C1q in hypocomplementemic urticarial vasculitis syndrome. Arthritis Rheum 1989;32:1119-27.
2. Uwatoko S, Aotsuka S, Okawa M, et al. Characterization of C1q-binding IgG complexes in systemic lupus erythematosus. Clin Immunol Immunopathol 1984;30:104-16.
3. Antes U, Heinz H-P, Loos M. Evidence for the presence of autoantibodies to the collagen-like portion of C1q in systemic lupus erythematosus. Arthritis Rheum 1988;31:457-64.
4. Uwatoko S, Mannik M. Low-molecular weight C1q-binding immunoglobulin G in patients with systemic lupus erythematosus consists of autoantibodies to the collagen-like region of C1q. J Clin Invest 1988;82:816-24.

5. Zeiss CR, Burch FX, Marder RJ, et al. A hypocomplementemic vasculitic urticarial syndrome. Report of four new cases and definition of the disease. Am J Med 1980;68:867-75.

C1q BINDING ASSAY FOR CIC

Changes in circulating immune complexes, as detected by C1q binding assay, correlate with changes in joint counts in rheumatoid arthritis.[1] In general, however, the clinical utility of this and other assays for CIC is, at best, dubious.[2-4] Although likely to improve comparability and reproducibility, the use of an international preparation of aggregated IgG[5] is not expected to make these assays more useful. Recently, the C1q and conglutinin binding assays for CIC were reported positive in serum and CSF respectively of patients with active multiple sclerosis.[6] Detection of CIC by the C1q binding assay may provide useful prognostic information at diagnosis and during remission of acute myelogenous leukemia.[7] Some authorities recommend the C1q binding assay and the conglutinin assay for detection of circulating immune complexes, because these assays "may be helpful for assessing and monitoring of disease activity in conditions such as rheumatoid arthritis and SLE".[4]

REFERENCES:
1. Reynolds WJ, Yoon SJ, Emin M, Chapman KR, Klein MH. Circulating immune complexes in rheumatoid arthritis: a prospective study using five immunoassays. J Rheumatol 1986;13:700-6.
2. McDougal JS, Hubbard M, Strobel PL, McDuffie FC. Comparison of five assays for immune complexes in the rheumatic diseases: performance characteristics of the assays. J Lab Clin Med 1982;100:705-19.
3. Lessard J, Nunnery E, Cecere F, McDuffy S, Pope RM. Relationship between the articular manifestations of rheumatoid arthritis and circulating immune complexes detected by three methods and specific classes of rheumatoid factors. J Rheumatol 1983;10:411-7.
4. IUIS/WHO Working Group. Laboratory investigations in clinical immunology: methods, pitfalls, and clinical indications: a second IUIS/WHO report. Clin Immunol Immunopathol 1988;49:478-97.
5. Nydegger UE, Svehag S-E. Improved standardization in the quantitative estimation of soluble immune complexes making use of an international reference preparation: results of a collaborative multicentre study. Clin Exp Immunol 1984;58:502-9.
6. Procaccia S, Lanzanova D, Caputo D, et al. Circulating immune complexes in serum and in cerebrospinal fluid of patients with multiple sclerosis. Acta Neurol Scand 1988;77:373-81.
7. Carpentier NA, Fiere DM, Schuh D, Lange GT, Lambert P-H. Circulating immune complexes and the prognosis of acute myeloid leukemia. N Engl J Med 1982;307:1174-80.

C3 AND C4 NEPHRITIC FACTOR (NFII/C3NeF; C4NeF)

The hypocomplementemia seen in approximately 60% of patients with idiopathic membranoproliferative glomerulonephritis (MPGN) is characterized by decreased levels of serum C3 and by the presence in serum of NFII which is an IgG autoantibody that stabilizes the amplification of C3 convertase (C3bBb) and causes a decrease in serum C3 but no decrease of other complement components.[1] NFII (C3bBb-stabilizing activity) is found in MPGN type II and in partial lipodystrophy and occasionally in MPGN type I.[2] C3 nephritic factors (C3NeF) express a common idiotype;[3] a simplified assay for C3NeF is available.[4] Just as C3NeF, an IgG autoantibody, often causes hypocomplementemia in MPGN II (but rarely in MPGN I) by binding to a neoantigen of the C3bBb complex from the alternative pathway, C4NeF is an autoantibody to the C4b2a complex, which is reported in acute post-injection GN and in MPGN I.[5] See also **PROPERDIN DEPENDENT NEPHRITIC FACTOR (NFI and II)**.

REFERENCES:
1. Jackson EC, McAdams AJ, Strife CF, Forristal J, Welch TR, West CD. Differences between membranoproliferative glomerulonephritis types I and III in clinical presentation, glomerular morphology, and complement perturbation. Am J Kidney Dis 1987;9:115-20.
2. Sissons JGP, West RJ, Fallows J, et al. The complement abnormalities of lipodystrophy. N Engl J Med 1976;294:461-5.
3. Tsokos GC, Stitzel AE, Patel AD, et al. Human polyclonal and monoclonal IgG and IgM complement 3 nephritic factors: evidence for idiotypic commonality. Clin Immunol Immunopathol 1989;53:113-22.

4. Ohi H, Watanabe S, Fujita T, Seki M, Hatano M. Detection of C3bBb-stabilizing activity (C3 nephritic factor) in the serum from patients with membranoproliferative glomerulonephritis. J Immunol Methods 1990;131:71-6.
5. Seino J, Kinoshita Y, Sudo K, et al. Quantitation of C4 nephritic factor by an enzyme-linked immunosorbent assay. J Immunol Methods 1990;128:101-8.

C3a, C4a, C5a AND ANAPHYLATOXINS; COMPLEMENT SPLIT PRODUCTS (C4d, Ba and C3dg)

Elevated levels of plasma C3a (average ∿180 ng/ml) are found in most patients with active SLE. The average level of plasma C3a rises to about 240 ng/ml 1-2 months before flares of SLE (e.g., nephritis, pericarditis, and/or cutaneous vasculitis). During flares, average plasma C3a is markedly increased to about 525 ng/ml. The highest levels (average ∿1300 ng/ml) are found in CNS lupus. Elevated levels of plasma C3a (∿320 ng/ml) are found in pregnant patients with SLE.[1] Expression of the complement receptor CR3 on neutrophil surfaces is increased in relatively direct proportion to the levels of the circulating anaphylatoxin C3a in plasma.[2] In general, however, the short half-lives of anaphylatoxins (C3a, C4a and C5a) in plasma[3] and the presence of high affinity receptors on phagocytes and mast cells[4] bode poorly for incisive clinical utility (cf. 5 for review). In addition to its reported, but as yet unconfirmed usefulness for predicting flares of SLE, serial estimation of plasma C3a is suggested to be helpful for monitoring response to therapy.[1] Plasma levels of complement split products (C4d, Ba and C3dg) are more promising although relatively inert biologically. Low concentrations can be detected in normal subjects; this is a distinct advantage for incisive clinical utilization of any assay. Some data indicate that these split products (especially C4d) are progressively elevated with increasing disease activity of SLE. Levels of C3dg are higher in patients with systemic sclerosis who have more severe diffuse cutaneous skin disease.[6-8] Levels of C3dg are greatly increased in plasma of patients with sepsis and the highest levels are associated with sepsis-related mortality.[9] For review of anaphylatoxins in disease, see 4 and 10. For discussion of CNS lupus, see also **NEURONAL ANTIBODIES, RIBOSOMAL P PROTEIN ANTIBODIES, FACTOR B** and **MEMBRANE ATTACK COMPLEX.**

REFERENCES:
1. Hopkins P, Belmont HM, Buyon J, Philips M, Weissmann G, Abramson SB. Increased levels of plasma anaphylatoxins in sytemic lupus erythematosus predict flares of the disease and may elicit vascular injury in lupus cerebritis. Arthritis Rheum 1988;31:632-41.
2. Buyon JP, Shadick N, Berkman R, et al. Surface expression of Gp165/95, the complement receptor CR3, as a marker of disease activity in systemic *Lupus erythematosus.* Clin Immunol Immunopathol 1988;46:141-9.
3. Charlesworth JA, Gwyn Williams D, Sherington E, et al. Metabolic studies of the third component of complement and the glycine rich beta glycoprotein in patients with hypocomplementemia. J Clin Invest 1974;53:1578-87.
4. Hugli TE. Structure and function of the anaphylatoxins. Springer Semin Immunopathol 1984;7:193-219.
5. Peakman M, Senaldi G, Vergani D. *Review:* Assessment of complement activation in clinical immunology laboratories: time for reappraisal? J Clin Pathol 1989;42:1018-25.
6. Senaldi G, Makinde VA, Vergani D, Isenberg DA. Correlation of the activation of the fourth component of complement (C4) with disease activity in systemic lupus erythematosus. Ann Rheum Dis 1988;47:913-17.
7. Senaldi G, Lupoli S, Vergani D, Black C. Activation of the complement system in systemic sclerosis. Relationship to clinical severity. Arthritis Rheum 1989;32:1262-7.
8. Senaldi G, Peakman M, Vergani D. New nephelometric techniques that measure C4d, Ba and C3d: clinical importance in the assessment of complement activation. Complement 1988;5:212.
9. Hack CE, Nuijens JH, Felt-Bersma RJF, et al. Elevated plasma levels of the anaphylatoxins C3a and C4a are associated with a fatal outcome in sepsis. Am J Med 1989;86:20-6.
10. Vogt W. Anaphylatoxins: possible roles in disease. Complement 1986;3:177-88.

C4 ALLOTYPES

In man there are two polymorphic, closely linked, structural loci for C4 (called C4A and C4B) on the short arm of chromosome 6. At each of these loci there are several possible expressed alleles (at least 13 recognized allelic products of the C4A locus and 21 products of the C4B locus), as well as unexpressed (null) alleles.[1] The presence and number of null alleles at C4A and C4B determine the expected reference range of serum C4 for a given individual.[2-8] The 15-45 mg/dL range, usually considered normal, does not take into account the fact that individuals with 0, 1, or 2 null alleles at the C4A and C4B loci (i.e., individuals with 4, 3, or 2 expressed alleles, respectively) will have greatly different levels of serum C4. With zero null alleles (4 expressed alleles) the 95% reference range for serum C4 is 22-50 mg/dL.[6] With one null allele (3 expressed alleles) the range is 13-38 mg/dL, and with two null alleles (2 expressed alleles) the 95% range for serum C4 is 10-16 mg/dL.[6] Note that in the normal population, 2.5% of individuals will have serum C4 levels below these allotype-adjusted reference ranges, and 2.5% will have the serum C4 levels above these allotype-adjusted reference ranges. Current data suggest that serum C4 levels in the 10-22 mg/dL range cannot be interpreted with respect to complement consumption unless complement allotyping is performed to estimate the number of null alleles, if any, and the appropriate serum C4 reference range (i.e., the C4 allotype-adjusted reference range).[3,4,6] For recent review, see 8. Null alleles at the C4 loci are associated with susceptibility to a number of autoimmune diseases, including SLE and drug-induced LE[9,10] (cf. 11 for review) and with a number of other abnormalities including IgA deficiency. Inhibition of C4 by hydralazine and isoniazid may be important in the pathogenesis of drug-induced lupus.[12] Quantification of C4 isotypes is also possible by ELISA.[13]

REFERENCES:
1. Awdeh ZL, Ochs HD, Alper CA. Genetic analysis of C4 deficiency. J Clin Invest 1981;67:260-3.
2. Uko G, Christiansen FT, Dawkins RL, McCann VJ. Reference ranges for serum C4 concentrations in subjects with and without C4 null alleles. J Clin Pathol 1986;39:573-6.
3. Christiansen FT, McCluskey J, Dawkins RL, Kay PH, Uko G, Zilko PJ. Complement allotyping in SLE: association with C4A null. Aust N Z J Med 1983;13:483-8.
4. Reveille JD, Arnett FC, Wilson RW, Bias WB, McLean RH. Null alleles of the fourth component of complement and HLA haplotypes in familial systemic lupus erythematosus. Immunogenetics 1985;21:299-311.
5. Uko G, Christiansen FT, Dawkins RL. Serum C4 concentration in the monitoring of systemic lupus erythematosus: requirement for C4 allotyping. Rheumatol Int 1986;6:111-4.
6. Welch TR, Beischel L, Berry A, Forristal J, West CD. The effect of null C4 alleles on complement function. Clin Immunol Immunopathol 1985;34:316-25.
7. Howard PF, Hochberg MC, Bias WB, Arnett FC Jr, McLean RH. Relationship between C4 null genes, HLA-D region antigens, and genetic susceptibility to sytemic lupus erythematosus in Caucasian and black Americans. Am J Med 1986;81:187-93.
8. Hauptmann G, Tappeiner G, Schifferli JA. Inherited deficiency of the fourth component of human complement. Immunodeficiency Rev 1988;1:3-22.
9. Fielder AHL, Walport MJ, Batchelor JR, et al. Family study of the major histocompatibility complex in patients with systemic lupus erythematosus: importance of null alleles of C4A and C4B in determining disease susceptibility. Br Med J 1983;286:425-8.
10. Speirs C, Fielder AHL, Chapel H, Davey NJ, Batchelor JR. Complement system protein C4 and susceptibility to hydralazine-induced systemic lupus erythematosus. Lancet 1989;1:922-3.
11. Dawkins RL, Christiansen FT, Kay PH, et al. Disease associations with complotypes, supratypes and haplotypes. Immunol Rev 1983;70:11-22.
12. Sim E, Gill EW. Drugs that induce systemic lupus erythematosus inhibit complement component C4. Lancet 1984;2:422-4.
13. Chrispeels J, Bank S, Rittner C, Bitter-Suermann D. Sandwich enzyme-linked immunosorbent assays for the quantification of the C4 isotypes (C4A and C4B) in human plasma. J Immunol Methods 1989;125:5-12.

CARDIOLIPIN ANTIBODIES

Anti-cardiolipin antibodies (ACA) are reported to be associated with thrombotic events,[1-6] thrombocytopenia[1,2,7,8] and recurrent fetal loss[2,9,10] in patients with SLE, but these associations have been challenged.[11-13] Positive results on a single determination of IgG, IgM and IgA antibodies to cardiolipin in 85 consecutive outpatients with SLE correlated with the predisposition to thrombosis, fetal loss and thrombocytopenia. There was no correlation with other clinical manifestations of SLE, including activity and severity of disease.[14] The presence of these antibodies is associated with a high prevalence of valve abnormalities in patients with SLE.[15] Data indicate that assays for ACA should include separate testing for ACA of the IgG, IgM and IgA isotypes.[14,16-18] Some assays for anti-cardiolipin antibodies[17] are quite unsatisfactory in precision and in the false-positive results which can be due to high levels of non-specific IgG and IgM in serum.[19-23] Some data indicate that LAC assays are more reliable predictors of risk for thrombosis, fetal loss and thrombocytopenia than are ACA assays.[24] Surprisingly, few objections have been voiced to the published associations of phospholipid antibodies with an astonishing variety of disorders. A moratorium on the description of such associations in unrefereed journals is undoubtedly overdue. For clinical management purposes, tests for ACA are probably indicated in patients with SLE who are pregnant or plan to become pregnant, as well as in all patients with SLE and a history of thrombosis[14] (cf. 25 for recent review). The fact that β_2-glycoprotein I (apolipoprotein H), which binds anionic phospholipids and is known to cause multiple inhibitory effects on coagulation pathways and platelet aggregation, is required for binding of cardiolipin antibodies may be important to the thrombotic effects of these antibodies.[26,27] The cofactor(s) important for ACA activity might react differently with cardiolipin antibodies associated with SLE than those associated with syphilis.[28] See also **PHOSPHOLIPID ANTIBODIES** and **LUPUS ANTICOAGULANT.**

REFERENCES:
1. Harris EN, Gharavi AE, Boey ML, et al. Anticardiolipin antibodies: detection by radioimmunoassay and association with thrombosis in systemic lupus erythematosus. Lancet 1983;2:1211-4.
2. Harris EN, Gharavi AE, Hughes GRV. Anti-phospholipid antibodies. Clin Rheum Dis 1985;11:591-609.
3. Petri M, Rheinschmidt M, Whiting-O'Keefe Q, Hellmann D, Corash L. The frequency of lupus anticoagulant in systemic lupus erythematosus: a study of sixty consecutive patients by activated partial thromboplastin time, Russell viper venom time, and anticardiolipin antibody level. Ann Intern Med 1987;106:524-31.
4. Trimble M, Bell DA, Brien W, et al. The antiphospholipid syndrome: prevalence among patients with stroke and transient ischemic attacks. Am J Med 1990;88:593-7.
5. Levine SR, Deegan MJ, Futrell N, Welch KMA. Cerebrovascular and neurologic disease associated with antiphospholipid antibodies: 48 cases. Neurology 1990;40:1181-9.
6. Brey RL, Hart RG, Sherman DG, Tegeler CH. Antiphospholipid antibodies and cerebral ischemia in young people. Neurology 1990;40:1190-6.
7. Harris EN, Asherson RA, Gharavi AE, Morgan SH, Derue G, Hughes GRV. Thrombocytopenia in SLE and related autoimmune disorders: association with anticardiolipin antibody. Br J Haematol 1985;59:227-30.
8. Harris EN, Gharavi AE, Hegde V, et al. Anticardiolipin antibodies in autoimmune thrombocytopenic purpura. Br J Haematol 1985;59:231-4.
9. Lockshin MD, Druzin ML, Goei S, et al. Antibody to cardiolipin as a predictor of fetal distress or death in pregnant patients with sytemic lupus erythematosus. N Engl J Med 1985;313:152-6.
10. Derue GJ, Englert HJ, Harris EN, et al. Fetal loss in systemic lupus: association with anticardiolipin antibodies. J Obstet Gynecol 1985;5:207-9.
11. Stimmler MM, McGehee WG, Quismorio FP Jr. A prospective study of anticardiolipin antibodies (ACA) in hospitalized SLE patients [Abstract]. Arthritis Rheum 1986;29:S44.
12. Fort JG, Cowchock FS, Abruzzo JL, Smith JB. Anticardiolipin antibodies in patients with rheumatic diseases. Arthritis Rheum 1987;30:752-60.
13. Sturfelt G, Nived O, Norberg R, et al. Anticardiolipin antibodies in patients with systemic lupus erythematosus. Arthritis Rheum 1987;30:382-8.
14. Kalunian KC, Peter JB, Middlekauff HR, et al. Clinical significance of a single test for anti-cardiolipin antibodies in patients with sytemic lupus erythematosus. Am J Med 1988;85:602-8.
15. Khamashta MA, Cervera R, Asherson RA, et al. Association of antibodies against phospholipids with heart valve disease in systemic lupus erythematosus. Lancet 1990;335:1541-4.
16. Mahmood T, Racis SP, Krey PR. Ig-A anticardiolipin antibody (aCLA) in systemic lupus erythematosus (SLE) [Abstract]. Arthritis Rheum 1990;3:R45.

17. Loizou S, McCrea JD, Rudge AC, Reynolds R, Boyle CC, Harris EN. Measurement of anti-cardiolipin antibodies by an enzyme-linked immunosorbent assay (ELISA): standardization and quantitation of results. Clin Exp Immunol 1985;62:738-45.
18. Qamar T, Levy RA, Sammaritano L, et al. Characteristics of high-titer IgG antiphospholipid antibody in systemic lupus erythematosus patients with and without fetal death. Arthritis Rheum 1990;33:501-4.
19. Peter JB. Cardiolipin antibody assays [Letter]. Lancet 1990;335:1405.
20. Hughes TP, Jones P, Rozenberg MC. Hypergammaglobulinemia and the anticardiolipin antibody test [Letter]. Arthritis Rheum 1989;32:813.
21. Fort JG, Cowchock S. Comment on the letter by Hughes et al. [Letter]. Arthritis Rheum 1990;33:607.
22. Cowchock S, Fort J, Munoz S, et al. False positive ELISA tests for anticardiolipin antibodies in sera from patients with repeated abortion, rheumatologic disorders and primary biliary cirrhosis: correlation with elevated polyclonal IgM and implications for patients with repeated abortion. Clin Exp Immunol 1988;73:289-94.
23. Palosuo T, Aho K. Technical falsely positive rheumatoid factor by ELISA in sera with elevated IgM levels. Med Biol 1983;61:203-7.
24. Derksen RHWM, Hasselaar P, Blokziji L, et al. Coagulation screen is more specific than the anticardiolipin antibody ELISA in defining a thrombotic subset of lupus patients. Ann Rheum Dis 1988;47:364-71.
25. Mackworth-Young C. Antiphospholipid antibodies: more than just a disease marker? Immunology Today 1990;11:60-5.
26. McNeil H, Simpson RJ, Chesterman CN, Krilis SA. Anti phospholipid antibodies are directed against a complex antigen that includes a lipid-binding inhibitor of coagulation: β_2-glycoprotein I (apolipoprotein H). Proc Natl Acad Sci USA 1990;87:4120-4.
27. Galli M, Comfurius P, Maassen C, et al. Anticardiolipin antibodies (ACA) directed not to cardiolipin but to a plasma protein cofactor. Lancet 1990;335:1544-7.
28. Matsuura E, Igarashi Y, Fujimoto M, Ichikawa Koike T. Anticardiolipin cofactor(s) and differential diagnosis of autoimmune disease [Letter]. Lancet 1990;2:177-8.

CENTRIOLE ANTIBODIES

Anti-centriole antibodies are found occasionally in sera with antibodies to mitotic-spindle apparatus (MSA) and are rarely detected in patients with evolving connective tissue diseases, including scleroderma[1-3] (cf. 4 for review). See also **KINETOCHORE ANTIBODIES.**

REFERENCES:
1. McCarty GA, Valencia DW, Fritzler MJ, Barada FA. Unique antinuclear antibody staining only the mitotic-spindle apparatus [Letter]. N Engl J Med 1981;305:703.
2. Osborn TG, Patel NJ, Ross SC, Bauer NE. Antinuclear antibody staining only centrioles in a patient with scleroderma [Letter]. N Engl J Med 1982;307:253-4.
3. Tuffanelli DL, McKeon F, Kleinsmith D'AM, Burnham TK, Kirschner M. Anticentromere and anticentriole antibodies in the scleroderma spectrum. Arch Dermatol 1983;119:560-6.
4. Moroi Y, Murata I, Takeuchi A, Kamatani N, Tanimoto K, Yokohari R. Human anticentriole autoantibody in patients with scleroderma and Raynaud's phenomenon. Clin Immunol Immunopathol 1983;29:381-90.

CENTROMERE ANTIBODIES

A centromere is a specialized domain at the primary constriction of a eucaryotic chromosome; a kinetochore is that region of the centromere with which spindle fibers are associated. Antibodies to centromeres/kinetochores are found in 22% of patients with systemic sclerosis, almost all of whom have limited scleroderma (an appellation more appropriate than CREST syndrome, because many patients with diffuse scleroderma have 4 or 5 features of CREST).[1] Positive anti-centromere antibodies (ACENAs) are found in about 12% of primary biliary cirrhosis (PBC) of whom about half have features of scleroderma.[2] On the other hand, scleroderma usually in its limited form (CREST), is present in 4-18% of PBC.[2] ACENA-positive, limited scleroderma is more often accompanied by calcinosis and telangiectasias and less often by pulmonary interstitial fibrosis than ACENA-negative, limited scleroderma. Survival and pulmonary hypertension in limited scleroderma are not influenced by ACENA positivity.[1-3] Antibodies to centromeres and to Scl-70 are rarely found in the same serum.[1] Positive ACENA in patients with Raynaud syndrome suggest a transition to limited scleroderma.[4]

Survival rates measured from time of first symptom(s) are much longer in ACENA-positive (and ACENA-negative) limited scleroderma than in anti-Scl-70-positive (and anti-Scl-70-negative) diffuse scleroderma.[1] The fact that these rates may not differ when measured from time of presentation to tertiary care centers reflects the long interval before severe disease in limited scleroderma. Causes of death differ in the ACENA-positive (pulmonary hypertension and scleroderma gastrointestinal disease) and in anti-Scl-70-positive patients (scleroderma-related heart, lung, kidney and gastrointestinal disease; cf. 1 for review). Levels of ACENA are stable for long periods.[5] Use of EIA with its more sensitive detection of ACENA promises improvements in laboratory evaluation of Raynaud syndrome.[6] Positive ACENA are reported rarely in chronic active hepatitis[7] and primary pulmonary hypertension.[8] Immunoblotting of ACENA-positive sera typically reveals IgG[9] (and sometimes IgA[10] and IgM[10,11]) bands at 17-18 kd (CENP-A), 80 kd (CENP-B) and 140 kd (CENP-C) and sometimes an $\sim$50 kd (CENP-D)[9] (cf. 12). The striking conservation of certain kinetochore proteins is manifest by staining of kinetochores of some plants by ACENA-positive sera.[13] See also **KINETOCHORE ANTIBODIES.**

REFERENCES:
1. Steen VD, Powell DL, Medsger TA Jr. Clinical correlations and prognosis based on serum autoantibodies in patients with systemic sclerosis. Arthritis Rheum 1988;31:196-203.
2. Powell FC, Winkelmann RK, Venencie-Lemarchand F, Spurbeck JL, Schroeter AL. The anticentromere antibody: disease specificity and clinical significance. Mayo Clin Proc 1984;59:700-6.
3. Steen VD, Ziegler GL, Rodnan GP, Medsger TA Jr. Clinical and laboratory associations of anticentromere antibody in patients with progressive systemic sclerosis. Arthritis Rheum 1984;27:125-31.
4. Sarkozi J, Bookman AAM, Lee P, Keystone EC, Fritzler MJ. Significance of anticentromere antibody in idiopathic Raynaud's syndrome. Am J Med 1987;83:893-8.
5. Tramposch HD, Smith CD, Senecal J-L, Rothfield N. A long-term longitudinal study of anticentromere antibodies. Arthritis Rheum 1984;27:121-4.
6. Rothfield N, Whitaker D, Bordwell B, Weiner E, Senecal J-L, Earnshaw W. Detection of anticentromere antibodies using cloned autoantigen CENP-B. Arthritis Rheum 1987;30:1416-9.
7. Devars du Mayne J-F, Yeni P, Harlé X, Chagnon J-P, Boulanger F, Brion N. Hépatite chronique active avec syndrome CRST incomplet: intéret des anticorps anti-centromIres. Gastroenterol Clin Biol 1982;6:949.
8. Seibold JR, Trontell MC. Anticentromere antibody and primary pulmonary hypertension. J Rheumatol 1982;9:607-9.
9. Earnshaw WC, Bordwell B, Marino C, Rothfield NF. Three human chromosomal autoantigens are recognized by sera from patients with anticentromere antibodies. J Clin Invest 1986;77:426-30.
10. Hildebrandt S, Weiner E, Senécal J-L, et al. The IgG, IgM, and IgA isotypes of antitopoisomerase I and anticentromere autoantibodies. Arthritis Rheum 1990;33:724-7.
11. McHugh NJ, James TE, Maddison PJ. Differential isotype recognition of two centromere associated polypeptides by immunoblotting in connective tissue disease. Clin Exp Immunol 1988;72:457-64.
12. Kingwell B, Rattner JB. Mammalian kinetochore/centromere composition: a 50 kDa antigen is present in the mammalian kinetochore/centromere. Chromosoma 1987;95:403-7.
13. Mole-Bajer J, Bajer AS, Zinkowski RP, et al. Autoantibodies from a patient with scleroderma CREST recognized kinetochores of the higher plant *Haemanthus*. Proc Natl Acad Sci USA 1990;87:3599-603.

CH50

Total complement hemolytic activity of the classical pathway (CP) is measured by CH50 assay with results expressed in units which represent the amount of serum required to lyse 50% of sheep cells sensitized with rabbit antibody (hemolysin).

A normal CH50 assay indicates that C1 through C9 are present in the serum being tested. However, even in the presence of a normal CH50, the absolute levels of some complement components (e.g., C4) can be significantly lower than normal, because normal serum contains C4 in substantial excess of that required to yield a normal result for CH50. Hence, CH50 can be used to assess the integrity of the classical pathway (i.e., the presence of complement components C1-C9), but can not be used as a sensitive test for *in vivo* fixation of complement (cf. 1 and 2 for review). The prognosis of lupus nephritis is better in patients with consistent normalization of CH50 than in patients with only short-term control or persistently decreased CH50 levels.[3] Whether a profile of tests measuring functional activity of CH50 and AH50 together with immunochemical assay of components or products of those pathways (C3, C4, B, C1-INH and C3d) is clinically useful is not yet known.[4] See also **AH50, C3a, C4a, C5a, and ANAPHYLATOXINS; COMPLEMENT SPLIT PRODUCTS (C4d, Ba and C3dg); C4 ALLOTYPES** and **MEMBRANE ATTACK COMPLEX.**

REFERENCES:
1. Dalmasso AP. Complement in the pathophysiology and diagnosis of human diseases. CRC Crit Review Clin Lab Sci 1986;24:123-83.
2. Tucker ES III. Complement activation in autoimmune disease. J Clin Immunoassay 1984;7:310-20.
3. Laitman RS, Glicklich D, Sablay LB, et al. Effect of long term normalization of serum complement levels on the course of lupus nephritis. Am J Med 1989;87:132-8.
4. Wiener F, Groth T, Nilsson U. A knowledge-based system for automatic interpretation of an analytical profile of complement factors. J Clin Lab Analysis 1989;3:287-95.

CHEMOTACTIC FACTORS
Chemotactic factors produced by smooth muscle cells[1] and malignant cells[2] have very similar amino acid sequences and may represent a family of proteins responsible for nonlatent monocyte chemotactic activity.

REFERENCES:
1. Graves DT, Jiang YL, Williamson MJ, Valente AJ. Identification of monocyte chemotactic activity produced by malignant cells. Science 1989;245:1490-3.
2. Valente AJ, Graves DT, Vialle-Valentin CE, Delgado R, Schwartz CJ. Purification of a monocyte chemotactic factor secreted by nonhuman primate vascular cells in culture. Biochemistry 1988;27:4162-8.

CIRCULATING IMMUNE COMPLEXES
The major varieties of circulating immune complexes (CIC) are detectable using a combination of tests including C1q binding assay, conglutinin solid phase assay, polyethylene glycol (PEG) assay and Raji cell assay. This combination has the merit of high sensitivity (conglutinin), detection of aggregated immunoglobulins (PEG) which often obfuscate results by other techniques, as well as the capacity to detect complexes of different Ag/Ab ratios (Ag excess [1q binding], Ab excess [large excess = Raji; slight excess = conglutinin]). Some authorities recommend a combination of the C1q binding assay and the conglutinin assay for detection of CIC, because these assays "may be helpful for assessing and monitoring of disease activity in conditions such as rheumatoid arthritis and SLE".[1] In general, more than a single technique is needed to detect the rather wide variety of CIC known to exist in various clinical conditions,[2-5] because no single test provides the spectrum needed. Overall disease activity in SLE correlates with reduced levels of C3 (predictive value of abnormal result is 82%, but 53% of those with normal C3 levels had active disease);[6,7] activity is also reflected by reduced CH50 as well as by CIC as detected by increased C1q binding.[7,8] Decreased CH50, however, has even lower diagnostic sensitivity than C3 but specificity is high[8] (cf. **CH50**). In about 1/3 of SLE patients testing can detect a variable (e.g., an assay for immune complexes or a complement component) which correlates with disease activity in a given patient; unfortunately, the variables which prove most useful must be established for each individual patient by serial samples and clinical correlation.[6] Additional longitudinal studies for CIC by a combination of techniques are needed.

Detection and characterization of CIC, which are often composed, at least in part, of polyreactive human natural antibodies,[9] will continue to be largely of research interest,[1,3-5,10-12] until studies of better design yield definitive data on the clinical utility of a well selected combination of assays for CIC. As regards screening, however, the lack of merit of isolated assays for CIC by a single technology is beyond doubt.

The presence of IgA-containing ICs correlates with hematuria in ankylosing spondylitis,[13] which is sometimes accompanied by IgA nephropathy.[14] IgA-fibronectin aggregates ("complexes") are commonly found in IgA nephropathy,[15,16] which is sometimes accompanied by sacroiliitis;[17] these aggregates are not found in ankylosing spondylitis.[16]

The presence of C1q-binding ICs (which are usually higher in arterial than venous blood in RA[17]) and of IgA-ICs correlates with seropositivity, disease activity and vasculitis in rheumatoid arthritis.[18] In RA, ICs induce PMN-mediated detachment of human endothelial cells in culture.[19] In SLE, complement-activating aggregates of IgG are cleaved slowly, bind less to patient erythrocytes and are taken up less by the spleen.[20]

Assay for products of complement activation are likely to be more useful clinically than are direct assays for circulating immune complexes.[21] The frequency of immune complexes detectable in serum of patients with diabetes mellitus correlates with complications,[22] but no data on predictive value are available. Antibodies to *Borrelia burgdorferi* are said to be sequestered in immune complexes in seronegative Lyme disease.[23] Antigens documented as present in ICs of relevant diseases include yersinia antigens in synovial fluid in yersinia-reactive arthritis,[24] HBsAg in cryoglobulins in urticarial vasculitis,[25] DNA in ICs in SLE,[26,27] in serum sickness due to serotherapy,[28] and many others. Small ICs formed *in vivo* in humans being treated for cancer cause decreases of C4, C3, CH50 and erythrocyte CR1 as well as binding of C4d and C3dg to erythrocyte.[29] These changes are very similar to abnormalities found in active SLE (cf. 29 for review). See **C1q BINDING ASSAY FOR CIC, CONGLUTININ SOLID PHASE ASSAY FOR CIRCULATING IMMUNE COMPLEXES, IgA-FIBRONECTIN AGGREGATES, POLYETHYLENE GLYCOL (PEG) ASSAY FOR CIC** and **RAJI CELL ASSAY FOR CIC.**

REFERENCES:
1. IUIS/WHO Working Group. Laboratory investigations in clinical immunology: methods, pitfalls, and clinical indications. A second IUIS/WHO report. Clin Immunol Immunopathol 1988;49:478-97.
2. Lambert PH, Dixon FJ, Zubler RH, et al. A WHO collaborative study for the evaluation of eighteen methods for detecting immune complexes in serum. J Clin Lab Immunol 1978;1:1-15.
3. Ritzmann SE, Daniels JC. Immune complexes: characteristics, clinical correlations, and interpretive approaches in the clinical laboratory. Clin Chem 1982;28:1259-71.
4. Puccetti A, Trovatello G, Cantarella S, Celada F. Circulating immune complexes in connective tissue diseases. Clin Immunol Newsletter 1987;8:1-5.
5. Migliorini P, D'Amelio R, Passaleva A, et al. Comparison of pathologic and normal sera by immune complex determination: five disease groups within 190 samples are discriminated by computer-selected combinations of 13 methods. Clin Immunol Immunopathol 1984;32:298-315.
6. Valentijn RM, van Overhagen H, Hazevoet HM, et al. The value of complement and immune complex determinations in monitoring disease activity in patients with systemic lupus erythematosus. Arthritis Rheum 1985;28:904-13.
7. Weinstein A, Bordwell B, Stone B, et al. Antibodies to native DNA and serum complement (C3) levels. Application to diagnosis and classification of systemic lupus erythematosus. Am J Med 1983;74:206-16.
8. Laitman RS, Glicklich D, Sablay LB, et al. Effect of long-term normalization of serum complement levels on the course of lupus nephritis. Am J Med 1989;87:132-8.
9. Reynolds WJ, Yoon SJ, Emin M, et al. Circulating immune complexes in rheumatoid arthritis: a prospective study using five immunoassays. J Rheumatol 1986;13:700-6.
10. Louzir H, Ternynck T, Gorgi Y, Ayed K, Avrameas S. Enzyme immunoassay analysis of antibody specificities present in the circulating immune complexes of selected pathological sera. J Immunol Methods 1988;114:145-53.
11. McDougal JS, Hubbard M, Strobel PL, McDuffie FC. Comparison of five assays for immune complexes in the rheumatic diseases: performance characteristics of the assays. J Lab Clin Med 1982;100:705-19.
12. Lessard J, Nunnery E, Cecere F, et al. Relationship between the articular manifestations of rheumatoid arthritis and circulating immune complexes detected by three methods and specific classes of rheumatoid factors. J Rheumatol 1983;10:411-7.

13. Peeters AJ, Warmold A, van den Wall Bake AWL, et al. IgA containing immune complexes and hematuria in ankylosing spondylitis. A prospective longitudinal study. J Rheumatol 1988;15:1662-7.
14. Jones DW, Mansell MA, Samuell CT, et al. Renal abnormalities in ankylosing spondylitis. Br J Rheumatol 1987;26:341-5.
15. Cederholm B, Wieslander J, Bygren P, Heinegård D. Circulating complexes containing IgA and fibronectin in patients with primary IgA nephropathy. Proc Natl Acad Sci USA 1988;85:4865-8.
16. Hollingsworth PN, Peter JB. Unpublished data.
17. van den Wall Bake AWL, Kroon HM, van der Linden SM, et al. Association of IgA nephropathy with minor radiological abnormalities of the sacroiliac joints. Clin Nephrol 1988;29:163-4.
18. Steven MM, Westedt M-L, Daha MR, et al. Comparison of immune complexes and complement components in arterial and venous blood of patients with rheumatoid arthritis. J Rheumatol 1986;13:74-8.
19. Westedt M-L, Daha MR, de Vries E, et al. IgA containing immune complexes in rheumatoid vasculitis and in active rheumatoid disease. J Rheumatol 1985;12:449-55.
20. Lobatto S, Daha MR, Breedveld FC, et al. Abnormal clearance of soluble aggregates of human immunoglobulin G in patients with systemic lupus erythematosus. Clin Exp Immunol 1988;72:55-9.
21. Dalmasso AP. Complement in the pathophysiology and diagnosis of human diseases. CRC Crit Rev Clin Lab Sci 1986;24:123-83.
22. Virella G, Wohltmann H, Sagel J, et al. Soluble immune complexes in patients with diabetes mellitus: detection and pathological significance. Diabetologia 1981;21:184-91.
23. Schutzer SE, Coyle PK, Belman AL, et al. Sequestration of antibody to *Borrelia burgdorferi* in immune complexes in seronegative Lyme disease. Lancet 1990;335:312-5.
24. Granfors K, Jalkanen S, von Essen R, et al. Yersinia antigens in synovial-fluid cells from patients with reactive arthritis. N Engl J Med 1989;320:216-21.
25. Heermann KH, Gerlich WH. Immunology of hepatitis B virus infections. Rheumatol Int 1989;9:167-73.
26. Stollar BD. The origin and pathogenic role of anti-DNA autoantibodies. Autoimmunity 1990;2:607-12.
27. Brinkman K, Termaat R, Berden JHM, Smeenk RJT. Anti-DNA antibodies and lupus nephritis: the complexity of crossreactivity. Immunol Today 1990;11:232-4.
28. Nielsen H, Sorensen H, Faber V, Svehag SE. Circulating immune complexes, complement activation kinetics and serum sickness following treatment with heterologous anti-snake venom globulin. Scand J Immunol 1978;7:25-33.
29. Davies KA, Hird V, Stewart S, et al. A study of in vivo immune complex formation and clearance in man. J Immunol 1990;144:4613-20.

CLASS I AND II ANTIGENS

The term "class I antigens" includes the gene products of the HLA-A, B and C genes. These glycoproteins can be found in normal serum as well as in their characteristic location on the surface of nucleated cells.[1] The term "class II antigens" includes HLA-DR, DP and DQ antigens. The "class III" or central genes include complement components C4, C2 and factor B as well as TNF, HSP and 21 hydroxylase. Increased expression of class II antigens on involved tissues is common in immunologically mediated diseases, including autoimmunity, transplant rejection and graft-versus-host disease. Serum (and urine) levels of class II antigens are being evaluated as immune monitors.[2] See also **MAJOR HISTOCOMPATIBILITY COMPLEX.**

REFERENCES:
1. Russo C, Fotino M, Carbonara A, Ferrone S. A double determinant immunoassay for HLA class I typing using serum as an antigen source. Hum Immunol 1987;19:69-77.
2. Thompson S, Wareham M, Pearson ADJ, et al. A preliminary study of serum class II levels in healthy individuals and bone-marrow transplant patients. Clin Chim Acta 1989;185:45-52.

CLUSTERS OF DIFFERENTIATION

Antigens of lymphocytes, monocytes, macrophages, platelets and other cells are now defined by their reactions with clusters of monoclonal antibodies. Hence, the antigens are referred to as clusters of differentiation (CD). The CDs listed below were defined by three international workshops as summarized previously.[1-4]

Clusters of Differentiation (1989)

CD	CLONES	CELL DISTRIBUTION/FUNCTION	ANTIBODY CLUSTERS
1	OKT6,Leu-6	Thymocytes	}
2	OKT11,Leu-5a	E-rosette receptor	}
3	OKT3,Leu-4	T receptor (TCR)-associated	}
4	OKT4,Leu-3a	T helper	}
5	OK-CLL,Leu-1, T101	T cells, B cell subset	}---T cell biased
6		Pan T cell	}
73	A1,Leu-9	Pan T cell, FcR(IgM receptor)(?)	}
8	OKT8,Leu-2a	T suppressor/cytotoxic	}
11A		Leucocyte function antigen (LFA-1) p150/90	}
11	BLeu-15,Mol, Mac-1	Complement receptor 3 (CR3), p165/95	}
11	CLeu-M5	p150/95	}
13	My7	Monocyte, granulocyte, early myeloid	}
14	My4	Monocyte, B cell	}---Myeloid biased
15	Leu-M1,My1	x-hapten	}
16	Leu-11a,b,c	FcRIII (IgG receptor)	}
17		Lactosyl ceramide	}
18		Leukocyte function antigen (LFA-1); beta chain	}
33	My9	Early myeloid	}
34	My10	Stem cell	}
9	Ba-2	Leukemia associated, p24 antigen (non-T, non-B ALL)	}
10	J5	Common acute lymphoblastic leukemia antigen (CALLA)	}
19		Leu-12,B4 B cell	}
20	Leu-16,B1	B cell	}
21		B-Complement receptor 2 (CR2), EBV receptor	}---B cell biased
22	Leu-14	B cell	}
3	B532	Activated B cell, FcRII (low affinity IgE receptor);IL-4 receptor (?)	}
24	BA1	B cell, granulocyte	}
25		TAC, IL-2R β chain, gp55, gp55d	}
w26	Ta-1	T cell activation	}
w29	4B4	Helper-inducer T cell	}
30	Ki-1	Reed-Sternberg cell	}
31		Platelet glycoprotein IIa	}
w32		FcRII (IgG receptor)	}---Miscellaneous
35		Complement receptor 1 (CR1)	}
38	OKT10,Leu-17	Thymocyte, null cell, stem cell, activated lymphocyte	}
39			}
w41		Platelet glycoprotein IIb/IIIa complex	}

CD	CLONES	CELL DISTRIBUTION/FUNCTION	ANTIBODY CLUSTERS
w42		Platelet glycoprotein Ib	}
44		Pgp-1, ECMIII	}
45	T200	Leukocyte common antigen (LCA)	}
45R	Leu-18,2H4	Restricted LCA	}
54		Intercellular adhesion molecule 1	}
55		Complement regulatory DAF protein	}---Miscellaneous
56	NKH1	N-CAM isoform (Neural-cell Adhesion Molecule)	}
58		LFA-3	}
71		Transferrin receptor	}
73		Ecto 5′-nucleotidase	}

NAME SPECIFICITY	MOLECULAR CHARACTERISTICS	HLA ALLELE	HLA SEROLOGICAL SPECIFICITY	HLA-DR
HLA-A	Class I α-chain	*101	A1	
HLA-B	Class I α-chain B	*27012 tlB		
		2706	B27	HLA-DR

REFERENCES:
1. Reinherz EL, Haynes BF, Nadler LM, Bernstein ID. Human T lymphocytes. New York: Springer-Verlag 1986;1:1-535.
2. Reinherz EL, Haynes BF, Nadler LM, Bernstein ID. Human B lymphocytes. New York: Springer-Verlag 1986;2:1-550.
3. Reinherz EL, Haynes BF, Nadler LM, Bernstein ID. Human myeloid and hematopoietic cells. New York: Springer-Verlag 1986;3:1-355.
4. Knapp W, Dorken B, Rieber P, Schmidt RE, Stein H, von dem Borne AEGKr. CD antigens 1989. Am J Pathol 1989;135:420-1.

COLLAGEN (TYPES I, II, III) ANTIBODIES

In rodents and monkeys, immunization with type II collagen produces anti-collagen antibodies which, in turn, induce arthritis in these animals[1,2] (cf. 3 for review). Autoantibodies to collagen types I, II and III are found in human rheumatic diseases such as adult and juvenile rheumatoid arthritis, but the frequency varies and the pathogenic role is not well established,[4] even though intra-articular synthesis of antibodies to denatured collagen has been demonstrated.[5,6] Autoantibodies to collagens are also found in other inflammatory, articular and bone diseases including psoriatic arthritis, ankylosing spondylitis, Reiter syndrome, gout, osteoarthritis, osteoporosis and Paget disease.[3-8] Antibodies to type II collagen are reported in autoimmune diseases including scleroderma and systemic lupus erythematosus;[8,9] heart and vascular diseases such as infective endocarditis[10] and thromboangiitis obliterans;[7] and periodontal diseases.[11] Antibodies to type II collagen epitopes which may be responsible for collagen-induced ear diseases might aid in diagnosis of Meniére disease, otosclerosis or autoimmune sensorineural hearing loss,[12-15] but only the association of antibodies to type II collagen with autoimmune sensorineural hearing loss has been confirmed to date.[15] Assays for antibodies to collagen types I, II and III are not of proven clinical utility at this time with the possible exception of antibodies to type II collagen in autoimmune sensorineural hearing loss.

REFERENCES:
1. Yoo TJ, Kim S-Y, Stuart JM, et al. Induction of arthritis in monkeys by immunization with type II collagen. J Exp Med 1988;168:777-82.
2. Stuart JM, Cremer MA, Townes AS, Kang AH. Type II collagen-induced arthritis in rats: passive transfer with serum and evidence that IgG anticollagen antibodies can cause arthritis. J Exp Med 1982;155:1-16.
3. Stuart JM, Watson WC, Kang AH. Collagen autoimmunity and arthritis. FASEB J 1988;2:2950-6.

4. Charriere G, Hartmann DJ, Vignon E, et al. Antibodies to types I, II, IX, and XI collagen in the serum of patients with rheumatic diseases. Arthritis Rheum 1988;31:325-32.
5. Rowley MJ, Williamson DJ, Mackay IR. Evidence for local synthesis of antibodies to denatured collagen in the synovium in rheumatoid arthritis. Arthritis Rheum 1987;30:1420-5.
6. Tarkowski A, Klareskog L, Carlsten H, et al. Secretion of antibodies to types I and II collagen by synovial tissue cells in patients with rheumatoid arthritis. Arthritis Rheum 1989;32:1087-92.
7. Adar R, Papa MZ, Halpern Z, et al. Cellular sensitivity to collagen in thromboangiitis obliterans. N Engl J Med 1983;308:1113-6.
8. Choi EKK, Gatenby PA, McGill NW, et al. Autoantibodies to type II collagen: occurrence in rheumatoid arthritis, other arthritides, autoimmune connective tissue diseases, and chronic inflammatory syndromes. Ann Rheum Dis 1988;47:313-22.
9. Gioud M, Meghlaoui A, Costa O, Monier JC. Antibodies to native type I and II collagens detected by an enzyme-linked immunosorbent assay (ELISA) in rheumatoid arthritis and systemic lupus erythematosus. Coll Relat Res 1982;2:557-64.
10. De Buyzere ML, De Scheerder IK, Delanghe JR, et al. Measurement of autoimmune response against collagen types I, III, and IV by enzyme-linked immunosorbent assay, and its application in infective endocarditis. Clin Chem 1989;35:246-50.
11. Ftis A, Singh G, Dolby AE. Antibody to collagen type I in periodontal disease. J Periodontol 1986;57:693-8.
12. McCabe BF. Autoimmune sensorineural hearing loss. Ann Otol Rhinol Laryngol 1979;88:585-9.
13. Yoo TJ, Stuart JM, Kang AH, et al. Type II collagen autoimmunity in otosclerosis and Meniere's disease. Science 1982:217:1153-5.
14. Yoo TJ, Nam SH, Ye XI, et al. Molecular characterization of epitope responsible for type II collagen induced ear disease. Third Annual Conference on Clinical Immunology Society, San Francisco, California 1988;11.
15. Helfgott SM, Mosciscki R, Sanmartine J, et al. Association of antibodies to type II collagen with idiopathic bilateral progessive sensorineural hearing loss. Clin Res 1989;37:411a.

COLLAGEN (TYPE IV) ANTIBODIES

Autoantibodies to basement membrane type IV collagen have been reported in several rheumatic diseases,[1] including progressive systemic sclerosis (PSS) and primary Raynaud phenomenon (PRP), but the clinical utility of such measurements has not been established. In one study,[2] the raw data suggested that antibodies to type IV collagen and laminin might be used to predict progression from PRP to PSS. Circulating antibodies reactive with the globular domain of type IV collagen are found in Goodpasture syndrome and are responsible for the rapidly progressive glomerulonephritis in these patients;[3,4] detection by EIA is the method of choice.[5] A succinct review of cartilage collagens and their possible involvement in articular disease is available.[6] In Alport syndrome, a hereditary glomerulonephritis with progressive loss of kidney function and hearing, there is absence or alteration of the noncollagenous domain of GBM type IV collagen due to mutations of the COL4A5 gene (located at Xq22), which controls synthesis of the $\alpha5(IV)$ gene.[7] Whether similar mutations cause familial or sporadic deafness or sporadic nephritis with or without deafness is not known. Autoantibodies have not been reported. See also **COLLAGEN (TYPES I, II, III) ANTIBODIES** and **GLOMERULAR BASEMENT MEMBRANE ANTIBODIES.**

REFERENCES:

1. Petty RE, Hunt DWC, Rosenberg AM. Antibodies to type IV collagen in rheumatic diseases. J Rheumatol 1986;13:246-53.
2. Gabrielli A, Montroni M, Rupoli S, et al. A retrospective study of antibodies against basement membrane antigens (type IV collagen and laminin) in patients with primary and secondary Raynaud's phenomenon. Arthritis Rheum 1988;31:1432-6.
3. Wieslander J, Bygren P, Heinegård D. Isolation of the specific glomerular basement membrane antigen involved in Goodpasture syndrome. Proc Natl Acad Sci USA 1984;81:1544-8.
4. Wieslander J, Barr JF, Butkowski RJ, et al. Goodpasture antigen of the glomerular basement membrane: localization to noncollagenous regions of type IV collagen. Proc Nat Acad Sci USA 1984;81:3838-42.

5. Peter JB, Shen GQ, Lin H-C. A sensitive enzyme immunoassay (EIA) for detection of antibodies to glomerular basement membranes (GBM) [Abstract]. Am J Clin Pathol 1989;91:367.
6. Mayne R. Cartilage collagens: what is their function, and are they involved in articular disease? Arthritis Rheum 1989;32:241-6.
7. Barker DF, Hostikka SL, Zhou J, et al. Identification of mutations in the COL4A5 collagen gene in Alport syndrome. Science 1990;248:1224-7.

COLON ANTIBODIES

Such antibodies are not reproducibly demonstrable in inflammatory bowel disease.[1]

REFERENCES:
1. Cantrell M, Prindiville T, Gershwin ME. Autoantibodies to colonic cells and subcellular fractions in inflammatory bowel disease: do they exist? J Autoimmunity 1990;3:307-20.

COLONY-STIMULATING FACTORS

Currently subsumed under the term "colony simulating factors" are four major human myeloid growth factors, including granulocyte CSF (G-CSF), macrophage CSF (M-CSF) granulocyte-macrophage CSF (GM-CSF) and interleukin-3 (IL-3). The molecular cloning, regulation of CSF gene expression, structure of recombinant CSFs, biological activities, *in vivo* activities and therapeutic applications have recently been reviewed.[1-5] Data on the therapeutic utility of CSFs and the clinical utility of assays for CSFs are developing rapidly.[4,6-8] Serum G-CSF is increased in the neutropenic phase of cyclic neutropenia as well as in a variable proportion of patients with idiopathic aplastic anemia (82%), *Fanconi anemia,* myelodysplastic syndromes (50%) and acute and chronic leukemias[9] (cf. 10 and 11 for review) of haemopoietic growth factors. GM-CSF causes profound decreases in serum cholesterol by mechanisms which are currently undefined.[12] Induction of synthesis and secretion of CSFs by endothelial cells exposed *in vitro* to modified low-density lipoproteins (which are thought to be important in formation of the foam cells characteristics of early atherosclerosis) could mediate recruitment of phagocytic cells to areas of arterial damage;[13] quantitation of mRNAs in artery walls will be of interest.[14] There is local production of GM-CSF in rheumatoid synovitis.[15]

REFERENCES:
1. Clark SC, Kamen R. The human hematopoietic colony-stimulating factors. Science 1987;236:1229-37.
2. Golde DW, Gasson JC. Hormones that stimulate the growth of blood cells. Sci Am 1988;259:62-70.
3. Groopman JE, Molina J-M, Scadden DT. Hematopoietic growth factors. Biology and clinical applications. N Engl J Med 1989;321:1449-59.
4. Auger MJ. Mononuclear phagocytes. Br Med J 1989;298:546-8.
5. Metcalf D. The molecular control of cell division, differentiation commitment and maturation in haemopoietic cells. Nature 1989;339:27-30.
6. Gasson JC, Golde DW. In vivo studies with granulocyte macrophage colony-stimulating factors. In: Weissbart RH, ed. Colony-stimulating factors and host defense. Ann Intern Med 1989;110:297-303.
7. Sieff CA. Hematopoietic growth factors. J Clin Invest 1987;79:1549-57.
8. Ganser A, Ottmann OG, Erdmann H, et al. The effect of recombinant human granulocyte-macrophage colony-stimulating factor on neutropenia and related morbidity in chronic severe neutropenia. Ann Intern Med 1989;111:887-92.
9. Watari K, Asano S, Shirafuji N, et al. Serum granulocyte colony-stimulating factors levels in healthy volunteers and patients with various disorders as estimated by enzyme immunoassay. Blood 1989;73:117-22.
10. Metcalf D. Haemopoietic growth factors 1. Lancet 1989;1:765-7.
11. Metcalf D. Haemopoietic growth factors 2: clinical applications. Lancet 1989;1:885-7.
12. Nimer SD, Champlin RE, Golde DW. Serum cholesterol-lowering activity of granulocyte-macrophage colony-stimulating factor. JAMA 1988;260:3297-300.
13. Rajavashisth TB, Andalibi A, Territo MC, et al. Induction of endothelial cell expression of granulocyte and macrophage colony-stimulating factors by modified low-density lipoproteins. Nature 1990;344:254-7.

14. Wang AM, Doyle MV, Mark DV. Quantitation of mRNA by the polymerase chain reaction. Proc Natl Acad Sci USA 1989;86:9717-21.
15. Xu WD, Firestein GS, Taetle R, et al. Cytokines in chronic inflammatory arthritis. II. Granulocyte-macrophage colony-stimulating factor in rheumatoid synovial effusions. J Clin Invest 1989;83:876-82.

COMPLEMENT COMPONENTS

Homozygous deficiencies of early components of the classical pathway (C1, C2 and C4) are largely associated with SLE and related autoimmune disorders.[1] Deficiencies of C5-C8,[2,3] properdin,[3] C3,[3] and C4B[4] are associated with predisposition to serious infections with *Neisseria spp*. C3 and C3b inactivator deficiencies predispose to life-threatening bacterial infections.[3] Association of given deficiencies with different clinical syndromes shows much more overlap than indicated by these three discrete groups (e.g., C5-C8 with SLE).[5] A reported association of IgG subclass deficiency with deficiencies of early components of complement has not yet been confirmed.[6] A review with excellent illustrations of complement pathways is available.[7] See **AH50, C3, C4, CH50** and **MEMBRANE ATTACK COMPLEX**.

REFERENCES:
1. Agnello V. Lupus diseases associated with hereditary and acquired deficiencies of complement. Springer Semin Immunopathol 1986;9:161-78.
2. Rother K, Rother U, eds. Hereditary and acquired complement deficiencies in animals and man. New York: Karger-Basel, 1986;39:1-396.
3. Fijen CAP, Kuijper EJ, Hannema AJ, et al. Complement deficiencies in patients over ten years old with meningococcal disease due to uncommon serogroups. Lancet 1989;2:585-8.
4. Rowe PC, McLean RH, Wood RA, et al. Association of homozygous C4B deficiency with bacterial meningitis. J Infect Dis 1989;160:448-51.
5. Ruddy S. The second component. In: Rother K, Rother U, eds. Hereditary and acquired complement deficiencies in animals and man. New York: Karger-Basel, 1986;39:250-66.
6. Bird P, Lachmann PJ. The regulation of IgG subclass production in man: low serum IgG4 in inherited deficiencies of the classical pathway of C3 activation. Eur J Immunol 1988;18:1217-22.
7. Tucker ES III. Complement activation in autoimmune disease. J Clin Immunoassay 1984;7:310-20.

COMPLEMENT RECEPTOR TYPE 1 (CR1,CD35)

Complement receptor type 1 (CR1,CD35) is decreased on circulating erythrocytes in SLE[1] (cf. 2 and 3 for review) as well as inautoimmune hemolytic anemias,[4] paroxysmal nocturnal hemoglobinuria,[5] AIDS[6] and lepromatous leprosy.[7] There is an inverse correlation between serum levels of IgG or IgM anti-cardiolipin antibodies and numbers of CR1 on erythrocytes, but only IgM anti-cardiolipin antibody levels in serum correlate with erythrocyte C4d and C3d numbers.[1] Recombinant soluble CR1 blocks complement activation in human serum by both the classical and alternate pathways.[8] Regulators of complement activation include three membrane proteins (CR1, decay-accelerated factor [DAF] and membrane co-factor protein [MCP] and two plasma proteins [factor H and C4-binding protein]); CR2 also has some complement regulatory activity but is fundamentally involved with activation of B cells (cf. 8). See also **C3a (SPLIT PRODUCT OF C3)**.

REFERENCES:
1. Hammond A, Rudge AC, Loizou S, Bowcock SJ, Walport MJ. Reduced numbers of complement receptor type 1 on erythrocytes are associated with increased levels of anticardiolipin antibodies. Arthritis Rheum 1989;32:259-64.
2. Walport MJ, Lachmann PJ. Erythrocyte complement receptor type 1, immune complexes, and the rheumatic diseases. Arthritis Rheum 1988;31:153-8.
3. Fearon DT. Complement, C receptors, and immune complex disease. Hosp Pract 1988;23:63-72.
4. Ross GD, Yount WJ, Walport MJ, et al. Disease-associated loss of erythrocyte complement receptors (CR$_1$, C3b receptors) in patients with systemic lupus erythematosus and other diseases involving autoantibodies and/or complement activation. J Immunol 1985;135:2005-14.

5. Pangburn MK, Schreiber RD, Trombold JS, Müller-Eberhard JH. Paroxysmal nocturnal hemoglobinuria: deficiency in factor H-like functions of the abnormal erythrocytes. J Exp Med 1983;157:1971-80.
6. Tausk FA, McCutchan JA, Spechko P, Schreiber RD, Gigli I. Altered erythrocyte C3b receptor expression, immune complexes, and complement activation in homosexual men in varying risk groups for acquired immune deficiency syndrome. J Clin Invest 1986;78:977-82.
7. Tausk FA, Hoffman T, Schreiber R, Gigli I. Leprosy: altered complement receptors in disseminated disease. J Invest Dermatol 1985;85(Suppl):58S-61S.
8. Weisman HF, Bartow T, Leppo MK, et al. Soluble human complement receptor type 1: in vivo inhibitor of complement suppressing post-ischemic myocardial inflammation and necrosis. Science 1990;249:146-51.

CONGLUTININ SOLID PHASE (Kg SP) ASSAY FOR CIRCULATING IMMUNE COMPLEXES

This assay measures iC3b-containing complexes which are capable of complement activation by the classical or alternative pathways.[1-3] Use of an international reference preparation of aggregated IgG is expected to improve reproducibility and comparability of results.[4] Some authorities recommend the C1q binding assay and the conglutinin assay for detection of circulating immune complexes because these assays "may be helpful for assessing and monitoring of disease activity in conditions such as rheumatoid arthritis and SLE".[5]

REFERENCES:
1. Ritzmann SE, Daniels JC. Immune complexes: characteristics, clinical correlations, and interpretive approaches in the clinical laboratory. Clin Chem 1982;28:1259-71.
2. Casali P, Bossus A, Carpentier NA, Lambert P-H. Solid-phase enzyme immunoassay or radioimmunoassay for the detection of immune complexes based on their recognition by conglutinin: conglutinin-binding test. Clin Exp Immunol 1977;29:342-54.
3. Araga S, Irie H, Takahashi K. Conglutinin microtiter plate ELISA system for detecting circulating immune complexes. J Neuroimmunol 1984;6:161-8.
4. Nydegger UE, Svehag S-E. Improved standardization in the quantitative estimation of soluble immune complexes making use of an international reference preparation. Results of a collaborative muticentre study. Clin Exp Immunol 1984;58:502-9.
5. IUIS/WHO Working Group. Laboratory investigations in clinical immunology: methods, pitfalls, and clinical indications. A second IUIS/WHO report. Clin Immunol Immunopathol 1988;49:478-97.

CORTICOTROPHIN RECEPTOR ANTIBODIES

These antibodies, which are a type of anti-adrenal antibody, are important in the pathogenesis of Addison disease. Anti-corticotrophin receptor antibodies (ACRA) of the blocking type act by inhibiting the binding of ACTH to its receptor on adrenal cortical cells.[1-3] This variety of AAA (i.e., ACRA) almost certainly explains the rather high sensitivity, specificity and predictive value of AAA for idiopathic Addison disease.[4] Cushing syndrome due to primary pigmented nodular adrenocortical disease is associated with ACRA of the stimulating variety as measured by increase of DNA synthesis and increase in % of cells in S-phase.[5]

REFERENCES:
1. Smith EM, Brosnan P, Meyer WJ III, Blalock JE. An ACTH receptor on human mononuclear leukocytes. N Engl J Med 1987;317:1266-9.
2. Kendall-Taylor P, Lambert A, Mitchell R, Robertson WR. Antibody that blocks stimulation of cortisol secretion by adrenocorticotrophic hormone in Addison's disease. Br Med J 1988;296:1489-91.
3. Wulffraat NM, Drexhage HA, Bottazzo G-F, et al. Immunoglobulins of patients with idiopathic Addison's disease block the in vitro action of adrenocorticotropin. J Clin Endocrinol Metab 1989;69:231-8.
4. Ahonen P, Miettinen A, Perheentupa J. Adrenal and steroidal cell antibodies in patients with autoimmune polyglandular disease type I and risk of adrenocortical and ovarian failure. J Clin Endocrinol Metab 1987;64:494-500.

5. Young WF Jr, Carney JA, Musa BU, et al. Familial Cushing's syndrome due to primary pigmented nodular adrenocortical disease. N Engl J Med 1989;321:1659-64.

CRYOFIBRINOGEN

Cryofibrinogenemia may be primary or secondary (tumors, necrosis, acute and chronic inflammation and lymphoproliferative and autoimmune disorders).[1,2] Although cryofibrinogenemia is common in IgA nephropathy,[3] its relationship to IgA antibodies reactive with fibronectin remains unknown[4] as does its relationship to IgA rheumatoid factor and polymeric IgA.[5]

REFERENCES:
1. Zlotnick A, Shahin W, Rachmilewitz EA. Studies in cryofibrinogenemia. Acta Haematol (Basel) 1969;42:8-17.
2. Hobbs JR. Cryoproteins. Ann Med Interne 1986;137:254-9.
3. Nagy J, Ambrus M, Paal M, et al. Cryoglobulinaemia and cryofibrinogenaemia in IgA nephropathy: a follow-up study. Nephron 1987;46:337-42.
4. Cederholm B, Wieslander J, Bygren P, Heinegård D. Circulating complexes containing IgA and fibronectin in patients with primary IgA nephropathy. Proc Natl Acad Sci USA 1988;85:4865-8.
5. Julian BA, Waldo FB, Rifai A, Mestecky J. IgA nephropathy, the most common glomerulonephritis worldwide: a neglected disease in the United States. Am J Med 1988;84:129-32.

CRYOGLOBULINS

Cryoglobulins are classified in three major varieties on the basis of their composition. Type I cryoglobulins are composed of a single cryoprecipitable monoclonal immunoglobulin of the IgG, IgM or IgA class without known antibody specificity or they are composed of monoclonal light chains (Bence Jones proteins). Type II (mixed) cryoglobulins are composed of a monoclonal immunoglobulin (usually IgM but sometimes IgG or IgA) with anti-globulin activity against polyclonal IgG. Type III cryoglobulins are not composed of monoclonal immunoglobulins but consist of one or more classes of polyclonal immunoglobulins and sometimes non-immunoglobulin molecules such as C3 or lipoproteins[1] (cf. 2 and 3 for review). In cryoglobulinemia, vascular purpura and petechiae, or papules which often occur in rashes, are the most common findings (60-100%) followed by Raynaud phenomenon ($\sim$50%), arthralgias (50-90%), especially in types II and III, skin necrosis including leg ulcers and distal necrosis (11-30% overall and most common in type I [30-70%]), and nephrosis or nephritis (10-60%) (cf. 2 for review). In cryoglobulinemia, the serum concentration of the cryoprecipitable immunoglobulin is usually in the 20-100 mg/dl range with cryocrits (which are not recommended) in the 1-70% range. Associated diseases include SLE,[4] PAN, Sjögren syndrome and other autoimmune diseases,[5,6] Kawasaki syndrome,[7] IgA nephropathy[8] and lymphoproliferative disorders (cf. 1-3 for review). Absolute quantitation of the amount of cryoglobulin on an immunoglobulin protein basis (as opposed to cryocrit) is useful for diagnosis and monitoring.

REFERENCES:
1. Brouet J-C, Clauvel J-P, Danon F, Klein M, Seligmann M. Biologic and clinical significance of cryoglobulins: a report of 86 cases. Am J Med 1974;57:775-88.
2. Montagnino G. Reappraisal of the clinical expression of mixed cryoglobulinemia. In: Lambert PH, ed. Cryoglobulins. Geneva: Springer International 1988;1-19. (Miescher PA, Spiegelberg HL, eds. Springer Seminars in Immunopathology; vol 10).
3. Gorevic PD, Kassab HJ, Levo Y, et al. Mixed cryoglobulinemia: clinical aspects and long-term follow-up of 40 patients. Am J Med 1980;69:287-308.
4. Gripenberg M, Teppo AM, Kurki P, Gripenberg G, Helve T. Autoantibody activity of cryoglobulins and sera in sytemic lupus erythematosus: association of IgM class rheumatoid factors with Raynaud's syndrome. Scand J Rheumatol 1988;17:249-54.
5. Ardiles Sandoval A, Bekavac Alcalde J, Varas de la Jara MA, et al. Cryoglobulins in rheumatologic patients: clinical and laboratory findings. Rev Clin Espanol 1988;82:7-11.
6. Tzioufas AG, Papadopoulos NM, Moutsopoulos NM. Monoclonal cryoglobulins in primary Sjögren's syndrome. Ter Arkh 1988;60:25-7.

7. Herold BC, Davis AT, Arroyave CM, Duffy E, Pachman LM, Shulman ST. Cryoprecipitates in Kawasaki syndrome: association with coronary artery aneurysms. Pediatr Infect Dis J 1988;7:255-7.
8. Nagy J, Ambrus M, Paal M, Trinn C, Burger T. Cryoglobulinaemia and cryofibrinogenaemia in IgA nephropathy: a follow-up study. Nephron 1987;46:337-42.

CSF CARCINOEMBRYONIC ANTIGEN

An elevated CSF carcinoembryonic antigen (CEA) Index (a determination which estimates intra-blood-brain barrier (IBBB) synthesis of CEA in analogy to estimation of IBBB synthesis of IgG by the IgG Index) is found in approximately 90% of leptomeningeal carcinomas but in only about 50% of intraparenchymal carcinomas.[1-3] An elevated CSF CEA without taking serum CEA into account is only 60% sensitive for detection of leptomeningeal carcinomatosis[4] and is subject to false positives when serum CEA is elevated and the blood-brain barrier is damaged (cf. 5). See also BETA 2-MICROGLOBULIN and BETA-GLUCURONIDASE.

REFERENCES:
1. Jacobi C, Reiber H, Felgenhauer K. The clinical relevance of locally produced carcinoembryonic antigen in cerebrospinal fluid. J Neurol 1986;233:358-61.
2. Reiber H, Jacobi C, Felgenhauer K. Sensitive quantitation of carcinoembryonic antigen in cerebrospinal fluid and its barrier-dependent differentiation. Clin Chim Acta 1986;156:259-70.
3. van Zanten AP, Twijnstra A, Ongerboer de Visser BW, Hart AA, Nooyen WJ. Tumour markers in the cerebrospinal fluid of patients with central nervous system metastases from extracranial malignancies. Clin Chim Acta 1988;175:157-66.
4. Twijnstra A, van Zanten AP, Nooyen WJ, Ongerboer de Visser BW. Sensitivity and specificity of single and combined tumour markers in the diagnosis of leptomeningeal metastasis from breast cancer. J Neurol Neurosurg Psychiatry 1986;49:1246-50.
5. Klee GG, Tallman RD, Goellner JR, Yanagihara T. Elevation of carcinoembryonic antigen in cerebrospinal fluid among patients with meningeal carcinomatosis. Mayo Clin Proc 1986;61:9-13.

CYCLOSPORINE

Cyclosporine (CS), a neutral, lipophilic, cyclic endecapeptide, selectively inhibits T-helper cell activation and adaptive immune responses in contrast to azathioprine which inhibits cell division and prednisone which inhibits cytokine generation. Routinely used in transplantation and widely evaluated in autoimmune diseases, CS causes many nonimmunologic toxic side effects.[1] Monitoring of trough levels in whole blood with appropriate adjustment of dosage in early post-transplant immunosuppression (∿4 months) and during stable, long-term maintenance minimizes nephrotoxicity.[2] Identification of the drug's precise molecular target should facilitate function-based monitoring. To date, combination with other agents which down regulate response to donor MHC has not resulted in tolerance of a transplant as defined by the absence of all immunosuppressive agents. Upregulation of class II antigen expression on epithelial cells and down-regulation on thymic medullary cells are probably important in CS-induced, organ-specific autoimmunity in neonatal mice[3] and in CS-induced syngeneic GVHD (CS-induced autoimmunity),[4] which is a murine model of the human GVHD-like condition sometimes seen as CS is tapered following organ allografting.[5-7] Cyclosporine-induced hypertension is associated with sympathetic neural activation.[8,9] FK 506, a macrolide immunosuppressant, was used successfully for liver, kidney and pancreas transplantation,[9] but additional studies of toxicity and long-term outcome are needed in transplantation and in treatment of glomerulonephritis.[10]

REFERENCES:
1. Kahan DB. Cyclosporine. N Engl J Med 1989;321:1725-38.
2. Moyer TP, Post GR, Sterioff S, Anderson CF. Cyclosporine nephrotoxicity is minimized by adjusting dosage on the basis of drug concentration in blood. Mayo Clin Proc 1988;63:241-7.
3. Sakaguchi S, Sakaguchi N. Organ-specific autoimmune disease induced in mice by elimination of T-cell subsets. V. Neonatal administration of cyclosporin A causes autoimmune disease. J Immunol 1989;142:471-80.

4. Glazier A, Tutschka PJ, Farmer ER, Santos GW. Graft-versus-host disease in cyclosporin A-treated rats after syngeneic and autologous bone marrow reconstitution. J Exp Med 1983;158:1-8.
5. Sliman GA, Beschorner WE, Baughman KL, et al. Graft-versus-host-like disease in a heart allograft recipient: a possible autoimmune phenomenon. Transplantation 1988;45:253-6.
6. Herman JG, Beschorner WE, Baughman KL, et al. Pseudo-graft-versus-host disease in heart and heart-lung recipients. Transplantation 1988;46:93-8.
7. Parfrey NA, Prud'homme GJ. Patterns of MHC antigenic modulation in cyclosporine-induced autoimmunity. Implications for pathogenesis. Am J Pathol 1990;136:479-86.
8. Scherrer U, Vissing SF, Morgan BJ, et al. Cyclosporine-induced sympathetic activation and hypertension after heart transplantation. N Engl J Med 1990;323:693-704.
9. Mark AL. Cyclosporine, sympathetic activity, and hypertension. N Engl J Med 1990;323:748-80.
10. Starzl TE, Todo S, Fung J, et al. FK 506 for liver, kidney, and pancreas transplantation. Lancet 1989;2:1000-4.
11. McCauley J, Tzakis AG, Fung JJ, et al. FK 506 in steroid-resistant focal sclerosing glomerulonephritis of childhood. Lancet 1990;1:674.

CYTOKINES

The cytokines, which include interleukins and interferons, are polypeptide members of a family of peptide regulatory factors which affect functions of specific cell types.[1-4] The terminology for cytokines (lymphokines/monokines/interleukins) is discussed in reference 2. Of the numerous responses of endothelial cells (ECs) to cytokines, the prothrombotic and proinflammatory effects of IL-1 and TNF; the stimulation of accessory cell function by IFN-γ; the migration/proliferation effects of certain CSFs and FGFs; and the down regulation of proinflammatory activities of ECs by TGF-β are all of great importance (cf. 3 for review) and are expected to result in useful assays for clinically important phenomena (cf. 5 and 6 for review). Cloned receptors for cytokines, including those for IL-2,[7] IL-3,[8] IL-4,[9,10] IL-6,[11] GM-CSF,[12] and erythropoietin,[13] reveal a common structural motif suggestive of a distinct family of receptors.[14] See **INTERLEUKIN-1** through **INTERLEUKIN-8, INTERFERONS, MACROPHAGE INFLAMMATORY PROTEINS** and **PEPTIDE REGULATORY FACTORS.**

REFERENCES:
1. Balkwill FR, Burke F. The cytokine network. Immunol Today 1989;10:299-304.
2. Green AR. Peptide regulatory factors: multifunctional mediators of cellular growth and differentiation. Lancet 1989;1:705-7.
3. Mantovani A, Dejana E. Cytokines as communication signals between leukocytes and endothelial cells. Immunol Today 1989;10:370-75.
4. Lipsky PE. The control of antibody production by immunomodulatory molecules. Arthritis Rheum 1989;32:1345-55.
5. Farrant J, Webster ADB. B cell-cytokine interactions: lessons from clinical immunology. Clin Exp Immunol 1989;78:321-22.
6. Durum SK, Mealy K. Hilton Head revisited - cytokine explosion of the 80s takes shape for the 90s. Immunol Today 1990;11:103-6.
7. Hatakeyama M, Tsudo M, Minamoto S, et al. Interleukin-2 receptor β chain gene: generation of three receptor forms by cloned human α and β chain cDNA's. Science 1989;244:551-6.
8. Itoh N, Yonehara S, Schreurs J, et al. Cloning of an interleukin-3 receptor gene: a member of a distinct receptor gene family. Science 1990;247:324-7.
9. Mosley B, Bechmann P, March CJ, et al. The murine interleukin-4 receptor: molecular cloning and characterization of secreted and membrane bound forms. Cell 1989;59:335-48.
10. Harada N, Castle BE, Gorman DM, et al. Expression cloning of a cDNA encoding the murine interleukin 4 receptor based on ligand binding. Proc Natl Acad Sci USA 1990;87:857-61.
11. Yamasaki K, Taga T, Hirata Y, et al. Cloning and expression of the human interleukin-6 (BSF-2/IFNβ 2) receptor. Science 1988;241:825-8.
12. Gearing DP, King JA, Gough NM, Nicola NA. Expression cloning of a receptor for human granulocyte-macrophage colony-stimulating factor. EMBO J 1989;8:3667-76.

13. D'Andrea AD, Lodish HF, Wong GG. Expression cloning of the murine erythropoietin receptor. Cell 1989;57:277-85.
14. Gorman DM, Itoh N, Kitamura T, et al. Cloning and expression of a gene encoding an interleukin 3 receptor-like protein: identification of another member of the cytokine receptor gene family. Proc Natl Acad Sci USA 1990;87:5459-63.

CYTOKINE ANTIBODIES AND CYTOKINE-α2-MACROGLOBULIN COMPLEXES

Antibodies to IL-1α and TNF-α are found in 24% and 48% of normal adults, respectively (cf. 1 for review). The function of these antibodies is unknown; serum levels increase during infections and other inflammation conditions.[1]

At least 10 cytokines are known to bind to α2-macroglobulin; the physiological and pathological significance of this binding is unknown.[2]

REFERENCES:
1. Bendtzen K, Svenson M, Jonsson V, Hippe E. Autoantibodies to cytokines - friends or foes? Immunol Today 1990;11:167-8.
2. James K. Interactions between cytokines and α2-macroglobulin. Immunol Today 1990;11:163-6.

DEFENSINS (HUMAN NEUTROPHIL PROTEINS 1-4)

These amphipathic, carbohydrate-free, cytotoxic, antimicrobial molecules, which are produced by neutrophils and macrophages, are chemotactic for monocytes (cf. 1 for review). Clinical studies will be of great interest.

REFERENCES:
1. Lehrer RI, Ganz T, Selsted ME. Defensins: natural peptide antibiotics from neutrophils. ASM News 1990;56:315-8.

DELAYED-TYPE HYPERSENSITIVITY

Delayed-type hypersensitivity (DTH) (type IV hypersensitivity of Gell and Coombs)[1] can be measured *in vivo* by skin tests and *in vitro* by proliferation of peripheral blood mononuclear cells in response to stimulation with antigen (PPD of tuberculin, tetanus toxoid, candida, trichophyton, etc.). The reproducibility of DTH responses to skin tests with individual, commercially available antigens is poor[2] compared with the "Multitest" system which permits rapid, simultaneous and reproducible application of seven recall antigens (tetanus toxoid, diphtheria, streptococcus, old tuberculin, candida, trichophyton, *Proteus mirabilis*) and a glycerol control in a relatively painless manner. The Multitest, an effective measure of cell-mediated immunity in man, yields a sum reflective of cumulative DTH reactivity with the [7] antigens; this sum correlates inversely with stage of disease in cancer,[3] is useful for assessing risk of serious infection and mortality in patients undergoing major surgery,[4,5] and is a reliable tool for nutritional assessment.[6,7] Normal values for DTH skin test responses by Multitest are well established in adults[8] and in children.[9,10] Significant decreases or increases in Multitest scores may be valuable for prognosis in HIV infection.[11] See also **LYMPHOCYTE ANTIGEN STIMULATION**.

REFERENCES:
1. Coombs RRA, Gell PGH. Classification of allergic reactions responsible for clinical hypersensitivity and disease. In: Gell PGH, Coombs RRA, Lachmann PJ, eds. Clinical aspects of immunology. Oxford: Blackwell Scientific Publications, 1975:761-81.
2. Grimsley G. The significance of tests of cell-mediated immunity: an evaluation of the utility of tests used for the assessment of cell-mediated immunity [Thesis]. Western Australia: The University of Western Australia, 1987:1-194.
3. Reuben JM, Hersh EM. Delayed hypersensitivity responses of cancer patients to recall antigens using a new "Multitest" applicator. Ann Allergy 1984;53:390-4.
4. Christou NV. Anergy testing in surgical patients. Inf Surg 1983;692-700.
5. Christou NV, Boisvert G, Broadhead M, Meakins JL. Two techniques of measurement of the delayed hypersensitivity skin test response for the assessment of bacterial host resistance. World J Surg 1985;9:798-806.

6. Kaminski MV Jr, Pinchcofsky-Devin GD, McCormick DC. DCH testing as a nutritional assessment tool. Nutritional Support Services 1985;5:21-3.
7. Pinchcofsky-Devin GD, Kaminski MV Jr, Pfeifer E. Mortality risk index for predicting futility of nutritional support. Nutritional Support Services 1986;6:14-6.
8. Kniker WT, Anderson CT, McBryde JL, Roumiantzeff M, Lesourd B. Multitest CMI for standardized measurement of delayed cutaneous hypersensitivity and cell-mediated immunity. Normal values and proposed scoring system for healthy adults in the USA. Ann Allergy 1984;52:75-82.
9. Corriel RN, Kniker WT, McBryde JL, Lesourd BM. Cell-mediated immunity in school children assessed for multitest skin testing. Am J Dis Child 1985;139:141-6.
10. Kniker WT, Lesourd BM, McBryde JL, Correil RN. Cell-mediated immunity assessed by multitest CMI skin testing in infants and preschool children. Am J Dis Child 1985;139:840-5.
11. Grimsley G, Dawkins RL. Personal communication. 1989.

DEOXYRIBONUCLEOPROTEIN ANTIBODIES

Antibodies to insoluble DNP (the exact antigen[s] are not known) are found in 60-70% of active SLE. They produce a homogeneous staining pattern and are responsible for the LE cell phenomenon which requires complement-fixing IgG anti-DNP antibodies.[1] Assay for these antibodies has been replaced by more reproducible, equally sensitive tests.

REFERENCES:
1. Dubois EL. Current status of the LE cell test. Arthritis Rheum 1971;1:97-115.

DOUBLE-STRANDED DNA ANTIBODIES (dsDNA)

Of the major methods for the detection of anti-double-stranded DNA (dsDNA) antibodies, the *Crithidia* IFA test is relatively specific but has poor sensitivity[1,2] (cf. 3 for review) and is unsatisfactory for routine use. Serial studies of elevated values of anti-dsDNA antibodies by Farr assay are useful for predicting activity of disease and for therapeutic monitoring especially in conjunction with measurement of serum C3 or C4 concentrations (cf. 4 for review). Doubling of levels of anti-dsDNA antibodies or increases greater than 30 IU/ml in less than 10 weeks is reliably predictive of exacerbations of SLE,[4,5] and decreases of serum C4 make the prediction even more reliable.[6] The methods of choice are the Farr (ammonium sulfate precipitation) technique[7,8] with the membrane filter assay a distant second.[2,9,10] Discrepant results by different techniques are quite common and for this reason, testing by more than one method is indicated.[1,2] In contrast to the Farr assay which detects high avidity antibodies to dsDNA,[11] assays which detect low avidity antibodies (e.g., *Crithidia*, EIA and PEG assays) are not useful for predicting exacerbations of renal or cerebral disease which are often associated with large increases in anti-dsDNA antibodies by the Farr technique.[12] An international standard is available and should lead to improvements in assay technique.[8] Antibodies against a cell surface protein cross-reactive with dsDNA are said to be detectable in active but not inactive disease. If confirmed, this assay could be a better tool for diagnosis and monitoring than anti-dsDNA antibodies.[13] Dysfunction of DNA receptors is reported in SLE.[14] The role of circulating oligonucleosomal DNA in the pathogenesis of SLE is under study.[15] In SLE, antibodies to single-stranded (ssDNA) and dsDNA are produced spontaneously by CD5+ cells and by CD5- cells after polyclonal B cell activation.[16] Assay for antibodies to ssDNA is not clinically useful. The role of DNA in the immunopathogenesis of SLE was usefully discussed.[17,18] The notion that cross-reactivity of anti-DNA antibodies plays a central role in SLE is very unlikely.[19]

The common anti-DNA idiotype (Id) designated 16/6, which is coded by a germ line gene, is found in SLE and other autoimmune diseases.[20] Immunization with hu MAb 16/6 (or with other antibodies with the 16/6 Id and diverse capacities for antigen binding), as well as with T-cell lines specific for the 16/6 Id, causes SLE-like disease in mice.[21]

REFERENCES:
1. Isenberg DA, Dudeney C, Williams W, et al. Measurement of anti-DNA antibodies: a reappraisal using five different methods. Ann Rheum Dis 1987;46:448-56.
2. McMillan SA, Fay AC. Evaluation of five commercial kits to detect dsDNA antibodies. J Clin Pathol 1988;41:1223-8.

3. Mackworth-Young C, Schwartz RS. Autoantibodies to DNA. In: Atassi MZ, ed. Critical reviews in immunology. Boca Raton: CRC Press, Inc., 1988;8:147-73.
4. Swaak AJG, Groenwold J, Bronsveld W. Predictive value of complement profiles and anti-dsDNA in systemic lupus erythematosus. Ann Rheum Dis 1986;45:359-66.
5. ter Borg EJ, Horst G, Hummel EJ, et al. Measurement of increases in anti-double-stranded DNA antibody levels as a predictor of disease exacerbation in systemic lupus erythematosus. A long-term, prospective study. Arthritis Rheum 1990;33:634-43.
6. Swaak AJG, Groenwold J, Aarden LA, et al. Prognostic value of anti-dsDNA in SLE. Ann Rheum Dis 1982;41:388-95.
7. Monier JC, Sault C, Veysseyre C, Bringuier JP. Discrepancies between two procedures for ds-DNA antibody detection: Farr test and indirect immunofluorescence on Crithidia luciliae. J Clin Lab Immunol 1988;25:149-52.
8. Feltkamp TEW, Kirkwood TBL, Maini RN, Aarden LA. The first international standard for antibodies to double stranded DNA. Ann Rheum Dis 1988;47:740-6.
9. Ginsberg B, Keiser H. A millipore filter assay for antibodies to native DNA in sera of patients with systemic lupus erythematosus. Arthritis Rheum 1973;16:199-207.
10. Fritzler MJ. Autoantibody testing: procedures and significance in systemic rheumatic diseases. In: Jasmin G, Simard R, eds. Nuclear submicroscopy. Methods Achiev Exp Pathol 1986;12:224-60.
11. Smeenk RJT, Van Rooijen A, Swaak TJG. Disassociation studies of DNA/anti-DNA complexes in relation to anti-DNA avidity. J Immunol Methods 1988;109:27-35.
12. Nossent JC, Huysen V, Smeenk RJT, Swaak AJG. Low avidity antibodies to double stranded DNA in systemic lupus erythematosus: a longitudinal study of their clinical significance. Ann Rheum Dis 1989;48:677-82.
13. Jacob L, Lety M-A, Choquette D, et al. Presence of antibodies against a cell-surface protein, cross-reactive with DNA, in systemic lupus erythematosus: a marker of the disease. Proc Natl Acad Sci USA 1987;84:2956-9.
14. Bennett RM, Kotzin BL, Merritt MJ. DNA receptor dysfunction in systemic lupus erythematosus and kindred disorders. Induction by anti-DNA antibodies, antihistone antibodies, and antireceptor antibodies. J Exp Med 1987;166:850-63.
15. Rumore PM, Steinman CR. Endogenous circulating DNA in systemic lupus erythematosus. Occurence as multimeric complexes bound to histone. J Clin Invest 1990;86:69-74.
16. Suzuki N, Sakane T, Engleman EG. Anti-DNA antibody production by CD5+ (and CD5−) B cells of patients with systemic lupus erythematosus. J Clin Invest 1990;85:238-47.
17. Pisetksy DS, Grudier JP, Gilkeson GS. A role for immunogenic DNA in the pathogenesis of systemic lupus erythematosus. Arthritis Rheum 1990;33:153-9.
18. Stollar BD. The origin and pathogenic role of anti-DNA autoantibodies. Autoimmunity 1990;2:607-12.
19. Brinkman K, Termaat R, Berden JHM, Smeenk RJT. Anti-DNA antibodies and lupus nephritis: the complexity of crossreactivity. Immunol Today 1990;11:232-4.
20. Shoenfeld Y, Teplizki H, Mendlovic S, et al. The role of human anti-DNA idiotype 16/6 in autoimmunity. Clin Immunol Immunopathol 1989;51:313-25.
21. Blank M, Krup M, Mendlovic S, et al. The importance of Pathogenic 16/6 idiotype in the induction of SLE in naive mice. Scand J Immunol 1990;31:45-52.

ENA ANTIBODIES

Subsumed under the term "anti-ENA" (which refers to antibodies to extractable nuclear antigens) are antibodies to RNP (ribonucleoprotein) which are now known as anti-U1 snRNP (or anti-U1 RNP) as well as antibodies to the Smith antigen which are now known as anti-Sm antibodies. The Sm antibodies, which are specific for SLE, react with the B, B', D, and E polypeptides that are shared by U1, U2 and U4-6 snRNP (small nuclear ribonucleoproteins). Anti-U1 snRNP antibodies in high titer are associated with mixed connective tissue disease and in low titer are associated with anti-Sm antibodies in patients with SLE (cf. 1-3 for review). See also **U1 snRNP ANTIBODIES** and **Sm ANTIBODIES**.

REFERENCES:
1. Hardin JA. The lupus autoantigens and the pathogenesis of systemic lupus erythematosus. Arthritis Rheum 1986;29:457-60.

2. Tan EM, Chan EKL, Sullivan KF, Rubin RL. Antinuclear antibodies (ANAs): diagnostically specific immune markers and clues toward the understanding of systemic autoimmunity. Clin Immunol Immunopathol 1988;47:121-41.
3. Sperling R. Autoantibodies against nuclear ribonucleoprotein (RNP) complexes. Isr J Med Sci 1988;24:358-62.

ENDOMETRIAL ANTIBODIES

Anti-endometrial antibodies are found in 66% of patients with endometriosis. These IgG antibodies react only with the glandular (epithelial) component and not the stromal component of normal epithelium without regard to phase of the menstrual cycle.[1] Some serum IgG antibodies in endometriosis sera are said to react on immunoblots with several proteins found only in endometrium and endometrial explants of endometriosis patients.[2] Patients with endometriosis commonly have lupus anticoagulant (45%) and elevated IgG levels; a few have IgG antibodies to phospholipids and histones.[3] Currently, the assay for anti-endometrial antibodies has no proven clinical utility.

REFERENCES:
1. Wild RA, Satyaswaroop PG, Shivers AC. Epithelial localization of antiendometrial antibodies associated with endometriosis. Am J Reprod Immunol Microbiol 1987;13:62-5.
2. Mathur S, Garza DE, Smith LF. Endometrial autoantigens eliciting immunoglobulin (Ig)G, IgA, and IgM responses in endometriosis. Fertil Steril 1990;54:56-63.
3. Gleicher N, El-Roeiy A, Confino E, Friberg J. Is endometriosis an autoimmune disease? Obstet Gynecol 1987;70:115-22.

ENDOMYSIAL ANTIBODIES

Anti-endomysial antibodies of the IgA subclass (IgA-AEmA), which react with the reticulin component of the endomysium of smooth muscle of primate tissue, are found in at least 60-70% of patients with dermatitis herpetiformis (DH) on a normal gluten-containing diet and in 100% of patients with celiac disease (gluten-sensitive enteropathy) with subtotal villous atrophy.[1-5] Others report sensitivities for IgA-AEmA of 91-100% for CD and 79-100% for DH with specificities of 96-100%.[6,7] In general, IgA-AGA have a higher positive predictive value for CD than IgA-AGA which have higher negative predictive value;[8] a positive IgA-AEmA is confirmatory evidence and is perhaps an indication for intestinal biopsy.[8] IgA-antigliadin antibodies (IgA-AGA) and IgA-R_1-anti-reticulin antibodies (IgA-R_1-ARA) are each found in about 25% of patients with DH[2] and in over 93% and 44% respectively of active celiac disease.[4]

The titers of IgA-AEmA, IgA-AGA and IgA-R1-ARA decrease to normal levels within a few months after introduction of a gluten-free diet (GFD), and change in titer of IgA-AEmA and IgA-AGA can be used to monitor compliance with GFD.[3] IgA-ARA decrease more slowly than IgA-AGA. IgA-AGA and IgG-AGA rise significantly during gluten challenge, sometimes several months before clinical relapse.[9] IgG-AEmA and IgG-AGA are especially useful in patients with IgA deficiency who have a 10-15 fold increased frequency of celiac disease.[10] Monitoring serum levels of antibodies to gliadin, endomysium, and reticulin as a test of compliance with a gluten-free diet (GFD) is important, because a GFD protects patients with CD against development of non-Hodgkin lymphomas and perhaps against cancer of the mouth, pharynx and esophagus.[11] Because lymphomas are also increased in dermatitis herpetiformis (DH), monitoring levels of these antibodies for compliance with a GFD is probably also worthwhile in DH.[12] IgA-ARA, like IgA anti-gliadin and IgA anti-endomysial antibodies, can be used to measure compliance with a GFD which requires an average of 2 years for clearing of DH.[13] In children, IgA-AGA, usually in relatively low amounts, are sometimes seen in bovine milk intolerance and post-infection malabsorption.[14] IgA antibodies to lactalbumin, casein or ovalbumin are elevated in approximately 50-90% of patients with celiac disease.[15] See also **GLIADIN ANTIBODIES** and **RETICULIN ANTIBODIES**.

REFERENCES:
1. Reunala T, Chorzelski TP, Viander M, et al. IgA anti-endomysial antibodies in dermatitis herpetiformis: correlation with jejunal morphology, gluten-free diet and anti-gliadin antibodies. Br J Dermatol 1987;117:185-91.

2. Kumar V, Lerner A, Valeski JE, et al. Endomysial antibodies in the diagnosis of celiac disease and the effect of gluten on antibody titers. Immunol Invest 1989;18:533-44.

3. Kapuscinska A, Zalewski T, Chorzelski TP, et al. Disease specificity and dynamics of changes in IgA class anti-endomysial antibodies in celiac disease. J Pediatr Gastroenterol Nutr 1987;6:529-34.

4. Volta U, Bonazzi C, Pisi E, et al. Antigliadin and antireticulin antibodies in coeliac disease and at onset of diabetes in children [Letters]. Lancet 1987;2:1034-5.

5. Volta U, Lenzi M, Lazzari R, et al. Antibodies to gliadin detected by immunofluorescence and a micro-ELISA method: markers of active childhood and adult coeliac disease. Gut 1985;26:667-71.

6. Hällström O. Comparison of IgA-class reticulin and endomysium antibodies in coeliac disease and dermatitis herpetiformis. Gut 1989;30:1225-32.

7. Peters MS, McEvoy MT. IgA antiendomysial antibodies in dermatitis herpetiformis. J Am Acad Dermatol 1989;21:1225-31.

8. Calabuig M, Torregosa R, Polo P, et al. Serological markers and celiac disease: a new diagnostic approach? J Pediatr Gastroenterol Nutr 1990;10:435-42.

9. Scott H, Ek J, Brandtzaeg P. Changes of serum antibody activities to various dietary antigens related to gluten withdrawal or challenge in children with coeliac disease. Int Archs Allergy Appl Immunol 1985;76:138-44.

10. Scott H, Brandtzaeg P. Gluten IgA antibodies and coeliac disease [Letter]. Lancet 1989;1:382-3.

11. Holmes GKT, Prior P, Lane MR, et al. Malignancy in coeliac disease--effect of a gluten free diet. Gut 1989;30:333-8.

12. Leonard JN, Tucker WFG, Fry JS, et al. Increased incidence of malignancy in dermatitis herpetiformis. Br Med J 1983;286:16-8.

13. Fry L, Seah PP, Riches DJ, Hoffbrand AV. Clearance of skin lesions in dermatitis herpetiformis after gluten withdrawal. Lancet 1973;1:288-91.

14. Lindberg T, Nilsson L-Å, Borulf S, et al. Serum IgA and IgG gliadin antibodies and small intestinal mucosal damage in children. J Pediatr Gastroenterol Nutr 1985;4:917-22.

15. Scott H, Fausa O, Ek J, Brandtzaeg P. Immune response patterns in coeliac disease. Serum antibodies to dietary antigens measured by an enzyme linked immunosorbent assay (ELISA). Clin Exp Immunol 1984;57:25-32.

ENDOPLASMIC RETICULUM ANTIBODIES (HALOTHANE-INDUCED)

These antibodies, which react with halothane-modified liver microsomal protein fractions, were found in sera of several patients with halothane-induced hepatitis.[1] The clinical utility of assay for these antibodies is unknown.

REFERENCES:
1. Satoh H, Martin BM, Schulick AH, Christ DD, Kenna JG, Pohl LR. Human anti-endoplasmic reticulum antibodies in sera of patients with halothane-induced hepatitis are directed against a trifluoroacetylated carboxylesterase. Proc Natl Acad Sci USA 1989;86:322-6.

ENDOTHELIAL CELL ANTIBODIES

AECA of the IgG subclass are detectable in the sera of patients with active SLE and may be responsible for immune injury to blood vessel walls.[1] The presence of AECA is not restricted to SLE. Cytotoxic antibodies to vascular endothelial cells and monocytes are found in patients with hyperacute rejection of cardiac allografts and compatible direct lymphocytotoxic cross match;[2] in patients with rejected renal allografts;[3] in patients with the hemolytic uremic syndrome[4] and in Kawasaki syndrome.[5] Non-cytolytic AECA are found in some patients with micropolyarteritis and Wegener's granulomatosis.[6] IgM AECA found in autoimmune hypoparathyroidism are reactive with bovine endothelial cells and are neither organ- nor species-specific.[7] Approximately ⅓ of patients with IgA nephropathy have serum antibodies which bind to vascular endothelial cells and some of these have anti-HLA class I specificity.[8] The relationships of AECA to anti-phospholipid antibodies[9,10] and heterophile antibodies[11] are not yet clear. Sera from some patients with scleroderma mediate antibody-dependent cellular cytotoxicity.[12] Cytokine-mediated activation of vascular endothelium may be important in the pathogenesis of antibody-mediated and cell-mediated damage to blood vessels.[13,14]

REFERENCES:
1. Cines DB, Lyss AP, Reeber M, Bina M, DeHoratius RJ. Presence of complement-fixing anti-endothelial cell antibodies in systemic lupus erythematosus. J Clin Invest 1984;73:611-25.
2. Trento A, Hardesty RL, Griffith BP, Zerbe T, Kormos RL, Bahnson HT. Role of the antibody to vascular endothelial cells in hyperacute rejection in patients undergoing cardiac transplantation. J Thorac Cardiovasc Surg 1988;95:37-41.
3. Paul LC, Carpenter CB. Antibodies against renal endothelial alloantigens. Transplant Proc 1980;12:43-8.
4. Leung DYM, Moake JL, Havens PL, Kim M, Pober JS. Lytic anti-endothelial cell antibodies in haemolytic-uraemic syndrome. Lancet 1988;2:183-6.
5. Leung DYM, Geha RS, Newburger JW, et al. Two monokines, interleukin 1 and tumor necrosis factor, render cultured vascular endothelial cells susceptible to lysis by antibodies circulating during Kawasaki syndrome. J Exp Med 1986;164:1958.
6. Ferraro G, Meroni PL, Tincani A, et al. Anti-endothelial cell antibodies in patients with Wegener's granulomatosis and micropolyarteritis. Clin Exp Immunol 1990;79:47-53.
7. Fattorossi A, Aurbach GD, Sakaguchi K, et al. Anti-endothelial cell antibodies: detection and characterization in sera from patients with autoimmune hypoparathyroidism. Proc Natl Acad Sci USA 1988;85:4015-9.
8. Yap HK, Sakai RS, Bahn L, et al. Anti-vascular endothelial cell antibodies in patients with IgA nephropathy: frequency and clinical significance. Clin Immunol Immunopathol 1988;49:450-62.
9. Vismara A, Meroni PL, Tincani A, et al. Relationship between anti-cardiolipin and anti-endothelial cell antibodies in systemic lupus erythematosus. Clin Exp Immunol 1988;74:247-53.
10. Baguley E, Harris EN, Brown KA, Haskard D, Hughes GRV. Failure of antiphospholipid antibodies to bind human endothelial cells. Lupus Arthritis Research Unit, St Thomas Hospital, London. Br J Rheumatol 1987;26:95.
11. Hawkins BR, McDonald BL, Dawkins RL. Characterization of immunofluorescent heterophile antibodies which may be confused with autoantibodies. J Clin Pathol 1977;30:299-307.
12. Marks RM, Czerniecki M, Andrews BS, Penny R. The effects of scleroderma serum on human microvascular endothelial cells. Arthritis Rheum 1988;31:1524-34.
13. Pober JS. Cytokine-mediated activation of vascular endothelium. Am J Pathol 1988;133:426-33.
14. Cavender DE, Edelbaum D, Ziff M. Endothelial cell activation induced by tumor necrosis factor and lymphotoxin. Am J Pathol 1989;134:551-60.

ENDOTHELIAL LEUKOCYTE ADHESION MOLECULE 1

Endothelial leukocyte adhesion molecule 1 (ELAM-1), a cytokine- and endotoxin-inducible molecule which mediates focal adhesion of leukocytes to the lining of blood vessels, is a member of the family of adhesion molecules.[1] ELAM-1 is expected to be very important in pathogenesis of infectious, autoimmune and atherosclerotic diseases[2,3] (cf. 4).

REFERENCES:
1. Hession C, Osborn L, Goff D, et al. Endothelial leukocyte adhesion molecule 1: direct expression cloning and functional interactions. Proc Natl Acad Sci USA 1990;87:1673-7.
2. Bevilacqua MP, Pober JS, Mendrick DL, et al. Identification of an inducible endothelial-leukocyte adhesion molecule. Proc Natl Acad Sci USA 1987;84:9238-42.
3. Bevilacqua MP, Stengelin S, Gimbrone MA Jr, Seed B. Endothelial leukocyte adhesion molecule 1: an inducible receptor for neutrophils related to complement regulatory proteins and lectins. Science 1989;243:1160-5.
4. Edelman GM. Topobiology. Sci Am 1989;260:76-88.

ENDOTHELINS

The endothelins, a family of structurally and pharmacologically distinct peptides, include human endothelin 1, which is a potent vasoconstrictor found in blood vessels as well as in the central and peripheral nervous systems.[1]

REFERENCES:
1. Giaid A, Gibson SJ, Ibrahim NB, et al. Endothelin 1, an endothelium-derived peptide, is expressed in neurons of the human spinal cord and dorsal root ganglia. Proc Natl Acad Sci USA 1989;86:7634-8.

EPIDERMAL GROWTH FACTOR

Epidermal growth factor EGF-like activities are probably important in wound healing and might alter cell growth in cancer (cf. 1 and 2 for review). Transforming growth factor-α (TGF-α), which is closely related to EGF, is produced in abnormal amounts in some tumor cells. The c-*neu* gene, which is amplified in certain breast and ovarian cancers which have a poor prognosis,[3] encodes a receptor similar to the EGF receptor. Truncated, autonomous (ligand-independent) growth factor receptors may be important in cancer. EGF and TGF-α are expected to be elevated in conditions with rapid turnover of cells. In genetic and streptozotocin-induced diabetes mellitus in rats, the low levels of EGF found in submandibular glands and plasma are reversed by insulin;[4] confirmation and similar studies in human IDDM are awaited. Assays for EGF itself are not yet of clinical importance.

REFERENCES:
1. Waterfield MD. Epidermal growth factor and related molecules. Lancet 1989;1:1243-6.
2. Fisher DA, Salido EC, Barajas L. Epidermal growth factor and the kidney. Annu Rev Physiol 1989;51:67-80.
3. Slamon DJ, Godolphin W, Jones LA, et al. Studies of the HER-2/*neu* proto-oncogene in human breast and ovarian cancer. Science 1989;244:707-12.
4. Kasayama S, Ohba Y, Oka T. Epidermal growth factor deficiency associated with diabetes mellitus. Proc Natl Acad Sci USA 1989;86:7644-8.

ERYTHROCYTE SEDIMENTATION RATE

In contrast to the ZSR (Zeta Sedimentation Ratio), the erythrocyte sedimentation rate (ESR) (or plasma viscosity) is greatly influenced by cell volume[1] and is preferred for monitoring chronic inflammation, including disease severity in rheumatoid arthritis.[2] Fibrinogen and alpha$_1$-acid glycoprotein are also useful for detection of chronic inflammatory disease. Because of its rapid response, reproducibility and sensitivity, CRP quantitation by rate nephelometry is recommended for detection and monitoring (e.g., response to antibiotics) of acute inflammation.[1-4] The ESR is more useful than the serum CRP for diagnosis and monitoring of PMR/GCA and is more frequently elevated during relapse. Normal values for ESR or CRP do not exclude a diagnosis of neither PMR or GCA, nor do normal values exclude relapse.[5]

REFERENCES:
1. Bull BS, Chien S, Dormandy JA, et al. Laboratory techniques: guidelines on selection of laboratory tests for monitoring the acute phase response. J Clin Pathol 1988;41:1203-12.
2. Bull BS, Westengard JC, Farr M, et al. Efficacy of tests used to monitor rheumatoid arthritis. Lancet 1989;2:965-7.
3. Bull BS, Brecher G. An evaluation of the relative merits of the Wintrobe and Westergren sedimentation methods, including hematocrit correction. Am J Clin Pathol 1974;62:502-10.
4. Reinhart WH. Blood sedimentation - a simple and useful test? Schweiz Med Wochenschr 1988;118:839-44.
5. Kyle V, Cawston TE, Hazelman BL. Erythrocyte sedimentation rate and C reactive protein in the assessment of polymyalgia rheumatica/giant cell arteritis on presentation and during follow up. Ann Rheum Dis 1989;48:667-71.

ERYTHROPOIETIN

After successful renal transplantation, slight increases in serum levels of endogenous erythropoietin induce erythropoiesis to the same extent as do large doses of exogenous erythropoietin in uremia.[1] Increased serum erythropoietin levels are also seen even after renal transplantation in erythrocytosis and iron-deficiency uremia.[1]

REFERENCES:
1. Sun CH, Ward HJ, Paul WL, et al. Serum erythropoietin levels after renal transplantation. N Engl J Med 1988;321:151-7.

EXTENDED HAPLOTYPES
(SUPRATYPES, ANCESTRAL HAPLOTYPES)
Autoimmune disorders are associated with individual polymorphisms of HLA class II glycoproteins and with nearby class III loci on chromosome 6 which code for complement proteins (C2, C4A, C4B, factor B) as well as TNF and HSP (heat-shock protein) 770. The products of this extended group with genes on the short arm of chromosome 6 are in linkage disequilibrium of these polymorphisms and/or deletions which, by one means or another, predispose to certain diseases. Highly conserved ancestral haplotypes are associated with predisposition to autoimmune diseases; the components of the ancestral haplotypes can vary from race to race but the association of ancestral haplotypes with certain diseases is uniformly observed (cf. 1-4 for review). Although the products of certain of these genes are of well recognized importance for solubilization and clearance of immune complexes[5] and for control of phagocytic activation,[6] the immediate relevance of the putative dysfunctions to the development of autoimmune diseases is entirely unclear.

REFERENCES:
1. Batchelor JR, McMichael AJ. Progress in understanding HLA and disease associations. Br Med Bull 1987;43:156-83.
2. Tokunaga K, Saueracker G, Kay PH, Christiansen FT, Anad R, Dawkins RL. Extensive deletions and insertions in different MHC supratypes detected by pulsed field gel electrophoresis. J Exp Med 1988;168:933-40.
3. Alper CA, Fleischnick E, Awdeh Z, Katz AJ, Yunis EJ. Extended major histocompatibility complex haplotyes in patients with gluten-sensitive enteropathy. J Clin Invest 1987;79:251-6.
4. Dawkins RL, Christiansen FT, Kay PH, et al. Disease associations with complotypes, supratypes and haplotypes. Immunol Rev 1983;70:5-22.
5. Schifferli JA, Ng YC, Peter DK. The role of complement and its receptor in the elimination of immune complexes. N Engl J Med 1986;315:488-95.
6. Polla BS. A role for heat shock proteins in inflammation? Immunol Today 1988;9:134-7.

FACTOR B
Plasma levels of factor B activation products (i.e., Ba and Bb which are members of the family of complement split products) are thought to be a better index of disease activity in SLE than C3 or C4.[1-5] The presence of activation products of Factor B (Ba) may be associated with poor short-term clinical outcome in SLE.[5] See **AH50, COMPLEMENT ACTIVATION** and **MEMBRANE ATTACK COMPLEX (SC5b9).**

REFERENCES:
1. Petri M, Kolb W, Morrow P, Tamerius J. Association of complement activation tests with clinical measures of lupus activity [Abstract]. Clin Res 1989;37(2):510A.
2. Kolb WP, Morrow PR, Tamerius JD. Ba and Bb fragments of factor B activation: fragment production, biological activities, neoepitope expression and quantitation in clinical samples. Complement Inflamm 1989;6:175-204.
3. Abramson SB, Weissmann G. Complement split products and the pathogenesis of SLE. Hosp Pract 1988;23:45-56.
4. Peakman M, Senaldi G, Vergani D. Review: assessment of complement activation in clinical immunology laboratories: time for reappraisal? J Clin Pathol 1989;42:1018-25.
5. Kerr LD, Adelsberg BR, Schulman P, Spiera H. Factor B activation products in patients with systemic lupus erythematosus. Arthritis Rheum 1989;32:1406-13.

FIBRILLARIN (ANTI-U3 RNP)
Approximately 8% of patients with scleroderma (both diffuse and limited) have antibodies to fibrillarin, a 34 kd protein component of U3 ribonucleoproteins (RNP).[1,2]

REFERENCES:
1. Reimer G, Pollard KM, Penning CA, et al. Monoclonal autoantibody from a (New Zealand black x New Zealand white) F_1 mouse and some human scleroderma sera target an M_r 34,000 nucleolar protein of the U3 RNP particle. Arthritis Rheum 1980;30:793-800.

2. Ochs RL, Lischwe MA, Spohn WH, Busch H. Fibrillarin: a new protein of the nucleolus identified by autoimmune sera. Biol Cell 1985;54;123-34.

FOLLICLE-STIMULATING HORMONE RECEPTOR ANTIBODIES

Inhibitors of follicle-stimulating hormone (FSH) binding to its receptor were reported in two patients with hypergonadotropic amenorrhea and myasthenia gravis[1] and in a male with polyostotic fibrous dysplasia, increased serum FSH and LH, primary gonadal failure and an IgM monoclonal gammopathy.[2]

REFERENCES:
1. Chiauzzi V, Cigorraga S, Escobar ME, et al. Inhibition of follicle-stimulating hormone receptor binding by circulating immunoglobulins. J Clin Endocrinol Metab 1982;54:1221-8.
2. Dias JA, Gates SA, Reichert LE. Evidence for the presence of follicle-stimulating hormone receptor antibody in human serum. Fertil Steril 1982;38:330-8.

FOOD HYPERSENSITIVITY REACTIONS

Immunologic responses to components (typically glycoproteins) of food which result in untoward reactions are called "food hypersensitivity reactions." The term "food allergy" is often used synonymously with food-hypersensitivity reactions and is unfortunately applied to the wide variety of untoward responses to food which are best characterized as food intolerance (i.e, the abnormal, non-immunologic effects of foods due to metabolic reactions of the host, pharmacologic reactions due to natural or added chemicals, and the toxic reactions due to components of the food or due to microbes within the food). Although spontaneous release of histamine by basophils (and presumably by mast cells of the skin) may be common in individuals with food-induced eczema or useful for detecting the presence of other relevant, but unsuspected food allergens in the diet, there are no data available on the clinical utility of the spontaneous histamine-release assay for assessing patient compliance with avoidance diets.[1,2] Food allergies mediated by non-IgE, antibody-mediated mechanisms[3] and the possible contribution of xenogeneic antibodies (e.g., from bovine milk) to atopic diseases[4] are controversial (cf. 5 for review). See also IgE IMMUNE COMPLEXES.

REFERENCES:
1. Sampson HA, Broadbent KR, Bernhisel-Broadbent J. Spontaneous release of histamine from basophils and histamine-releasing factor in patients with atopic dermatitis and food hypersensitivity. N Engl J Med 1989;321:228-32.
2. Metcalf DD. Diseases of food hypersensitivity [Editorial]. N Engl J Med 1989;321:255-7.
3. Halpern GM, Scott JR. Non-IgE antibody mediated mechanisms in food allergy. Ann Allergy 1987;58:14-27.
4. Collins AM. Xenogeneic antibodies and atopic disease. Lancet 1988;1:734-7.
5. Schreiber RA, Walker WA. Food allergy: facts and fiction. Mayo Clin Proc 1989;64:1381-91.

GASTRIC CELL c-AMP STIMULATING ANTIBODIES

These antibodies, a recent addition to the list of anti-receptor antibodies, are typically found in young males with long duration of duodenal ulcer disease, a family history thereof and a poor response to anti-H2-R drugs.[1] See also GASTRIN-PRODUCING CELL ANTIBODIES and PARIETAL CELL ANTIBODIES.

REFERENCES:
1. De Lazzari F, Mirakian R, Hammond L, et al. Gastric cell c-AMP stimulating autoantibodies in duodenal ulcer disease. Gut 1988;29:94-100.

GASTRIN-PRODUCING CELL ANTIBODIES

Anti-gastrin-producing cell antibodies (AGPCA) are found in approximately 8-16% of patients with antral (type B) chronic atrophic gastritis.[1,2] In type B gastritis, the antral mucosa is mainly affected; parietal cell antibodies are absent and there is no association with pernicious anemia or polyendocrinopathy;[3] (cf. 4 for review) of type A and type B gastritis. AGPCA probably explain the lower rates of gastrin secretion and the lower counts of gastrin-producing cells in antral gastritis.[5] AGPCA and their associated type B gastritis differ from anti-parietal cell antibodies (which react with parietal cells in the gastric fundus) and their associated atrophy of the fundal mucosa (type A gastritis). In a recent population study, isolated fundal gastritis was limited to those with anti-parietal cell antibodies (APCA) and/or anti-thyroid antibodies.[5] APCA were found only in those with normal antral mucosa.[6] AGPCA, on the other hand, were found only in those with normal antral mucosa or mild antral gastritis and not in those with moderate or severe antral gastritis.[5] Hence, the relationship of AGPCA to antral gastritis needs further longitudinal evaluation.[6] The association of *Campylobacter pylori* with antral (Type B) gastritis and pepticulcer disease (especially duodenal ulcer) is well established as is the increased frequency of antibodies to *C. pylori* in patients with gastritis and ulcer disease (cf. 7-11 for review). Antibodies to *C. pylori* or to *C. pylori* urease are not, however, useful for monitoring.[10-12] The confusing terminology for this bacterium (first *Campylobacter pyloridis*, then *Campylobacter pylori* and recently, *Helicobacter pylori*) has finally been resolved.[13] A thorough review is available.[14] See also **GASTRIN RECEPTOR ANTIBODIES, PARIETAL CELL ANTIBODIES** and **GASTRIC CELL c-AMP STIMULATING ANTIBODIES.**

REFERENCES:
1. Vandelli C, Bottazzo GF, Doniach D, Franceschi F. Autoantibodies to gastrin-producing cells in antral (type B) chronic gastritis. N Engl J Med 1979;300:1406-10.
2. Uibo RM, Krohn KJ. Demonstration of gastrin cell autoantibodies in antral gastritis with avidin-biotin complex antibody technique. Clin Exp Immunol 1984;58:341-7.
3. Korman MG, Strickland RG, Hansky J. The functional 'G' cell mass in atrophic gastritis. Gut 1972;13:349-51.
4. Strickland RG, Mackay IR. A reappraisal of the nature and significance of chronic atrophic gastritis. Am J Dig Dis 1973;18:426-40.
5. Stockbrügger R, Larsson L-I, Lundqvist G, Angervall L. Antral gastrin cells and serum gastrin in achlorhydria. Scand J Gastroenterol 1977;12:209-13.
6. Uibo R, Krohn K, Villako K, Tammur R, Tamm A. The relationship of parietal cell, gastrin cell, and thyroid autoantibodies to the state of the gastric mucosa in a population sample. Scand J Gastroenterol 1984;19:1075-80.
7. Marshall BJ, Goodwin CS, Warren JR, et al. Prospective double-blind trial of duodenal ulcer relapse after eradication of Campylobacter pylori. Lancet 1988;2:1437-42.
8. Goodwin CS. Duodenal ulcer, Campylobacter pylori, and the "leaking roof" concept. Lancet 1988;2:1467-9.
9. Dwyer B, Nanxiong S, Kaldor J, et al. Antibody response to *Campylobacter pylori* in an ethnic group lacking peptic ulceration. Scand J Infect Dis 1988;20:63-8.
10. Newell DG, Rathbone BJ. The serodiagnosis of *Campylobacter pylori* infection. Serodiag Immunother Infect Dis 1989;3:1-6.
11. Bolton FJ, Hutchinson DN, Hinchliffe PM, Holt AV. Distribution in various clinical groups of antibody to *C. pylori* detected by enzyme-linked immunosorbent assay, complement fixation and microagglutination tests. Serodiag Immunother Infect Dis 1989;3:41-50.
12. Dent JC, McNulty CAM, Uff JS, Gear MWL, Wilkinson SP. *Campylobacter pylori* urease: a new serological test. Lancet 1988;1:1002.
13. Anonymous. *Campylobacter pylori* becomes *Helicobacter pylori* [Editorial]. Lancet 1989;2:1019-20.
14. Dooley CP, Cohen H. The clinical significance of *Campylobacter pylori*. Ann Intern Med 1988;108:70-9.

GASTRIN RECEPTOR ANTIBODIES

Anti-gastrin receptor antibodies (AGRA) are found in about 30% of patients with pernicious anemia.[1] These antibodies are capable of blocking gastrin binding and have been shown by a number of techniques to bind to gastric parietal cells.[1-4] The contribution of autoantibodies to peptic ulcer disease is being widely explored both theoretically[5] and in the laboratory.[6] See also **PARIETAL CELL ANTIBODIES, GASTRIN-PRODUCING CELL ANTIBODIES** and **GASTRIC CELL c-AMP STIMULATING ANTIBODIES.**

REFERENCES:

1. De Aizpurua HJ, Ungar B, Toh B-H. Autoantibody to the gastrin receptor in pernicious anemia. N Engl J Med 1985;313:479-83.
2. De Aizpurua HJ, Toh BH, Ungar B. Parietal cell surface reactive autoantibody in pernicious anaemia demonstrated by indirect membrane immunofluorescence. Clin Exp Immunol 1983;52:341-9.
3. De Aizpurua HJ, Ungar B, Toh BH. Flow microfluorimetric analysis of autoantibody reactions with parietal cell surface membranes in pernicious anaemia. Clin Exp Immunol 1983;54:405-10.
4. De Aizpurua HJ, Cosgrove LJ, Ungar B, Toh B-H. Autoantibodies cytotoxic to gastric parietal cells in serum of patients with pernicious anemia. N Engl J Med 1983;309:625-9.
5. Kirk RM. Hypothesis: could chronic peptic ulcers be localised areas of acid susceptibility generated by autoimmunity? Lancet 1986;1:772-3.
6. De Lazzari F, Mirakian R, Hammond L, et al. Gastric cell c-AMP stimulating autoantibodies in duodenal ulcer disease. Gut 1988;29:94-100.

GENE REARRANGEMENT

Recent data in human (MS and rheumatoid arthritis) and experimental animals (EAE) suggest that specific combinations of genes from the variable region of the TCR (i.e., limited use of V_α and V_β genes) are important in the genesis of T-cell-mediated diseases.[1] Similar studies show unexpected use of specific combinations of immunoglobulin variable region genes in a number of diseases.[2] These observations led to the V-region disease hypothesis as an explanation for autoimmune diseases (see below and 1 for review).

Rearrangement of the *bcr* gene results from the reciprocal translocation of DNA between chromosomes 9 and 22 in which the distal portion of the long arm, including the *abl* locus of chromosome 9 is translocated to the "breakpoint cluster region" (*bcr*) on chromosome 22.[3-8] Most of these translocations give rise to a shorter chromosome 22, the Philadelphia (Ph[1]) chromosome. These translocations occur in approximately 95% of patients with CML, 5-10% of patients with ALL and in 1-2% of patients with acute myelogenous leukemia.[9-13] Ph[1]-positive CML and ALL differ from Ph[1]-negative CML and ALL in response to therapy and survival.[12] For example, patients with Ph[1]-negative CML have a shorter median survival than patients with Ph[1]-positive CML.[14] The *bcr* gene rearrangement assay has several distinct advantages over traditional cytogenic analysis in that it evaluates about 3×10^6 cells and has a high degree of sensitivity, detecting the molecular marker even when Ph[1] is absent by cytogenetics. This is particularly useful, because rearrangements of the *bcr* gene are also known to occur in CML which is cytogenetically negative for Ph[1],[15,16] (cf. also 17 and 18). Monitoring of minimum residual disease in CML by detection of *bcr* gene rearrangement with PCR is possible, but its clinical utility is not established.[19] Progeny of mice transgenic for a *bcr/abl* p190 DNA construct are either moribund or die of acute leukemia.[20]

Assays for rearrangement of the immunoglobulin heavy and light chain genes (IgH and IgL) and assays for rearrangement of the beta and gamma T cell receptor genes (β TCR & α TCR) allow classification of nearly all ALLs as either T, pre-B type, or B. These assays are also valuable for confirming pathological and immunological diagnoses in difficult cases of T and B cell lymphomas. In ALL and acute phase CML, rearrangement of IgH genes, which occurs early in B cell differentiation, is strong evidence of B cell lineage when accompanied by the presence of Ia (HLA-DR), CD19 (B4), CD10 (CALLA) and CD20 (B1), even in the absence of rearrangement of the IgL genes.[21-29] Lack of TCR gene rearrangement also supports a B lineage, even though rare B cell clones will contain rearrangement in the β TCR & α TCR genes. Some ALLs were previously referred to as "non-T, non-B" ALL because the leukemic cells lacked surface Ig, failed to rosette with sheep red cells and did not react with monoclonal antibodies to T cell antigens.[22] Essentially all of the "non-T, non-B leukemias" are now recognized to be pre-B in type, because they have rearranged IgH genes. Furthermore, half of the "non-T, non-B" leukemias have rearranged IgL genes. In pre-B ALL, IgH gene rearrangement and the expression of Ia and CD19 generally precede IgL gene rearrangements and appearance of CD10 (CALLA) and CD20.[30] Eighty to 90% of cases of non-Hodgkin lymphoma (NHL) are of B cell lineage. Over 90% of B-lineage neoplasms manifest immunophenotypic abnormalities which distinguish them from benign, reactive lymphoid processes.[31] Light chain immunophenotyping and clonal excess analysis by flow cytometry are

42

sufficiently sensitive and specific to confirm histologic diagnoses in the vast majority of surface Ig positive B cell NHL.[32]

Ig and TCR gene rearrangements result from the shuffling (rearrangement) of DNA segments of genes encoding variable portions of the IgH, IgL and TCR chains. This shuffling occurs when the genes for the different chains of Ig and TCR on different chromosomes are reorganized during differentiation of B and T lymphocytes. Rearrangements of Ig and TCR genes result in diversity of antibodies and antigen receptors in B cells and T cells, respectively (see 24, 33-35 for review). In addition to the prototypic TCR-$\alpha\beta$ heterodimer, a second TCR heterodimer (TCR-$\gamma\delta$), which is also associated with the CD3 complex on some CD3$^+$ T lymphocytes,[36] might be important in recognition of antologous stress proteins.[37] The β-chain genes of the TCR of synovial fluid lymphocytes from patients with RA show distinct, restricted rearrangements which suggest selective activation of a dominant population of T cells or the relative absence of cells with a broader capability for TCR rearrangements.[38] Similar restricted rearrangements (activations) of the Vα gene expression in brain lesions of patients with MS may have therapeutic implications,[39] because 1) *in vivo* treatment of mice with experimental allergic encephalomyelitis (EAE) with monoclonal antibodies to a predominant TCR V region product reverses paralytic disease[40-43] and 2) EAE is prevented by immunization with inactivated encephalitogenic T cells[44] as well as with synthetic peptides corresponding to the preferentially rearranged TCR V regions of encephalitogenic clones.[45,46] Restricted shared use of TCR V$_\beta$ genes is also found in PBMC of patients with MS[47] and Crohn disease.[48]

In addition to their well-known contribution to diversity by reassorting gene segments (TCR and IgR), gene rearrangements are also important in nature for alteration of gene copy number by amplification and by deletion and for controlled expression (via DNA inversion and transposition) of sets of genes that code for similar functions.[49] Expression control allows antigenic variation and hence capacity for avoidance of host defence by some unicellular organisms (including *Trypanosoma, Borrelia, Neisseria* and certain viruses). See also **MYELIN BASIC PROTEIN.**

REFERENCES:
1. Heber-Katz E, Acha-Orbea H. The V-region disease hypothesis: evidence from autoimmune encephalomyelitis. Immunology Today 1989;10:164-9.
2. Taussig MJ, Sims MJ, Krawinkel U. Regulation of immunoglobulin gene rearrangement and expression. Immunology Today 1989;10:143-6.
3. Heisterkamp N, Stephenson JR, Groffen J, et al. Localization of the c-*abl* oncogene adjacent to a translocation breakpoint in chronic myelocytic leukemia. Nature 1983;306:329-42
4. Heisterkamp N, Stam K, Groffen J, et al. Structural organization of the *bcr* gene and its role in the Ph^1 translocation [Letter]. Nature 1985;315:758-61.
5. Shtivelman E, Lifshitz B, Gale RP, Canaani E. Fused transcript of *abl* and *bcr* genes in chronic myelogenous leukaemia. Nature 1985;315:550-4.
6. Ben-Neriah Y, Daley GQ, Mes-Masson A-M, et al. The chronic myelogenous leukemia-specific P210 protein is the product of the *bcr/abl* hybrid gene. Science 1986;233:212-9.
7. Konopka JB, Watanabe SM, Witte ON. An alteration of the human c-*abl* protein in K562 leukemia cells unmasks associated tyrosine kinase activity. Cell 1984;37:1035-42.
8. Kloetzer W, Kurzrock R, Smith L, et al. The human cellular *abl* gene product in the chronic myelogenous leukemia cell line K562 has an associated tyrosine protein kinase activity. Virology 1985;140:230-8.
9. Rowley JD. A new consistent chromosomal abnormality in chronic myelogenous leukaemia identified by quinacrine fluorescence and Giemsa staining. Nature 1973;243:290-3.
10. Third International Workshop on Chromosomes in Leukemia: Chromosomal abnormalities and their clinical significance in acute lymphoblastic leukemia. Cancer Res 1983;43:111.
11. First International Workshop on Chromosomes in Leukaemia: Chromosomes in acute non-lymphocytic leukaemia. Br J Haematol 1978;39:311-6.
12. Bloomfield CD, Goldman AL, Alimena G, et al. Chromosomal abnormalities identify high-risk and low-risk patients with acute lymphoblastic leukemia. Blood 1986;67:415-20.
13. Kurzrock R, Gutterman JU, Talpaz M. The molecular genetics of Philadelphia chromosome-positive leukemias. N Engl J Med 1988;319:990-8.

14. Kurzrock R, Blick HB, Talpag M. Rearrangement in the Breakpoint Cluster Region and the clinical course in Philadelphia-negative chronic myelogenous leukemia. J Intern Med 1986;105:673-9.
15. Ganesan TS, Rassool F, Guo A-P, et al. Rearrangement of the *bcr* gene in Philadelphia chromosome-negative chronic myeloid leukemia. Blood 1986;68:957-60.
16. Dreazen O, Klisak I, Rassool F, et al. Do oncogenes determine clinical features in chronic myeloid leukaemia? Lancet 1987;1:1402-5.
17. Anonymous. *bcr-abl* in chronic myeloid leukaemia [Editorial]. Lancet 1986;2:258-9.
18. Anonymous. Molecular biology and chronic granulocytic leukaemia [Editorial]. Lancet 1986;2:666-8.
19. Sawyers CL, Timson L, Kawasaki ES, et al. Molecular relapse in chronic myelogenous leukemia patients after bone marrow transplantation detected by polymerase chain reaction. Proc Natl Acad Sci USA 1990;87:563-7.
20. Heisterkamp N, Jenster G, ten Hoeve J, et al. Acute leukemia in *bcr/abl* transgenic mice. Nature 1990;344:251-3.
21. Felix CA, Wright JJ, Poplack DG, et al. T cell receptor α-, β- and γ-genes in T cell and pre-B cell acute lymphoblastic leukemia. J Clin Invest 1987;80:545-56.
22. Chessells JM, Hardisty RM, Rapson NT, Greaves MF. Acute lymphoblastic leukaemia in children: classification and prognosis. Lancet 1977;2:1307-9.
23. Cleary ML, Chao J, Warnke R, Sklar J. Immunoglobulin gene rearrangement as a diagnostic criterion of B-cell lymphoma. Proc Natl Acad Sci USA 1984;81:593-7.
24. Korsmeyer SJ, Waldmann TA. Immunoglobulin genes: rearrangement and translocation in human lymphoid malignancy. J Clin Immunol 1984;4:1-11.
25. Cleary ML, Warnke R, Sklar J. Monoclonality of lymphoproliferative lesions in cardiac-transplant recipients. N Engl J Med 1984;310:477-82.
26. Schwartz RS. From molecular biology to the bedside: the example of immunoglobulin genes [Editorial]. N Engl J Med 1984;310:521-3.
27. Cleary ML, Sklar J. Lymphoproliferative disorders in cardiac transplant recipients are multiclonal lymphomas. Lancet 1984;2:489-93.
28. Aisenberg AC, Wilkes BM, Jacobson JO, Harris NL. Immunoglobulin gene rearrangements in adult non-Hodgkin's lymphoma. Am J Med 1987;82:738-44.
29. Finger LR, Harvey RC, Moore RCA, et al. A common mechanism of chromosomal translocation in T- and B-cell neoplasia. Science 1986;234:982-5.
30. Korsmeyer SJ, Arnold A, Bakhshi A, et al. Immunoglobulin gene rearrangement and cell surface antigen expression in acute lymphocytic leukemias of T cell and B cell precursor origins. J Clin Invest 1983;71:301-13.
31. Picker LJ, Weiss LM, Medeiros JL, et al. Immunophenotypic criteria for the diagnosis of non-Hodgkin's lymphoma. Am J Pathol 1987;128:181-201.
32. Berliner N, Ault KA, Martin P, Weinberg DS. Detection of clonal excess in lymphoproliferative disease by $\varkappa/\lambda$ analysis: correlation with immunoglobulin gene DNA rearrangement. Blood 1986;67:80-5.
33. Kronenberg M, Siu G, Hood LE, Shastri N. The molecular genetics of the T-cell antigen receptor and T-cell antigen recognition. Annu Rev Immunol 1986;4:529-91.
34. Cossman J, Uppenkamp M, Sundeen J, et al. Molecular genetics and the diagnosis of lymphoma. Arch Pathol Lab Med 1988;112:117-27.
35. Knowles DM II, Pelicci P-G, Dalla-Favera R. Immunoglobulin and T cell receptor beta chain gene DNA probes in the diagnosis and classification of human lymphoid neoplasia. Mol Cell Probes 1987;1:15-31.
36. Hochstenbach F, Brenner MB. Newly identified $\gamma\delta$ and $\beta\delta$ T-cell receptors. J Clin Immunol 1990;10:1-18.
37. Raulet DH. Antigens for γ/δ T cells. Nature 1989;339:342-3.
38. Miltenburg AMM, van Laar JM, Daha MR, et al. Dominant T-cell receptor β-chain gene rearrangements indicate clonal expansion in the rheumatoid joint. Scand J Immunol 1990;31:121-6.
39. Oksenberg JR, Stuart S, Begovich AB, et al. Limited heterogeneity of rearranged T-cell receptor Vα transcripts in brains of multiple sclerosis patients. Nature 1990;345:344-6.
40. Acha-Orbea H, Mitchell DJ, Timmermann L, et al. Limited heterogeneity of T cell receptors from lymphocytes mediating autoimmune encephalomyelitis allows specific immune intervention. Cell 1988;54:263-73.

41. Urban JL, Kumar V, Kono DH, et al. Restricted use of T cell receptor V genes in murine autoimmune encephalomyelitis raises possibilities for antibody therapy. Cell 1988;54:577-92.
42. Sakai K, Sinha AA, Mitchell DJ, et al. Involvement of distinct murine T-cell receptors in the autoimmune encephalitogenic response to nested epitopes of myelin basic protein. Proc Natl Acad Sci USA 1988;85:8608-12.
43. Janeway CA. Immunotherapy by peptides? Nature 1989;341:482-3.
44. Acha-Orbea H, McDevitt HO. The first external domain of the nonobese diabetic mouse class II I-A beta chain is unique. Proc Natl Acad Sci USA 1987;84:2435-9.
45. Vandenbark AA, Hashim G, Offner H. Immunization with a synthetic T-cell receptor V-region peptide protects against experimental autoimmune encephalomyelitis. Nature 1989;341:541-4.
46. Howell MD, Winters ST, Olee T, et al. Vaccination against experimental allergic encephalomyelitis with T cell receptor peptides. Science 1989;246:668-70.
47. Wucherpfennig KW, Ota K, Endo N, et al. Shared human T cell receptor V_β usage to immunodominant regions of myelin basic protein. Science 1990;248:1016-19.
48. Posnett DN, Schmelkin I, Burton DA, et al. T cell antigen receptor V gene usage. In: Increases in $V\beta8^+$ T cells in Crohn's disease. J Clin Invest 1990;85:1770-76.
49. Borst P, Greaves DR. Programmed gene rearrangements altering gene expression. Science 1987;235:658-67.

GLIADIN ANTIBODIES

IgA-AGA are found in approximately 25% of patients with dermatitis herpetiformis,[1,2] in essentially all patients with celiac disease (CD, gluten-sensitive enteropathy) not on a gluten-free diet (GFD),[3] and in only a few patients with other gastrointestinal and/or autoimmune diseases.[4] The titer of IgA-AGA decreases with a GFD[5,6] as do titers of IgA-anti-endomysial and IgA-anti-R$_1$ reticulin antibodies.[7] IgA-AGA and IgG-AGA rise significantly during gluten challenge, sometimes several months before clinical relapse.[8] IgG-AEmA and IgG-AGA are especially useful in patients with IgA deficiency who have a 10-15 fold increased frequency of CD.[9] In children, IgA-AGA, usually in relatively low amounts, are sometimes seen in bovine milk intolerance and post-infection malabsorption.[10] IgA antibodies to lactalbumin, casein or ovalbumin are elevated in approximately 50-90% of patients with CD.[11] A two-stage model of CD, which includes a latent period with documented anti-gliadin antibodies in jejunal secretions,[12] might help explain wide differences in incidence of CD[13] and might be useful for evaluation of possibly affected relatives,[14] as well as gluten-sensitive diarrhea without overt enteropathy[15] and idiopathic oral ulceration.[16] The vast majority of Norwegian children with CD share the same cis- or trans-encoded HLA-DQα/β heterodimer, i.e., they share DQA1 and DQB1 genes which are arranged in cis position on the DR3DQw2 haplotype and in trans position in DR5DQw7/DR7DQw2 heterozygous individuals.[17] Positive tests for AGA are useful for detection of CD in children with short stature even in the absence of gastrointestinal symptoms[18] (cf. also 19 and 20). The frequency of CD is increased in children with IgA deficiency.[21] The clinical utility of rectal gluten challenge for the diagnosis of CD is dubious.[22,23] In general, IgA-AGA have a higher positive predictive value for CD than IgA-AGA which have higher negative predictive value;[24] a positive IgA-AEmA is confirmatory evidence and is perhaps an indication for intestinal biopsy.[24] Monitoring serum levels of AGA as a test for compliance with a gluten-free diet (GFD) is important, because the GFD protects patients with CD against development of non-Hodgkin lymphomas and perhaps against cancer of the mouth, pharynx and esophagus.[25] Because the frequency of lymphomas is also increased in dermatitis herpetiformis, monitoring IgA-AGA levels as well as IgA-ARA and IgA-AEmA is probably worthwhile. See also **ENDOMYSIAL ANTIBODIES** and **RETICULIN ANTIBODIES.**

REFERENCES:
1. Kumar V, Jain N, Beutner EH, Chorzelski TP. Detection of antigliadin antibodies in bullous diseases and their recognition of similar antigenic polypeptides. Int Archs Allergy Appl Immunol 1987;83:155-9.
2. Mäki M, Hällström O, Vesikari T, Visakorpi JK. Evaluation of a serum IgA-class reticulin antibody test for the detection of childhood celiac disease. J Pediatr 1984;105:901-5.

3. Volta U, Lenzi M, Lazzari R, et al. Antibodies to gliadin detected by immunofluorescence and a micro-ELISA method: markers of active childhood and adult coeliac disease. Gut 1985;26:667-71.

4. Ståhlberg M-R, Savilahti E, Viander M. Antibodies to gliadin by ELISA as a screening test for childhood celiac disease. J Pediatr Gastroenterol Nutr 1986;5:726-9.

5. Unsworth DJ, Walker-Smith JA, Holborow EJ. Gliadin and reticulin antibodies in childhood coeliac disease [Letter]. Lancet 1983;1:874-5.

6. Savilahti E, Viander M, Perkkiö M, Vainio E, Kalimo K, Reunala T. IgA antigliadin antibodies: a marker of mucosal damage in childhood coeliac disease. Lancet 1983;1:320-2.

7. Kapuscinska A, Zalewski T, Chorzelski TP, Sulej J, Beutner EH, Kumar V, Rossi T. Disease specificity and dynamics of changes in IgA class anti-endomysial antibodies in œliac disease. J Pediatr Gastroenterol Nutr 1987;6:529-34.

8. Scott H, Ek J, Brandtzaeg P. Changes of serum antibody activities to various dietary antigens related to gluten withdrawal or challenge in children with coeliac disease. Int Archs Allergy Appl Immunol 1985;76:138-44.

9. Scott H, Brandtzaeg P. Gluten IgA antibodies and coeliac disease [Letter]. Lancet 1989;1:382-3.

10. Lindberg T, Nilsson L-Å, Borulf S, et al. Serum IgA and IgG gliadin antibodies and small intestinal mucosal damage in children. J Pediatr Gastroenterol Nutr 1985;4:917-22.

11. Scott H, Fausa O, Ek J, Brandtzaeg P. Immune response pattens in coeliac disease. Serum antibodies to dietary antigens measured by an enzyme linked immunosorbent assay (ELISA). Clin Exp Immunol 1984;57:25-32.

12. O'Mahony S, Vestey JP, Ferguson A. Similarities in intestinal humoral immunity in dermatitis herpetiformis without enteropathy and in coeliac disease. Lancet 1990;335:1487-90.

13. Logan RFA, Rifkind EA, Busuttil A, et al. Prevalence and "incidence" of celiac disease in Edinburgh and the Lothian region of Scotland. Gastroenterology 1986;90:334-42.

14. Marsh MN, Bjarnason I, Shaw J, et al. Studies of intestinal lymphoid tissue. XIV-HLA status, mucosal morphology, permeability and epithelial lymphocyte populations in first degree relatives of patients with coeliac disease. Gut 1990;31:32-6.

15. Cooper BT, Holmes GKT, Ferguson R, et al. Gluten-sensitive diarrhea without evidence of celiac disease. Gastroenterology 1980;79:801-6.

16. Wray D. Gluten-sensitive recurrent aphthous stomatitis. Dig Dis Sci 1981;26:737-40.

17. Sollid LM, Markussen G, Ek J, Gjerde H, Vartdal F, Thorsby E. Evidence for a primary association of celiac disease to a particular HLA-DQ α/β heterodimer. J Exp Med 1989;169:345-50.

18. Cacciari E, Salardi S, Volta U, et al. Can antigliadin antibody detect symptomless coeliac disease in children with short stature? Lancet 1985;1:1469-71.

19. Stenhammar L, Kilander AF, Nilsson LÅ, et al. Serum gliadin antibodies for detection and control of childhood coeliac disease. Acta Paediatr Scand 1984;73:657-63.

20. Stenhammar L, Fälhström SP, Jansson G, et al. Coeliac disease in children with short stature without gastrointestinal symptoms. Eur J Pediatr 1986;145:185-6.

21. Savilahti E, Pelkonen P, Visakorpi JK. IgA deficiency in children. A clinical study with special reference to intestinal findings. Arch Dis Child 1971;46:665-70.

22. Loft DE, Marsh MN, Crowe PT. Rectal gluten challenge and diagnosis of coeliac disease. Lancet 1990;1:1293-5.

23. Salazar de Sousa J. Rectal gluten challenge and diagnosis of coeliac disease [Letter]. Lancet 1990;2:323.

24. Calabuig M, Torregosa R, Polo P, et al. Serological markers and celiac disease: a new diagnostic approach? J Pediatr Gastroneterol Ntur 1990;10:435-42.

25. Holmes GKT, Prior P, Lane MR, et al. Malignancy in coeliac disease--effect of a gluten-free diet. Gut 1989;30:333-8.

26. Leonard JN, Tucker WFG, Fry JS, et al. Increased incidence of malignancy in dermatitis herpetiformis. Br Med J 1983;286:16-8.

GLOMERULAR BASEMENT MEMBRANE ANTIBODIES

These antibodies to the non-collagenous portion (NC1) of type IV collagen[1] are detected by EIA in all patients with classical, untreated, biopsy-proved Goodpasture syndrome.[2-4] Alternatively, the IFA technique, which is less specific than EIA, is positive at most, in only 75% of confirmed Goodpasture syndrome.[5] The occurrence of false positives can be a problem if the human kidney employed for the IFA contains sufficient non-specific IgG to make detection of anti-GBM antibodies difficult because of background. Long remissions are sometimes seen in rapidly progressive glomerulonephritis (RPGN).[6] Expeditious testing for anti-glomerular basement membrane (GBM) and anti-neutrophil cytoplasm antibodies is indicated for evaluation of RPGN which these antibodies, can sometimes be present simultaneously[7] or sequentially.[8] Although deficiency of C6 delays the onset of glomerular injury in anti-GBM nephritis in rabbits, a more severe glomerular injury ultimately develops because of delayed clearance of the glomerular immune deposits.[9]

REFERENCES:
1. Butkowski RJ, Langeveld JPM, Wieslander J, Hamilton J, Hudson BG. Localization of the Goodpasture epitope to a novel chain of basement membrane collagen. J Biol Chem 1987;262:7874-7.
2. Wieslander J, Bygren P, Heinegård D. Antiglomerular basement membrane antibody: antibody specificity in different forms of glomerulonephritis. Kidney Intl 1983;23:855-61.
3. Peter JB, Shen GQ, Lin H-C. A sensitive enzyme immunoassay (EIA) for detection of antibodies to glomerular basement membranes (GBM) [Abstract]. Am J Clin Pathol 1989;91:367.
4. Saxena R, Isaksson B, Bygren P, Wieslander J. A rapid assay for circulating anti-glomerular basement membrane antibodies in Goodpasture syndrome. J Immunol Methods 1989;118:73-8.
5. McPhaul JJ Jr, Dixon FJ. Characterization of human anti-glomerular basement membrane antibodies eluted from glomerulonephritic kidneys. J Clin Invest 1970;49:308-17.
6. Bruns FJ, Adler S, Fraley DS, Segel DP. Long-term follow-up of aggressively treated idiopathic rapidly progressive glomerulonephritis. Am J Med 1989;86:400-6.
7. Wahls TL, Bonsib SM, Schuster VL. Coexistent Wegener's granulomatosis and anti-glomerular basement membrane disease. Hum Pathol 1987;18:202-5.
8. O'Donoghue DJ, Short CD, Brenchley PE, et al. Sequential development of systemic vasculitis with anti-neutrophil cytoplasmic antibodies complicating anti-glomerular basement membrane disease. Clin Nephrol 1989;32:251-5.
9. Groggel GC, Terreros DA. Role of the terminal complement pathway in accelerated autologous anti-glomerular basement membrane nephritis. Am J Pathol 1990;136:533-50.

GLUTAMIC ACID DECARBOXYLASE ANTIBODIES

Autoantibodies to glutamic acid decarboxylase (GAD), an enzyme concentrated in GABA-ergic neurons (which control muscle tone and exteroreceptive spinal reflexes) and in pancreatic beta cells, are found in about 60% of patients of stiff-man syndrome.[1,2] The contribution of GAD antibodies to IDDM is unknown, as is the frequency of these antibodies in IDDM.

REFERENCES:
1. Solimena M, Folli F, Denis-Donini S, et al. Autoantibodies to glutamic acid decarboxylase in a patient with stiff-man syndrome, epilepsy, and type I diabetes mellitus. N Engl J Med 1988;318:1012-20.
2. Solimena M, Folli F, Aparisi R, et al. Autoantibodies to GABA-ergic neurons and pancreatic beta cells in stiff-man syndrome. N Engl J Med 1990;322:1555-60.

GM₁ ANTIBODIES

Ganglioside-monosialic acid (GM_1), a glycolipid present in both axolemma and myelin sheath,[1] is concentrated at synaptic terminals and accessible to an immune response.[2] IgM autoantibodies to GM_1 are detected in some patients with lower motor neuron diseases,[3-6] multifocal neuropathies,[7] IgM paraproteinemias with neuropathy[3,8] and systemic lupus erythematosus with central nervous system involvement.[9] Low titers of anti-GM_1 antibodies are detected in other neurologic diseases (e.g., multiple sclerosis and amyotrophic lateral sclerosis) and in some normal individuals.[10] Treatment of patients with lower motor neuron disease to lower anti-GM$_1$ antibody titer has resulted in clinical improvements.[7] Sensitivities, specificities and predictive values of assays for anti-GM$_1$ antibodies are not satisfactorily defined.

REFERENCES:
1. Devries GH, Zmachinski CJ. The lipid composition of rat CNS axolemma-enriched fractions. J Neurochem 1980;34:424-30.
2. Fabian RH. Uptake of antineuronal IgM by CNS neurons: comparison with antineuronal IgG. Neurology 1990;40:419-22.
3. Freddo L, Yu RK, Latov N, et al. Gangliosides GM$_1$ and GD$_{1b}$ are antigens for IgM M-protein in a patient with motor neuron disease. Neurology 1986;36:454-8.
4. Nardelli E, Steck AJ, Barkas T, et al. Motor neuron syndrome and monoclonal IgM with antibody activity against gangliosides GM1 and GD1b. Ann Neurol 1988;23:524-8.
5. Gzesh D, Evans VA, Heiman-Patterson TD, et al. Specificity of anti-GM1 antibodies in patients with motor neuron syndromes. Neurology 1989;39(Suppl 1):402.
6. Salazar-Grueso EF, Routbort MJ, Variakojis R, et al. Serum anti-ganglioside antibodies (AGA) in patients with motor neuron disease (MND) and MND variants. Neurology 1989;39(Suppl 1):402.
7. Pestronk A, Cornblath DR, Ilyas AA, et al. A treatable multifocal motor neuropathy with antibodies to GM1 ganglioside. Ann of Neurol 1988;24:73-8.
8. Miyatani N, Baba H, Sato S, et al. Antibody to sialosyllactosaminylparagloboside in a patient with IgM paraproteinemia and polyradiculoneuropathy. J Neuroimmunol 1987;14:189-96.
9. Hirano T, Hashimoto H, Shiokawa Y, et al. Antiglycolipid autoantibody detected in the sera from systemic lupus erythematosus patients. J Clin Invest 1980;66:1437-40.
10. Sadiq SA, Thomas FP, Kilidireas K, et al. The spectrum of neurologic disease associated with anti-GM$_1$ antibodies. Neurology 1990;40:1067-72.

GRANULOCYTE ANTIBODIES

Anti-granulocyte antibodies are pathogenetically important in febrile transfusion reactions,[1] isoimmune neonatal neutropenia,[2] drug-induced neutropenia,[3,4] and the neutropenias of several autoimmune disorders[5] (Felty syndrome[6,7]), Evans syndrome,[8] Graves disease,[9] primary autoimmune neutropenia of early childhood[10] and SLE[11]). Flow cytometry is the method of choice for detection and quantitation of anti-granulocyte antibodies.[12-14] Assays for antibodies mediating pure white cell aplasia are also recognized.[15] The clinical significance of granulocyte antigen systems and antibodies was recently reviewed.[16,17] See also **ANTINEUTROPHIL CYTOPLASM ANTIBODIES.**

REFERENCES:
1. Clay ME, Kline WE. Detection of granulocyte antigens and antibodies: current perspectives and approaches. In: Garraty G, ed. Transfusion therapy. Virginia: American Association of Blood Banks, 1985:183-265.
2. Lalezari P. Neutrophil antigens: immunology and clinical implications. In: Greenwalt TJ, Jamieson GA, eds. The granulocyte: function and clinical utilization. New York: Alan R. Liss Inc., 1977;209-25.
3. Weitzman SA, Stossel TP, Desmond M. Drug-induced immunological neutropenia. Lancet 1978;1:1068-71.
4. Chong BH, Berndt MC, Koutts J, Castaldi PA. Quinidine-induced thrombocytopenia and leukopenia: demonstration and characterization of distinct antiplatelet and antileukocyte antibodies. Blood 1983;62:1218-23.
5. Logue GL, Shimm DS. Autoimmune granulocytopenia. Annu Rev Med 1980;31:191-200.
6. Petersen J, Wiik A. Lack of evidence for granulocyte specific membrane-directed auto-antibodies in neutropenic cases of rheumatoid arthritis and in autoimmune neutropenia. Acta Pathol Microbiol Immunol Scand 1983;91:15-22.
7. Fiechtner JJ, Miller DR, Starkebaum G. Reversal of neutropenia with methotrexate treatment in patients with Felty's syndrome. Arthritis Rheum 1989;32:194-201.
8. Pegels JG, Helmerhorst FM, van Leeuwen EF, van de Plas-van Dalen C, Engelfriet CP, von dem Borne AEG Kr. The Evans syndrome: characterization of the responsible autoantibodies. Br J Haematol 1982;51:445-50.

9. Weitzman SA, Stossel TP, Harmon DC, Daniels G, Maloof F, Ridgway EC. Anti-neutrophil autoantibodies in Graves' disease: implications of thyrotropin binding to neutrophils. J Clin Invest 1985;75:119-23.
10. Madyastha PR, Glassman AB. Characterization of neutrophil agglutinins in primary autoimmune neutropenia of early childhood. Ann Clin Lab Sci 1988;18:367-73.
11. Rustagi PK, Currie MS, Logue GL. Complement-activating antineutrophil antibody in systemic lupus erythematosus. Am J Med 1985;78:971-7.
12. Lape ML, Baker JA, Chan JK. A comparison of immunofluorescent assays to detect anti-granulocyte antibodies. Am J Clin Pathol 1985;84:464-8.
13. Lucas GF, Saunders PWG, Waters AH. Report of the platelet and granulocyte serology working group, 1986. Clin Lab Haematol 1987;9:307-11.
14. Robinson JP, Duque RE, Boxer LA, Ward PA, Hudson JL. Measurement of anti-neutrophil antibodies by flow cytometry: simultaneous detection of antibodies against monocytes and lymphocytes. Diagn Clin Immunol 1987;5:163-70.
15. Currie MS, Weinberg JB, Rustagi PK, Logue GL. Antibodies to granulocyte precursors in selective myeloid hypoplasia and other suspected autoimmune neutropenias: use of HL-60 cells as targets. Blood 1987;69:529-36.
16. McCullough J. Granulocyte antigen systems and antibodies and their clinical significance. Hum Pathol 1983;14:228-34.
17. Madyastha PR, Glassman AB. Neutrophil antigens and antibodies in the diagnosis of im-mune neutropenias. Ann Clin Lab Sci 1989;19:146-54.

GRANULOCYTE-SPECIFIC ANTINUCLEAR ANTIBODIES

So-called granulocyte-specific anti-nuclear antibodies (GS-ANA) are found in approximately 75% of active RA and in approximately 90-95% of autoimmune neutropenia.[1] GS-ANA (the exact non-histone antigens have not yet been identified) correlate better with erosive joint disease than do organ-nonspecific ANA or negative ANA.[2]

REFERENCES:
1. Wiik A. Granulocyte-specific antinuclear antibodies: possible significance for the pathogenesis, clinical features and diagnosis of rheumatoid arthritis. Allergy 1980;35:263-89.
2. De Carvalho A, Graudal H. Radiographic progression of rheumatoid arthritis related to some clinical and laboratory parameters. Acta Radiol [Diagn] 1980;21:551-5.

GUANOSINE ANTIBODIES

The usefulness of these antibodies as a marker for procainamide-induced lupus (PIL) was not confirmed in a study relating antibodies to the H2A/H2B histone complex to PIL.[1,2]

REFERENCES:
1. Weisbart RH, Yee WS, Colburn KK, Whang SH, Heng MK, Boucek RJ. Antiguanosine antibodies: a new marker for procainamide-induced systemic lupus erythematosus. Ann Intern Med 1986;104:310-3.
2. Totoritis MC, Tan EM, McNally EM, Rubin RL. Association of antibody to histone complex H2A-H2B with symptomatic procainamide-induced lupus. N Engl J Med 1988;318:1431-6.

H2A-H2B HISTONE COMPLEX

IgG antibodies to H2A-H2B histones are found in nearly all patients with symptomatic procainamide-induced lupus, in about 19% of asymptomatic procainamide-treated individuals and in approximately 20% of SLE patients. Sensitivity of 100% for symptomatic procainamide-induced lupus and specificity of 94% are claimed when the antibodies are shown to react more strongly with the native H2A-H2B dimer than to the heat-denatured dimer,[1] but these striking results are not yet confirmed (cf. 2).

In SLE, antibodies react with multiple intact histones but not with trypsin-resistant fragments, whereas the antibodies to H2A, H2B and H2A-H2B complex in procainamide-induced lupus react strongly with such fragments. In hydralazine-induced lupus, antihistone antibodies react primarily with H3 and H4 and their trypsin-resistant fragments.[3] The clinical utility of various anti-histone antibodies is still under intense investigation,[4,5] but their clinical utility is dubious.

REFERENCES:

1. Totoritis MC, Tan EM, McNally EM, Rubin RL. Association of antibody to histone complex H2A-H2B with symptomatic procainamide-induced lupus. N Engl J Med 1988;318:1431-6.
2. Hess E. Drug-related lupus. N Engl J Med 1988;318:1460-2.
3. Portanova JP, Arndt RE, Tan EM, Kotzin BL. Anti-histone antibodies in idiopathic and drug-induced lupus recognize distinct intrahistone regions. J Immunol 1987;138:446-51.
4. Shoenfeld Y, Segol G, Segol O, et al. Detection of antibodies to total histones and their subfractions in systemic lupus erythematosus patients and their asymptomatic relatives. Arthritis Rheum 1987;30:169-75.
5. Rubin RL, Waga S. Antihistone antibodies in systemic lupus erythematosus. J Rheumatol 1987;14(Suppl 13):118-26.

HEAT SHOCK PROTEIN ANTIBODIES

The heat shock proteins (hsps) expressed by mycobacteria are arthritogenic in adjuvant arthritis.[1] These proteins, which have sequence similarities in bacteria, animals and man, are important in inflammation.[2] IgM, IgG and IgA antibodies to a 73 kd member of the hsp70 family are found in about 40% of SLE, 10-20% of RA, and less frequently in other rheumatic and infectious diseases.[3,4] The significance of these interesting findings remains to be determined. T cells reactive with a 65 kd mycobacterial hsp are found in RA synovial fluid in inverse proportion to the duration of disease,[5] but the findings have not been independently confirmed and definitive data relating this activity to exogenous or endogenous antigens are not yet available. Elevated levels of the human hsp90 found in lymphocytes of about 15% of patients with SLE[6] may reflect T cell activation. Mycobacterial proteins are mitogenic for the CD4⁻ CD8⁻, γ/δ TCR T cells in RA synovial fluid.[7] See 8 for review of bacterial hsps and serodiagnosis and references 9 and 10 for hsps, immune response and immunopathology.

REFERENCES:

1. van Eden W, Thole JER, van der Zee R, et al. Cloning of the mycobacterial epitope recognized by T lymphocytes in adjuvant arthritis. Nature 1988;331:171-3.
2. Polla BS. A role for heat shock proteins in inflammation? Immunol Today 1988;9:134-7.
3. Minota S, Cameron B, Welch WJ, Winfield JB. Autoantibodies to the constitutive 73-kD member of the hsp70 family of heat shock proteins in systemic lupus erythematosus. J Exp Med 1988;168:1475-80.
4. Tsoulfa G, Rook GAW, Van-Embden JDA, et al. Raised serum IgG and IgA antibodies to mycobacterial antigens in rheumatoid arthritis. Ann Rheum Dis 1989;48:118-23.
5. Res PCM, Schaar CG, Breedveld FC, et al. Synovial fluid T cell reactivity against 65 kD heat shock protein of mycobacteria in early chronic arthritis. Lancet 1988;2:478-9.
6. Norton PM, Isenberg DA, Latchman DS. Elevated levels of the 90 kd heat shock protein in a proportion of SLE patients with active disease. J Autoimmunity 1989;2:187-95.
7. Holoshitz J, Koning F, Coligan JE, et al. Isolation of CD4⁻ CD8⁻ mycobacteria-reactive T lymphocyte clones from rheumatoid arthritis synovial fluid. Nature 1989;339:226-9.
8. Pallen M. Bacterial heat-shock proteins and serodiagnosis. Serodiag Immunother Infect Dis 1989;3:149-59.
9. Kaufmann SHE. Heat shock proteins and the immune response. Immunol Today 1990;11:129-36.
10. Lydyard PM, van Eden W. Heat shock proteins: immunity and immunopathology. Immunol Today 1990;11:218-9.

HEMOCHROMATOSIS

Following the demonstration of HLA-associations with hemochromatosis, it became clear that this disease is dependent upon a common recessive gene which occurs in approximately 10% of the population. Since the inheritance is recessive and since other factors affect expression, the observed data are consistent with a prevalence of at least 1 per thousand.[1] Males are more likely to develop the disease but family studies have shown that females and children frequently have minor abnormalities which are now known to reflect homozygosity rather than heterozygosity as previously thought.

The hemochromatosis gene is carried by several MHC haplotypes but most notably HLA A3,B7 and A3,B14. Thus, 73% of patients have A3 compared with 30% of controls. It follows that HLA typing is of limited value in the individual case, but family studies are extremely valuable for tracking the gene through a family. The typing of an affected case allows the identification of carrier haplotypes which often (but not necessarily) contain A3. It should be emphasized that the recessive gene is common so that it will not be unusual to find 3 or more carrier haplotypes in one family.

Numerous family studies have indicated that the gene is within the MHC and probably between HLA-A and B. Recombination between the putative gene and HLA-A occurs with the frequency of less than 1%.The nature of the hemochromatosis gene has not been established (for a discussion of possibilities, see 2-4), but the same gene appears to be common in sporadic porphyria cutanea tarda and may be responsible for the hepatic siderosis which occurs in this condition.[5]

In undertaking family studies, it is generally sufficient to type for HLA-A, B and C without the need for class II typing. C4 allotyping will assist in the identification of the haplotypes and is recommended as a part of the initial family study.

Genotyping of the family is straightforward if the family tree is provided.

REFERENCES:
1. Edwards Q, Griffen LM, Goldgar D, et al. Prevalence of hemochromatosis in 11,065 presumably healthy blood donors. N Engl J Med 1988;318:1355-62.
2. Bothwell TH, Charlton RW, Motulsky AG. Hemochromatosis. In: Scriver CR, Beaudet AL, Sly WS, Valle D, eds. The metabolic basis of inherited disease. New York: McGraw-Hill, Inc., 1989:1433-62.
3. Flanagan PR, Lam D, Bajerjee D, Valberg LS. Ferritin release by mononuclear cells in hereditary hemochromatosis. J Lab Clin Med 1989;113:145-50.
4. David V, Papadopoulos P, Yaouang J, et al. Ferritin H gene polymorphism in idiopathic hemochromatosis. Hum Genet 1989;81:123-6.
5. Edwards CQ, Griffen LM, Goldgar DE, et al. HLA-linked hemochromatosis alleles in sporadic porphyria cutanea tarda. Gastroenterology 1989;97:972-81.

HETEROPHILE

The term "heterophile", i.e., "other loving", which is employed to describe antibodies giving rise to distinctive patterns of reactivity on indirect fluorescent antibody (IFA) studies with various tissues,[1] is useful for calling attention to antibodies which can otherwise be misidentified (cf. 1 for review). The appellation "heterophile", which is so useful in the context of IFA work for description of antibodies associated with blood transfusions and other alloimmunizations,[1] should not be confused with the heterophile agglutinin antibodies of infectious mononucleosis or serum sickness. See also **BRUSH BORDER ANTIBODIES.**

REFERENCES:
1. Hawkins BR, McDonald BL, Dawkins RL. Characterization of immunofluorescent heterophile antibodies which may be confused with autoantibodies. J Clin Pathol 1977;30:299-307.

HERPES GESTATIONIS ANTIBODIES

These antibodies to a 180 kd epidermal protein, which are not found in normal pregnancy, are detected in 89% of IFA-positive HG sera and in 47% of bullous pemphigoid sera;[1] (cf. 2 and 3 for review) of anti-skin antibodies. IgG antibodies to basement membrane zone (BMZ) are detected by DIF in approximately 30-50%, whereas C3 is found at the BMZ in essentially 100% of HG. By indirect immunofluorescence IgG antibodies to BMZ are detected in only 20% but when assessed with anti-C3 are detected in approximately 50% of HG.[3] Immunoblotting, a more sensitive method, allows detection of serum antibodies to hemidesmosomal components of the BMZ in approximately 90% of patients with herpes gestationis.[1] See also **SKIN ANTIBODIES.**

REFERENCES:
1. Morrison LH, Labib RS, Zone JJ, et al. Herpes gestationis autoantibodies recognize a 180-kD human epidermal antigen. J Clin Invest 1988;81:2023-6.

2. Stanley JR. Pemphigus and pemphigoid as paradigms of organ-specific, autoantibody-mediated diseases. J Clin Invest 1989;83:1443-8.
3. Jablonska S, Chorzelski TP, Beutner EH. Uses for immunofluorescence tests of skin and sera.

HETEROGENEOUS NUCLEAR RIBONUCLEOPROTEIN (hnRNP) ANTIBODIES

Heterogeneous nuclear ribonucleoprotein (hnRNP) is composed of heterogeneous nuclear RNA and at least 20 associated proteins designated A1 through U. Some of these proteins contain an octapeptide motif in their highly conserved RNA-binding domains. Because these proteins bind single-stranded polynucleotides, sometimes in a specific manner, their function resembles that of DNA-binding zinc-finger and homeobox motifs in eucaryotic transcriptions factors (cf. 1 for review). Patients with mixed connective tissue disease (MCTD) have antibodies to hnRNP antigens and approximately 54% of SLE patients with anti-U1 snRNP antibodies also have antibodies to hnRNP. At this time, anti-hnRNP antibodies offer no diagnostic help beyond what is currently available from anti-U1 snRNP antibodies.[1,2] Antibodies to the A1 protein component of hnRNP particles are found in about 25% of SLE and ∼50% of RA;[3] anti-keratin antibodies (which are present in ∼50% of RA[4]) cross-react with an A1 epitope. A different epitope is reactive in SLE (cf. 3).

REFERENCES:
1. Burd CG, Swanson MS, Görlach M, Dreyfuss G. Primary structures of the heterogeneous nuclear ribonucleoprotein A2, B1, and C2 proteins: a diversity of RNA binding proteins is generated by small peptide inserts. Proc Natl Acad Sci USA 1989;86:9788-92.
2. Gelpi C, Rodriguez-Sanchez JL, Hardin JA. Purification of hnRNP form HeLa cells with a monoclonal antibody and its application in ELISA: detection of autoantibodies. Clin Exp Immunol 1988;71:281-8.
3. Montecucco C, Caporali R, Negri C, et al. Antibodies from patients with rheumatoid arthritis and systemic lupus erythematosus recognize different epitopes of a single heterogeneous nuclear RNP core protein. Possible role of cross-reacting antikeratin antibodies. Arthritis Rheum 1990;33:180-6.
4. Kirstein H, Mathiesen FR. Anti-keratin antibodies in rheumatoid arthritis: methods and clinical significance. Scand J Rheumatol 1987;16:331-7.

Hu (NEURONAL NUCLEAR) ANTIBODIES

Hu antibodies, also known as anti-neuronal nuclear antibodies (ANNA), are reactive with 36-42 kd proteins of all neuronal nuclei. These antibodies are found in serum and CSF of patients with small cell lung cancers (and rarely with breast and prostate carcinomas) complicated by paraneoplastic sensory neuropathy and/or paraneoplastic encephalomyelitis. Increased IBBB synthesis of anti-Hu IgG is documented in these patients.[1-4] These antibodies give a homogeneous pattern of staining on nuclei of neurons but not on glial, endothelial or other non-neuronal nuclei.[1-6] ANNA are found in patients with various paraneoplastic neurologic syndromes including subacute sensory neuronopathy and paraneoplastic encephalomyelitis. ANNA were recently described in a patient with Lambert-Eaton syndrome and small-cell lung carcinoma;[7] in this patient, antibodies to voltage-gated-calcium channels would have been expected. In addition to Hu autoantibodies, Yo autoantibodies reactive with Purkinje cell cytoplasm and other antibodies with distinctive patterns of reactivity are being recognized in paraneoplastic serological diseases. The frequency and type of neurological involvement in patients with Hu antibodies was reviewed.[2,8] See also PURKINJE CELL (Yo) ANTIBODIES and VOLTAGE-GATED-CALCIUM CHANNEL ANTIBODIES.

REFERENCES:
1. Graus F, Elkon KB, Lloberes P, et al. Neuronal antinuclear antibody (anti-Hu) in paraneoplastic encephalomyelitis simulating acute polyneuritis. Acta Neurol Scand 1987;75:249-52.
2. Anderson NE, Rosenblum MK, Graus F, Wiley RG, Posner JB. Autoantibodies in paraneoplastic syndromes associated with small-cell lung cancer. Neurology 1988;38:1391-7.

3. Jaeckle KA, Greenlee JE. Immunohistological patterns of antibody response in paraneoplastic neurological syndromes correlate with specific syndromes and with tumor types. Ann Neurol 1988;24:121.
4. Furneaux HF, Reich L, Posner JB. Autoantibody synthesis in the central nervous system of patients with paraneoplastic syndromes. Neurology 1990;40:1085-91.
5. Grisold W, Drlicek M, Popp W, Jellinger K. Antineuronal antibodies in small cell lung carcinoma - a significance for paraneoplastic syndromes? Acta Neuropathol 1987;75:199-202.
6. Kimmel DW, O'Neill BP, Lennon VA. Subacute sensory neuronopathy associated with small cell lung carcinoma: diagnosis aided by autoimmune serology. Mayo Clin Proc 1988;63:29-32.
7. Dropcho EJ, Stanton C, Oh SJ. Neuronal antinuclear antibodies in a patient with Lambert-Eaton myasthenic syndrome and small-cell lung carcinoma. Neurology 1989;39:249-51.
8. Posner JB, Dalmau J, Furneaux HM, Graus F. Paraneoplastic "anti-Hu" syndrome: a clinical study of 47 patients [Abstract]. Neurology 1990; 40(Suppl 1):165.

HYALURONAN

Serum levels of this polysaccharide can be elevated as a result of increased production during inflammatory diseases, (e.g., rheumatoid arthritis,[1,2] scleroderma[3] and psoriasis[4]), as well as in certain cancers, (e.g., mesotheliomas[5] and Wilms tumors[6]). Serum levels are also elevated due to decreased uptake and catabolism in hepatic cirrhosis for which hyaluronan may be a better marker than procollagen III N-peptide.[7]

REFERENCES:
1. Engström-Laurent A, Laurent TC. Hyaluronan as a clinical marker. In: Lindh E, ed. Clinical impact of bone and connective tissue markers. Uppsala: Academic Press Ltd., 1989.
2. Engström-Laurent A, Hällgren R. Circulating hyaluronic acid levels vary with physical activity in healthy subjects and in rheumatoid arthritis patients. Relationship to synovitis mass and morning stiffness. Arthritis Rheum 1987;30:1333-8.
3. Horslev-Petersen K, Ammitzboll T, Engström-Laurent A, et al. Serum and urinary aminoterminal type III procollagen peptide in progressive systemic sclerosis: relationship to sclerodermal involvement, serum hyaluronan and urinary collagen metabolites. J Rheumatol 1988;15:460-7.
4. Lundin A, Engström-Laurent A, Michaëlsson G, Tengblad A. High levels of hyaluronate in suction blister fluid from active psoriatic lesions. Br J Dermatol 1987;116:335-40.
5. Smedsrod B, Einarsson M, Pertoft H. Tissue plasminogen activator is endocytosed by mannose and galactose receptors of rat liver cells. Thromb Haemost 1988;59:480-4.
6. Wu AHB, Parker OS, Ford L. Hyperviscosity caused by hyaluronic acid in serum in a case of Wilms' tumor. Clin Chem 1984;30:914-6.
7. Nyberg A, Engström-Laurent A, Lööf L. Serum hyaluronate in primary biliary cirrhosis - a biochemical marker for progressive liver damage. Hepatology 1988;8:142-6.

HYPERIMMUNOGLOBULIN E RECURRENT INFECTION (JOB) SYNDROME

Hyperimmunoglobulin E recurrent infection syndrome (HIERIS) is a congenital disorder characterized by high serum IgE, chronic eczematoid dermatitis, recurrent skin and sinopulmonary infections and increased *Staphylococcus aureus*-specific IgE.[1] IFN-γ, which is produced in normal amounts by mitogen stimulation of PBMC in HIERIS, inhibits spontaneous production of IgE (as well as IgG1, 3 and 4) by B-cell preparations from patients with HIERIS who have high spontaneous production of IgE *in vitro. IFN-γ* decreases serum IgE in HIERIS.[2]

REFERENCES:
1. Leung DY, Geha RS. Clinical and immunologic aspects of the hyperimmunoglobulin E syndrome. Hematol Oncol Clin North Am 1988;2:81-100.
2. King CL, Gallin JI, Malech HL, et al. Regulation of immunoglobulin production in hyperimmunoglobulin E recurrent-infection syndrome by interferon γ. Proc Natl Acad Sci USA 1989;86:10085-9.

iC3b-NEO

Plasma levels of iC3b-NEO are said to correlate with clinical disease activity and renal histologic activity in SLE,[1] but whether they are more reliable than levels of C4 and CH50[2] is not known.

REFERENCES:
1. Negoro N, Okamura M, Takeda T, et al. The clinical significance of iC3b neoantigen expression in plasma from patients with systemic lupus erythematosus. Arthritis Rheum 1989;32:1233-42.
2. Swaak AJG, Groenwold J, Bronsveld W. Predictive value of complement profiles and anti-dsDNA in systemic lupus erythematosus. Ann Rheum Dis 1986;45:359-66.

IgA

Serum IgA and secretory IgA (sIgA) are independently derived from two different sources, i.e., bone marrow/lymph nodes and mucosa.[1] In blood, IgA1 and IgA2, antigenically distinct subclasses, normally exist largely in monomeric form at a ratio of about 80-90% IgA1 and 10-20% IgA2.[2,3] In external secretions, IgA1 and IgA2 exist as homopolymers in nearly equal proportions.[4] Neither monomeric nor polymeric IgA from blood contribute significantly (less than 2%) to total sIgA, which is synthesized in secretory glands (including mammary) and in the lamina propria of the gastrointestinal and respiratory tracts. The frequency of IgA1 or IgA2 plasma cells in bone marrow and lymph nodes (80-95% IgA1 positive) and in lamina propria (50% IgA1 positive) corresponds to the concentrations of IgA1 and IgA2 in blood and external excretions, respectively.[5,6]

Polymeric IgA is found in serum in a variety of circumstances, including parenchymal liver damage which is thought to impair clearance,[1,7] untreated celiac disease in which there is spillover from intestine to circulation as reflected in the presence of sIgA in serum[8] and in IgA nephropathy.[9] Increased serum IgA is common in patients with chronic bronchial suppuration[10] and in ARC or AIDS.[11] Total deficiency of IgA can be selective (at a frequency of 1:700 in caucasians) or accompanied by deficiency of IgG2 and/or IgG4;[12] it also occurs in ataxia-telangiectasia and congenital rubella. Allergies are common in IgA deficient patients, but the mechanism (failure of immune exclusion[13] at mucosal barriers) is unknown.[14] IgA deficiency is commonly inherited with the ancestral haplotype which includes A1, B8 and DR3 (cf. 15) and, as expected from this association, is sometimes accompanied by autoimmune disease[16] but prevalence of autoantibodies is not increased in IgA deficient blood donors.[17] Selective deficiency of IgA2 but not of IgA1 has been reported.[18] Deficiency of IgA induced phenytoin[19] and sulfa salazine[20] is well recognized. Treatment of IgA-deficient individuals with parenteral preparations, occasionally including IV IgG, can lead to anaphylactoid reactions associated with production of IgE and/or IgG antibodies to IgA,[21] but preparations depleted of IgA have been used successfully in IgA deficient patients who have anti-IgA autoantibodies.[22] The clinical immunology of IgA deficiency has been expertly reviewed.[23]

REFERENCES:
1. Conley ME, Delacroix DL. Intravascular and mucosal immunoglobulin A: two separate but related systems of immune defense? Ann Intern Med 1987;106:892-9.
2. Mestecky J, Russell MW. IgA subclasses. Monogr Allergy 1986;19:277-301.
3. Mestecky J, Russell MW, Jackson S, Brown TA. The human IgA system: a reassessment. Clin Immunol Immunopathol 1986;40:105-14.
4. Underdown BJ, Schiff JM. Immunoglobulin A: strategic defense initiative at the mucosal surface. Annu Rev Immunol 1986;4:389-417.
5. Skvaril F, Morell A. Distribution of IgA subclasses in sera and in bone marrow. Adv Exp Med Biol 1975;45:433-5.
6. Kett K, Brandtzaeg P, Radl J, Haaijman JJ. Different subclass distribution of IgA-producing cells in human lymphoid organs and various secretory tisues. J Immunol 1986:136:3631-5.
7. Delacroix DL, Elkon KB, Geubel AP, et al. Changes in size, subclass, and metabolic properties of serum immunoglobulin A in liver diseases and in other diseases with high serum immunoglobulin A. J Clin Invest 1983;71:358-67.

8. Volta U, Molinaro N, Fratangelo D, Bianchi FB. IgA subclass antibodies to gliadin in serum and intestinal juice of patients with coeliac disease. Clin Exp Immunol 1990;80:192-5.
9. Hernando P, Egido J, de Nicolas R, Sancho J. Clinical significance of polymeric and monomeric IgA complexes in patients with IgA nephropathy. Am J Kidney Dis 1986;8:410-6.
10. Horan MA, Leahy BC, Fox RA, et al. Immunological abnormalities in patients with chronic bronchial suppuration: a possible relationship with endotoxaemia. Br J Dis 1984;78:66-74.
11. Fling JA, Fischer JR, Baswell RN, Reid MJ. The relationship of serum IgA concentration to human immunodeficiency virus (HIV) infection: a cross sectional study of HIV-seropositive individuals detected by screening in the United States Air Force. J Allergy Clin Immunol 1988;82:965-70.
12. Björkander J, Bengtsson U, Oxelius V-A, Hanson LÅ. Symptoms in patients with lowered levels of IgG subclasses, with or without IgA deficiency, and effects of immunoglobulin prophylaxis. In: Hanson LÅ, Söderström T, Oxelius V-A, eds. Immunoglobulin subclass deficiencies. New York: Karger, 1985:157-63. (Dukor P, Kallós P, Trnka Z, Waksman BH, eds. Monographs in Allergy; vol 20).
13. Childers NK, Bruce MG, McGhee, JR. Molecular mechanisms of immunoglobulin A defense. Annu Rev Microbiol 1989;43:503-36.
14. Soothill J. Food intolerance. Practitioner 1989;233:596-8.
15. Dawkins RL, Christiansen FT, Kay PH, et al. Disease associations with complotypes, supratypes and haplotypes. Immunol Rev 1983;70:1-22.
16. Waldmann TA. Immunodeficiency diseases: primary and acquired. In: Samter M, ed. Immunological diseases. 4th Ed. Boston/Toronto: Little, Brown, and Company, Inc. 1988;1:411-65.
17. Koistinen J, Sarna S. Immunological abnormalities in the sera of IgA-deficient blood donors. Vox Sang 1975;29:203-13.
18. van Loghem E, Zegers BJM, Bast EJEG, Kater L. Selective deficiency of immunoglobulin A2. J Clin Invest 1983;72:1918-23.
19. Burks AW, Charlton R, Casey P, et al. Immune function in patients treated with phenytoin. J Child Neurol 1989;4:25-9.
20. Leickly FE, Buckley RH. Development of IgA and IgG2 subclass deficiency after sulfasalazine therapy. J Pediatr 1986;108:481-2.
21. Burks AW, Sampson HA, Buckley RH. Anaphylactic reactions after gamma globulin administration in patients with hypogammaglobulinemia. Detection of IgE antibodies to IgA. N Engl J Med 1986;314:560-4.
22. Cunningham-Rundles C, Wong S, Björkander J, Hanson LA. Use of an IgA-depleted intravenous immunoglobulin in a patient with an anti-IgA antibody. Clin Immunol Immunopathol 1986;38:141-9.
23. French MAH, Dawkins RL. Central MHC genes, IgA deficiency and autoimmune disease. Immunol Today 1990;11:271-4.

IgA-FIBRONECTIN AGGREGATES

Approximately 50% of all cases of IgA nephropathy (IgAN), the most common form of glomerulonephritis worldwide,[1] are characterized by large amounts of circulating aggregates ("complexes") containing IgA and fibronectin.[2] Other abnormalities include high serum concentrations of IgA and immune complexes containing IgA rheumatoid factor and autologous IgG;[3] (cf. 1 and 4 for review of IgAN and reference 5 for review of fibronectin biology). IgG antibodies to unidentified glomerular antigens (distinct from Goodpasture antigen) are also reported.[6] The association of IgA nephropathy and ankylosing spondylitis/sacroiliitis is unexplained.[7] The fact that normal human IgG contains binding sites for fibronectin[8] complicates interpretation of the IgA-fibronectin aggregates described in IgAN, as does the fact that high serum concentrations of IgA increase the apparent levels of circulating aggregates of IgA-fibronectin.[9] In spite of these complexities, assays which detect IgA-fibronectin aggregates are useful in the investigation of hematuria and suspected glomerulonephritis and, if cut offs for the indeterminate range are appropriately adjusted, negative results are strong evidence against IgAN and positive results are strong evidence for IgAN.[9]

REFERENCES:
1. Julian BA, Waldo FB, Rifai A, Mestecky J. IgA nephropathy, the most common glomerulonephritis worldwide: a neglected disease in the United States? Am J Med 1988;84:129-32.
2. Cederholm B, Wieslander J, Bygren P, Heinegård D. Circulating complexes containing IgA and fibronectin in patients with primary IgA nephropathy. Proc Natl Acad Sci USA 1988;85:4865-8.
3. Czerkinsky C, Koopman WJ, Jackson S, et al. Circulating immune complexes and immunoglobulin A rheumatoid factor in patients with mesangial immunoglobulin A nephropathies. J Clin Invest 1986;77:1931-8.
4. Julian BA, ed. First National Symposium on IgA Nephropathy. Washington, DC: Grune & Stratton, 1988:337-453.
5. Ruoslahti E. Fibronectin and its receptors. Annu Rev Biochem 1988;57:375-413.
6. Ballardie FW, Brenchley PEC, Williams S, O'Donoghue DJ. Autoimmunity in IgA nephropathy. Lancet 1988;2:588-92.
7. Béné MC, Faure G. IgA nephropathy. Springer Semin Immunopathol 1987;9:387-94.
8. Rostagno AA, Frangione B, Gold LI. Biochemical characterization of the fibronectin binding sites for IgG. J Immunol 1989;143:3277-82.
9. Hollingsworth PN, Peter JB. Unpublished data.

IgA INDEX

The IgA Index, a measure of intra-blood-brain-barrier (IBBB) synthesis of total IgA, is elevated in approximately 18% of patients with multiple sclerosis and is more frequently abnormal when the IBBB synthesis of dimeric IgA is assessed.[1] The IgA Index is also abnormal in some patients with viral meningitis (e.g., due to mumps)[1-3] and in some with CNS lupus.[4] In contrast to the IgG Index and IgM Index, the IgA Index is characteristically normal in patients with borrelial disease of the CNS.[5] When the blood-brain barrier is leaky, however, as manifest by an Albumin Index greater than 9,[6-8] the only reliable measurements of IBBB synthesis of IgG, IgM, and IgA are provided by determinations of IgG(loc), IgM(loc) and IgA(loc) which represent, at a minimum, the local [i.e., (loc) or IBBB] synthesis of these immunoglobulins.[9] See **IgG(loc)**, **IgM(loc)** and **IgA(loc)**.

REFERENCES:
1. Sindic CJM, Delacroix DL, Vaerman JP, et al. Study of IgA in the cerebrospinal fluid of neurological patients with special reference to size, subclass and local production. J Neuroimmunol 1984;7:65-75.
2. Frydén A, Link H, Norrby E. Cerebrospinal fluid and serum immunoglobulins and antibody titers in mumps meningitis and aseptic meningitis of other etiology. Infect Immunity 1978;21:852-61.
3. Schuller E, Delasnerie N, Reboul J, Lefevre M. Serum and CSF IgA. Prot Biol Fluids 1978;25:881-5.
4. Hirohata S, Hirose S, Miyamoto T. Cerebrospinal fluid IgM, IgA, and IgG indexes in systemic lupus erythematosus. Arch Intern Med 1985;145:1843-6.
5. Henriksson A, Link H, Cruz M, Stiernstedt G. Immunoglobulin abnormalities in cerebrospinal fluid and blood over the course of lymphocytic meningoradiculitis (Bannwarth's syndrome). Ann Neurol 1986;20:337-45.
6. Tibbling G, Link H, Öhman S. Principles of albumin and IgG analyses in neurological disorders. I. Establishement of reference values. Scand J Clin Lab Invest 1977;37:385-90.
7. Rust RS Jr, Dodson WE, Trotter JL. Cerebrospinal fluid IgG in childhood: the establishment of reference values. Ann Neurol 1988;23:406-10.
8. Reiber H, Felgenhauer K. Protein transfer at the blood cerebrospinal fluid barrier and the quantitation of the humoral immune response within the central nervous system. Clin Chim Acta 1987;163:319-28.

IgE ANTIBODIES

Anti-IgE antibodies, which are said to be present in about 25% of normal children and adults, are not greatly elevated in patients with asthma or atopic eczema.[1] In young mice, both passive transfer of syngeneic polyclonal anti-IgE antibodies and immunization with syngeneic IgE cause prolonged inhibition of synthesis of IgE.[2] Suppression of synthesis of all immunoglobulin isotypes results from treatment of neonatal mice with xenogenicantic anti-μ chain antibodies,[3] whereas treatment with noncytotoxic MAbs to allotypic μ chain determinants causes tolerized B cells which produce mainly IgG3 on immunization. The presence of IgG anti-IgE antibodies can cause decreased results for total IgE and antigen-specific IgE.[4]

REFERENCES:
1. Twena DM, Marshall JS, Haeney MR, Bell EB. A survey of nonatopic and atopic children and adults for the presence of anti-IgE autoantibodies. Clin Immunol Immunopathol 1989;53:40-51.
2. Cooper MD, Kearney JF, Gathings WE, Lawton AR. Effects of anti-Ig antibodies on the development and differentiation of B cells. Immunol Rev 1980;52:29-53.
3. Gause A, Yoshida N, Kappen C, Rajewsky K. In vivo generation and function of B cells in the presence of a monoclonal anti-IgM antibody: implications for B cells tolerance. Eur J Immunol 1987;17:981-90.
4. Paganelli R, Quinti I, D'Offizi GP, et al. Studies on the *in vitro* effects of auto-anti-IgE. Inhibition of total and specific serum IgE detection by a human IgG autoantibody to IgE. J Clin Lab Immunol 1988;26:153-7.

IgE IMMUNE COMPLEXES

IgE complexes are found in many atopic diseases in which as much as 50% of circulating IgE may be in complexed form. It is unknown whether these complexes have a role in atopic diseases or in food allergy (cf. 1 for review).

REFERENCES:
1. Carini C. IgE immune complexes in food allergy: significance, pathogenicity and clinical considerations. Clin Allergy 1987;17:485-97.

IgG INDEX

The IgG Index [(CSF IgG/Serum IgG)/(CSF Albumin/Serum Albumin)] is an alternative method (to the IgG Synthesis Rate) for estimating the intra-blood-brain-barrier (IBBB) synthesis of IgG, which is less aptly termed the "intrathecal synthesis of IgG" or the "CNS IgG Synthesis Rate".[1-3] The IgG Index is elevated in a variety of infectious, inflammatory and neoplastic conditions of the CNS.[1] In addition to the IgG Index[1] and the IBBB IgG Synthesis Rate,[2] IBBB synthesis of immunoglobulins can be assessed by the IgM Index[4-6] and IgA Index.[7] However, when the blood-brain barrier is leaky, as manifest by an Albumin Index greater than 9,[8,9] the only reliable measurements of IBBB synthesis of IgG, IgM and IgA are provided by determination of IgG(loc), IgM(loc) and IgA(loc), which represent at a minimum, the local [i.e., (loc) or IBBB] synthesis of these immunoglobulins.[10-12] IgG(loc), IgM(loc) and IgA(loc) (each in mg/liter) correct for even major changes in permeability of the blood-brain barrier. Recommendations that the IgG Index be abandoned in favor of the IBBB IgG Synthesis Rate[13] are inadvisable because of the well known effect of increased blood-brain barrier permeability on the IBBB IgG Synthesis Rate.[10-12] See also **IgG SYNTHESIS RATE; IgM INDEX; IgA INDEX; IgG(loc), IgM(loc), IgA(loc);** and **OLIGOCLONAL IMMUNOGLOBULINS.**

REFERENCES:
1. Lefvert AK, Link H. IgG production within the central nervous system: a critical review of proposed formulae. Ann Neurol 1985;17:13-20.
2. Tourtellotte WW, Staugaitis SM, Walsh MJ, et al. The basis of intra-blood-brain-barrier IgG synthesis. Ann Neurol 1985;17:21-7.
3. Whitaker JN. Quantitation of the synthesis of immunoglobulin G within the central nervous system. Ann Neurol 1985;17:11-2.
4. Sindic CJM, Cambiaso CL, Depré A, Laterre EC, Masson PL. The concentration of IgM in the cerebrospinal fluid of neurological patients. J Neurol Sci 1982;55:339-50.
5. Forsberg P, Henriksson A, Link H, Öhman S. Reference values for CSF-IgM, CSF-IgM/S-IgM ratio and IgM index, and its application to patients with multiple sclerosis and aseptic meningoencephalitis. Scand J Clin Lab Invest 1984;44:7-12.

6. Williams AC, Mingioli ES, McFarland HF, Tourtellotte WE, McFarlin DE. Increased CSF IgM in multiple sclerosis. Neurology 1978;28:996-8.
7. Sindic CJM, Delacroix DL, Vaerman JP, Laterre EC, Masson PL. Study of IgA in the cerebrospinal fluid of neurological patients with special reference to size, subclass and local production. J Neuroimmunol 1984;7:65-75.
8. Tibbling G, Link H, Öhman S. Principles of albumin and IgG analyses in neurological disorders. I. Establishement of reference values. Scand J Clin Lab Invest 1977;37:385-90.
9. Rust RS Jr, Dodson WE, Trotter JL. Cerebrospinal fluid IgG in childhood: the establishment of reference values. Ann Neurol 1988;23:406-10.
10. Wurster U. Comparison of formulas for the calculation of intrathecal IgG. In: Pedersen E, Clausen J, Oades L, eds. Actual problems in multiple sclerosis research. Copenhagen: FADL 1983:298-301.
11. Peter JB, Bowman RL, Bowman RL Jr, Tourtellotte WW. Blood or plasma contamination of CSF: effect on CNS IgG synthesis rate and IgG Index [Abstract]. Am J Clin Pathol 1987;87:422.
12. Reiber H, Felgenhauer K. Protein transfer at the blood cerebrospinal fluid barrier and the quantitation of the humoral immune response within the central nervous system. Clin Chim Acta 1987;163:319-28.
13. Matteson EL, Flagler DG, Mesara BW. IgG synthesis rate in evaluation of multiple sclerosis in a community hospital. Neurology 1987;37:847-9.

IgG(loc), IgM(loc) and IgA(loc)

Intra-blood-brain-barrier ("intrathecal", CNS or CSF) synthesis of IgG, IgM and IgA cannot be reliably determined when the blood-brain barrier is leaky.[1-3] All commonly used methods, including IBBB IgG Synthesis Rate, IgG Index, IgM Index and IgA Index can be falsely elevated when the blood-brain barrier is leaky as documented by an Albumin Index greater than 9.[3-5] Increased IBBB synthesis of IgG or IgM or IgA can, however, be accurately quantified by IgG(loc), IgM(loc) and IgA(loc) which represent at a minimum, the local [i.e., (loc) or IBBB] synthesis of IgG, IgM and IgA in the CSF. IgG(loc), IgM(loc) and IgA(loc) (each in mg/liter) correct for even major changes in permeability of the blood-brain barrier.[2] See also **IgG SYNTHESIS RATE** and **IgG INDEX**.

REFERENCES:
1. Wurster U. Comparison of formulas for the calculation of intrathecal IgG. In: Pedersen E, Clausen J, Oades L, eds. Actual problems in multiple sclerosis research. Copenhagen: FADL 1983:298-301.
2. Reiber H, Felgenhauer K. Protein transfer at the blood cerebrospinal fluid barrier and the quantitation of the humoral immune response within the central nervous system. Clin Chim Acta 1987;163:319-28.
3. Peter JB, Bowman RL, Bowman RL Jr, Tourtellotte WW. Blood or plasma contamination of CSF: effect on CNS IgG synthesis rate and IgG index [Abstract]. Am J Clin Pathol 1987;87:422.
4. Tibbling G, Link H, Öhman S. Principles of albumin and IgG analyses in neurological disorders. I. Establishment of reference values. Scand J Clin Lab Invest 1977;37:385-90.
5. Rust RS Jr, Dodson WE, Trotter JL. Cerebrospinal fluid IgG in childhood: the establishment of reference values. Ann Neurol 1988;23:406-10.

IgG SUBCLASSES

A normal level of serum total IgG does not rule out a clinically important deficiency of one or more IgG subclasses, because compensatory increases can occur in serum levels of other IgG subclasses. Selective deficiencies of one or more IgG subclasses are associated with sinusitis, recurrent otitis media and/or asthma,[1,2] recurrent respiratory tract infections,[3-6] impaired lung function with or without IgA deficiency,[7,8] chronic chest symptoms in nonallergic children,[8] recurrent meningococcemia,[9] recurrent pneumococcal bacteremia,[10,11] unusual allergies, chronic and recurrent acute otitis and sinusitis,[12,13] and failure to respond to polysaccharide antigens of certain encapsulated bacteria[1,2,12,14-16] (see 17-22 for review). Individuals with IgA deficiency should have at least one determination of their IgG subclasses because of the association of impaired lung function with IgG subclass deficiency with (or without) IgA deficiency.[7,8,23] Patients with deficiency of one of the early components of the classical complement pathway should also be evaluated for deficiency of IgG subclasses because of recent data which suggest an increased frequency of IgG4 deficiency in patients with deficiencies of C3 or C1-C4.[24]

The absolute amount of IgG4 and of phospholipase PLA-specific IgG4 is greatly increased in beekeepers and in individuals immunized with PLA.[25] IgG4 is also greatly increased in certain chronic parasitic diseases (e.g., *Schistosoma mansoni*),[26] but the proportion of schistosoma-specific IgG is very similar ($\sim$10-15%) in each of the IgG subclasses.[27]

Some children with IgG2 levels 2SD below the appropriate age-adjusted means show no evidence of increased susceptibility to infection.[28] Some IgA-deficient patients with normal IgG2 levels and subnormal responses to pneumococcal polysaccharides are susceptible to pneumococcal sepsis.[29] Likewise, invasive *Hib* disease occurs despite vaccination with *Hib*-PRP in some children with normal IgG2 levels.[30,31] Although the frequency of failure to respond to polysaccharide antigens is seemingly associated with increased bacterial sepsis,[32-34] no epidemiologically acceptable data are available, as is also the case for the relationship of recurrent bacterial infections to deficiencies of IgG subclasses.

REFERENCES:
1. Umetsu DT, Ambrosino DM, Quinti I, Siber GR, Geha RS. Recurrent sinopulmonary infection and impaired antibody response to bacterial capsular polysaccharide antigen in children with selective IgG-subclass deficiency. N Engl J Med 1985;313:1247-51.
2. Timens W, Poppema S, et al. Impaired immune response to polysaccharides [Letters]. N Engl J Med 1987;317:837-9.
3. Beck CS, Heiner DC. Selective immunoglobulin G_4 deficiency and recurrent infections of the respiratory tract[1]. Am Rev Respir Dis 1981;124:94-6.
4. Stanley PJ, Corbo G, Cole PJ. Serum IgG subclasses in chronic and recurrent respiratory infections. Clin Exp Immunol 1984;58:703-8.
5. Shackelford PG, Polmar SH, Mayus JL, Johnson WL, Corry JM, Nahm MH. Spectrum of IgG2 subclass deficiency in children with recurrent infections: prospective study. J Pediatr 1986;108:647-53.
6. Leickly FE, Buckley RH. Development of IgA and IgG2 subclass deficiency after sulfasalazine therapy. J Pediatr 1986;108:481-2.
7. Björkander J, Bake B, Oxelius V-A, Hanson LÅ. Impaired lung function in patients with IgA deficiency and low levels of IgG2 or IgG3. N Engl J Med 1985;313:720-4.
8. Smith TF, Morris EC, Bain RP. IgG subclasses in nonallergic children with chronic chest symptoms. J Pediatr 1984;105:896-900.
9. Bass JL, Nuss R, Mehta KA, Morganelli P, Bennett L. Recurrent meningococcemia associated with IgG_2-subclass deficiency [Letter]. N Engl J Med 1983;309:430.
10. Matter L, Wilhelm JA, Angehrn W, Skvaril F, Schopfer K. Selective antibody deficiency and recurrent pneumococcal bacteremia in a patient with Sjögren's syndrome, hyperimmunoglobulinemia G, and deficiencies of IgG2 and IgG4. N Engl J Med 1985;312:1039-42.
11. Slade HB, Schwartz SA. Selective antibody deficiency and recurrent pneumococcal bacteremia in a patient with Sjögren's syndrome, hyperimmunoglobulinemia G, and deficiencies of IgG2 and IgG4 [Letter]. N Engl J Med 1985;313:891.
12. Freijd A, Hammarström L, Persson MAA, Smith CIE. Plasma anti-pneumococcal antibody activity of the IgG class and subclasses in otitis prone children. Clin Exp Immunol 1984;56:233-8.
13. Freijd A, Oxelius V-Å, Rynnel-Dagöö B. A prospective study demonstrating an association between plasma IgG2 concentrations and susceptibility to otitis media in children. Scand J Infect Dis 1985;17:115-20.
14. Ambrosino DM, Siber GR, Chilmonczyk BA, Jernberg JB, Fineberg RW. An immunodeficiency characterized by impaired antibody responses to polysaccharides. N Engl J Med 1987;316:790-3.
15. Ambrosino DM, Siber GR, Chilmonczyk BA, Jernberg JB, Fineberg RW. Impaired response to polysaccharides [Letter]. N Engl J Med 1987;317:838-9.
16. Siber GR, Schur PH, Aisenberg AC, Weitzman SA, Schiffman G. Correlation between serum IgG-2 concentrations and the antibody response to bacterial polysaccharide antigens. N Engl J Med 1980;303:178-82.
17. Heiner DC. Significance of immunoglobulin G subclasses. Am J Med 1984;76:1-6.
18. Oxelius V-A. Immunoglobulin G (IgG) subclasses and human disease. Am J Med 1984;76:7-18.
19. Shakib F, Stanworth DR. Human IgG subclasses in health and disease (A review) - Part I. La Ricerca Clin Lab 1980;10:463-79.

20. Stiehm ER, Ashida E, Kim KS, et al. Intravenous immunoglobulins as therapeutic agents. Ann Intern Med 1987;107:367-82.

21. Ochs HD, Wedgwood RJ. IgG subclass deficiencies. Annu Rev Med 1987;38:325-40.

22. Jefferis R, Kumararatne DS. Selective IgG subclass deficiency: quantification and clinical relevance. Clin Exp Immunol 1990;81:357-67.

23. Björkander J, Bengtsson U, Oxelius V-A, Hanson LÅ. Symptoms in patients with lowered levels of IgG subclasses, with or without IgA deficiency, and effects of immunoglobulin prophylaxis. In: Hanson LA, Söderström T, Oxelius V-A, eds. Immunoglobulin subclass deficiencies. New York: Basel & Karger, 1986:157-63.

24. Bird P, Lachmann PJ. The regulation of IgG subclass production in man: low serum IgG4 in inherited deficiencies of the classical pathway of C3 activation. Eur J Immunol 1988;18:1217-22.

25. Aalberse RC, van der Gaag R, van Leeuwen J. Serologic aspects of IgG4 antibodies. J Immunol 1983;130:722-6.

26. Iskander R, Das PK, Aalberse RC. IgG4 antibodies in Egyptian patients with schistosomiasis. Int Arch Allergy Appl Immunol 1981;66:200.

27. Boctor FN, Peter JB. IgG subclasses in human chronic schistosomiasis overproduction of schistosome-specific and non-specific IgG4. Clin Exp Immunol 1990;82:In press.

28. Shackelford PG, Granoff DM, Madassery JV, et al. Clinical and immunologic characteristics of healthy children with subnormal serum concentrations of IgG2. Pediatr Res 1990;27:16-21.

29. Lane PJL, MacLennan ICM. Impaired IgG2 anti-pneumococcal antibody responses in patients with recurrent infection and normal IgG2 levels but no IgA. Clin Exp Immunol 1986;65:427-33.

30. Granoff DM, Shackelford PG, Suarez BK, Collaborative Group. *Haemophilus influenzae* type b disease in children vaccinated with type b polysaccharide vaccine. N Engl J Med 1986;315:1584-90.

31. Granoff DM, Sheetz KE, Nahm MH, et al. Further immunologic evaluation of children who develop *Haemophilus* disease despite previous vaccination with type b polysaccharide vaccine. Mongr Allergy 1986;23:256.

32. Ambrosino DM, Umetsu DT, Siber GR, et al. Selective defect in antibody response to *Haemophilus influenzae* type b in children with recurrent infections and normal serum IgG subclass levels. J Allergy Clin Immunol 1988;81:1175-9.

33. Geha RS. IgG antibody response to polysaccharides in children with recurrent infections. Monogr Allergy 1988;23:97-102.

34. Knutsen AP. Patients with IgG subclass and/or selective antibody deficiency to polysaccharide antigens: initiation of a controlled clinical trial of intravenous immune globulin. J Allergy Clin Immunol 1989;84:640-5.

IgG SYNTHESIS RATE (IBBB IgG SYNTHESIS RATE)

Increased intra-blood-brain-barrier (IBBB) synthesis of IgG is found in a wide variety of infectious, inflammatory and neoplastic conditions of the CNS[1] (see **OLIGOCLONAL IMMUNOGLOBULINS** for additional references). The majority (93%[2] to 99%[1]) of patients with clinically definite multiple sclerosis will have CSF abnormalities including oligoclonal immunoglobulins by isoelectric focusing and increased IBBB synthesis of IgG.[1] Methods for determination of IBBB (sometimes referred to as "intrathecal") synthesis of IgG have major limitations in the presence of a leaky blood-brain barrier.[1-3] When the barrier is leaky as manifest by an Albumin Index greater than 9, the most reliable measurements of IBBB synthesis of IgG and IgM and IgA are provided by determination of IgG(loc), IgM(loc) and IgA(loc) which define the minimum amount of local [i.e., (loc) or IBBB] synthesis, because these three results (mg/liter) correct for even major changes in permeability of the blood-brain barrier.[4] Recommendations that the IgG Index be abandoned in favor of the IBBB IgG synthesis rate[5] are inadvisable because of the well known effect of increased blood-brain barrier permeability on the IBBB IgG synthesis rate.[2,4,6] An elevated IBBB IgG synthesis rate accompanied by oligoclonal immunoglobulins is said to be common in CNS lupus,[7] but not all data are in agreement.[8] See also **IgG(loc), IgM(loc), IgA(loc)** and **OLIGOCLONAL IMMUNOGLOBULINS**.

REFERENCES:
1. Tourtellotte WW, Walsh MJ, Baumhefner RW, Staugaitis SM, Shapshak P. The current status of multiple sclerosis intra-blood-brain-barrier IgG synthesis. In: Scheinberg L, Raine CS, eds. Multiple sclerosis: experimental and clinical aspects. New York: NY Academy of Sciences, 1984;436:52-67.
2. Wurster U. Comparison of formulas for the calculation of intrathecal IgG. In: Pedersen E, Clausen J, Oades L, eds. Actual problems in multiple sclerosis research. Copenhagen: FADL, 1983:298-301.
3. Tourtellotte WW, Potvin AR, Walsh MJ. Measurement of intra-blood-brain-barrier IgG synthesis in multiple sclerosis. A review: multiple sclerosis east and west. Kuroiwa Y, Kurland TL, eds. Fukuoka: Kyushu University Press, 1982.
4. Reiber H, Felgenhauer K. Protein transfer at the blood cerebrospinal fluid barrier and the quantitation of the humoral immune response within the central nervous system. Clin Chim Acta 1987;163:319-28.
5. Matteson EL, Flagler DG, Mesara BW. IgG synthesis rate in evaluation of multiple sclerosis in a community hospital. Neurology 1987;37:847-9.
6. Peter JB, Bowman RL, Bowman RL Jr, Tourtellotte WW. Blood or plasma contamination of CSF: effect on CNS IgG synthesis rate and IgG index. Am J Clin Pathol 1987;87:422.
7. Ernerudh J, Olsson T, Lindström F, Skogh T. Cerebrospinal fluid immunoglobulin abnormalities in systemic lupus erythematosus. J Neurol Neurosurg Psychiatry 1985;48:807-13.
8. Peter JB, Bowman RL. Intra-blood-brain-barrier synthesis of IgG: comparison of IgG synthesis formulae in a computer model and in 1629 consecutive specimens. Unpublished data, 1989.

IgM INDEX

The IgM Index, a measure of intra-blood-brain-barrier (IBBB) synthesis of total IgM (as distinguished from organism-specific IgM), is characteristically abnormal in patients with infectious meningoencephalitis,[1-3] including bacterial meningitis[4] and CNS infection by *Borrelia burgdorferi*.[5-7] Occasionally, patients with multiple sclerosis[2,3] or with CNS lupus[8] will have an elevated IgM Index even when the IgG Index is normal and oligoclonal immunoglobulins are absent. When the blood-brain barrier is leaky, however, as manifest by an Albumin Index greater than 9,[9,10] the only reliable measurements of IBBB synthesis of IgG, IgM and IgA are provided by determination of IgG(loc), IgM(loc) and IgA(loc) which yields the local [i.e., (loc) or IBBB] synthesis of these immunoglobulins.[11] The combination of a raised IgG index and/or IgM index with an elevated cell count and positive CSF VDRL has a positive predictive value of about 100% for the presence of (asymptomatic) neurosyphilis and a near perfect true negative rate of 1, i.e., essentially all latent syphilitic patients without CNS involvement do not have this combination of positive results.[12,13] Titers are expected to fall fourfold at three months and eightfold at six months with successful treatment. Failure to fall at this rate suggests treatment failure or reinfection. Monitoring permits identification of treatment failures or reinfections at the earliest possible time.[14] See also **IgG INDEX; IgG(loc), IgM(loc), IgA(loc)** and **ORGANISM-SPECIFIC ANTIBODY INDEX.**

REFERENCES:
1. Williams AC, Mingioli ES, McFarland HF, Tourtellotte WW, McFarlin DE. Increased CSF IgM in multiple sclerosis. Neurology 1978;28:996-8.
2. Sindic CJM, Cambiaso CL, Depré A, Laterre EC, Masson PL. The concentration of IgM in the cerebrospinal fluid of neurological patients. J Neurol Sci 1982;55:339-50.
3. Forsberg P, Henriksson A, Link H, Öhman S. Reference values for CSF-IgM, CSF-IgM/S-IgM ratio and IgM index, and its application to patients with multiple sclerosis and aseptic meningoencephalitis. Scand J Clin Lab Invest 1984;44:7-12.
4. Forsberg P, Frydén A, Link H. Immunoglobulin abnormalities in the cerebrospinal fluid during bacterial meningitis. J Neuroimmunol 1986;12:299-310.
5. Boeer A, Schipper HI, Prange HW. Local IgM production in meningoradiculitis Bannwarth and neurosyphilis. J Neuroimmunol 1988;20:315-6.
6. Henriksson A, Link H, Cruz M, Stiernstedt G. Immunoglobulin abnormalities in cerebrospinal fluid and blood over the course of lymphocytic meningoradiculitis (Bannwarth's syndrome). Ann Neurol 1986;20:337-45.

7. Kristoferitsch W, Lanschützer H. Oligoklonales immunoglobulin M im liquor cerebrospinalis von patienten mit meningopolyneuritis Garin-Bujadoux-Bannwarth. Wien Klin Wochenschr 1986;98:386-8.
8. Hirohata S, Hirose S, Miyamoto T. Cerebrospinal fluid IgM, IgA, and IgG indexes in systemic lupus erythematosus. Their use as estimates of central nervous system disease activity. Arch Intern Med 1985;145:1843-6.
9. Tibbling G, Link H, Öhman S. Principles of albumin and IgG analyses in neurological disorders. I. Establishment of reference values. Scand J Clin Lab Invest 1977;37:385-90.
10. Rust RS Jr, Dodson WE, Trotter JL. Cerebrospinal fluid IgG in childhood: the establishment of reference values. Ann Neurol 1988;23:406-10.
11. Reiber H, Felgenhauer K. Protein transfer at the blood cerebrospinal fluid barrier and the quantitation of the humoral immune response within the central nervous system. Clin Chim Acta 1987;163:319-28.
12. Wolters EC, Hische EAH, Tutuarima JA, et al. Central nervous system involvement in early and late syphilis: the problem of asymptomatic neurosyphilis. J Neurol Sci 1988;88:229-39.
13. van Kamp GJ, Wolters ECh. CSF-IgM measurement in neurovenereological disease. Clin Chim Acta 1989;183:295-300.
14. Brown ST, Zaidi A, Larsen SA, et al. Serological response to syphilis treatment. J Am Med Assoc 1985;253:1296-9.

IMMUNOBLOTS

This is a technique for separation of proteins by electrophoresis on solid supports (e.g., agarose) followed by electric- or osmotic-driven transfer to nitrocellulose strips or a similar material. Proteins transferred to the strips can be identified by antibodies of known specificity. In a common usage, strips containing a variety of proteins from a specific tissue (e.g., rabbit thymus) are used to identify serum antibodies to a specific proteins. These include antibodies to the 70 kd component of U1 RNP in MCTD and antibodies to the 28/29 kd proteins (B'/B) in SLE. Inefficient transfer of nuclear proteins to blotting material renders immunoblotting unreliable as a primary screening method (or confirmatory method) unless controls of appropriate antibody activity are routinely included to ensure adequate sensitivity and specificity.[1] Similar methods used for transfer of nucleic acids to strips followed by hybridization are known as Southern blots (DNA hybridization) and as Northern blots (transfer of RNA to strips followed by hybridization with specific DNA probes) (see 1-4 for review).

REFERENCES:
1. Van Dam AP, Van den Brink HG, Smeenk RJT. Technical problems concerning the use of immunoblots for the detection of antinuclear antibodies. J Immunol Methods 1990;129:63-70.
2. Burnette WN. "Western blotting": electrophoretic transfer of proteins from sodium dodecyl sulfate-polyacrylamide gels to unmodified nitrocellulose and radiographic detection with antibody and radioiodinated protein A. Anal Biochem 1981;112:195-203.
3. Bjerrum OJ, Heegaard NHH, eds. CRC handbook of immunoblotting of proteins. Volume I. Technical descriptions. Boca Raton, Florida, CRC Press, Inc., 1988.
4. Bjerrum OJ, Heegaard NHH, eds. CRC handbook of immunoblotting of proteins. Volume II. Experimental and clinical applications. Boca Raton, Florida, CRC Press, Inc., 1988.

INSULIN ANTIBODIES; aka INSULIN AUTOANTIBODIES

Current evidence indicates that IAA (insulin autoantibodies) (i.e., insulin autoantibodies found in sera of patients never treated with insulin as opposed to insulin antibodies found in sera of patients treated with insulin), like islet-cell antibodies (ICA), are markers of ongoing destruction of pancreatic β-cell and may be useful for screening.[1-3] However, discrepant results in different assays for IAA remain a serious problem unless precision and detection limits are considered; systematic variance can be reduced by using a standard curve with common derived units, a single species of ligand, a single assay type, and by control of nonspecific binding.[4,5] In addition to IDDM, insulin autoantibodies (typically in the absence of ICA) are also found in the insulin autoimmune syndrome, after treatment with penicillamine or methimazole and in patients with multiple autoimmune problems. The predictive value of combined testing for IAA and ICA in first degree relatives of patients with IDDM are being defined.[6,7] In contrast to the low frequency (0.03 ± 0.03% of IgG-producing cell precursors in peripheral blood), low affinity ($K_d \sim 10^{-5}$-10^{-6} moles/L), polyreactive IgG MAbs to insulin derived from normal peripheral blood cells, MAbs to insulin derived from B cells of patients with IDDM are high frequency (0.21 ± 0.14%), high affinity ($\sim 10^{-7}$ moles/L) and monoreactive.[8] See also **ISLET CELL ANTIBODIES.**

REFERENCES:

1. Palmer JP, Clemons P, Lyen K, Tatpati O, Raghu PK, Paquette TL. Insulin antibodies in insulin-dependent diabetics before insulin treatment. Science 1983;222:1337-9.
2. Vardi P, Dib SA, Tuttleman M, et al. Competitive insulin autoantibody assay: prospective evaluation of subjects at high risk for development of type I diabetes mellitus. Diabetes 1987;36:1286-91.
3. Dean BM, Becker F, McNally JM, et al. Insulin autoantibodies in the pre-diabetic period: correlation with islet cell antibodies and development of diabetes. Diabetologia 1986;29:339-42.
4. Kurtz AB, DiSilvio L, Bosi E. The determination of detection limits for insulin antibody assays. Diabetologia 1988;31:395-9.
5. Wilkin TJ, Schoenfeld SL, Diaz J-L, Kruse V, Bonifacio E, Palmer JP. Systematic variation and differences in insulin-autoantibody measurements. Diabetes 1989;38:172-81.
6. Ziegler AG, Ziegler R, Vardi P, et al. Life-table analysis of progression to diabetes of anti-insulin autoantibody-positive relatives of individuals with type 1 diabetes. Diabetes 1989;38:1320-5.
7. Dean BM, McNally JM, Bonifacio E, et al. Comparison of insulin autoantibodies in diabetes-related and healthy populations by precise displacement ELISA. Diabetes 1989;38:1275-81.
8. Casali P, Nakamura M, Ginsberg-Fellner F, Notkins AL. Frequency of B cells committed to the production of antibodies to insulin in newly diagnosed patients with insulin-dependent diabetes mellitus and generation of high affinity human monoclonal IgG to insulin. J Immunol 1990;144:3741-7.

INSULIN-LIKE GROWTH FACTOR I RECEPTOR ANTIBODIES

Two species of antibodies to IGF-I receptor are found in sera. One variety reacts with a site distinct from that for IGF-I binding. The other, which blocks IGF-I binding to its receptor and causes IGF-I resistance, has been found in several patients with rheumatic diseases (4/31), polycystic ovary syndrome (1/7), IDDM (1/52) and NIDDM (3/48). Two of these patients had elevated serum levels of IGF-I, but neither had glucose intolerance.[1] Antibodies to insulin-like growth factor 1 receptor inhibit growth of Wilms tumor in tissue culture and in nude mice.[2] See also **PEPTIDE GROWTH FACTORS.**

REFERENCES:

1. Tappy L, Fujita-Yamaguchi Y, LeBon TR, Boden G. Antibodies to insulin-like growth factor I receptors in diabetes and other disorders. Diabetes 1988;37:1708-14.
2. Gansler T, Furlanetto R, Gramling TS, et al. Antibody to type 1 insulinlike growth factor receptor inhibits growth of Wilms' tumor in culture and in athymic mice. Am J Pathol 1989;135:961-6.

INSULIN RECEPTOR ANTIBODIES

Insulin resistance due to anti-insulin receptor antibodies (type B insulin resistance) has been described in over twenty patients. This syndrome is often accompanied by acanthosis nigricans and evidence of autoimmune disease.[1] Hypoglycemia due to insulin-receptor antibodies is occasionally seen in autoimmune diseases and Hodgkin disease.[2-4] Antibodies that react with the insulin receptor at sites other than the insulin binding site are found in a few patients with IDDM and NIDDM.[5] Among first-degree relatives of patients with IDDM, detection of IAA and ICA has a predictive value of 60-77% for development of IDDM within 5-10 years.[6,7] See also **INSULIN-LIKE GROWTH FACTOR I RECEPTOR ANTIBODIES.**

REFERENCES:
1. Bloise W, Wajchenberg BL, Moncada VY, Marcus-Samuels B, Taylor SI. Atypical anti-insulin receptor antibodies in a patient with type B insulin resistance and scleroderma. J Clin Endocrinol Metab 1989;68:227-31.
2. Selinger S, Tsai J, Pulini M, Saperstein A, Taylor S. Autoimmune thrombocytopenia and primary biliary cirrhosis with hypoglycemia and insulin receptor autoantibodies. Ann Intern Med 1987;107:686-8.
3. Braund WJ, Naylor BA, Williamson DH, et al. Autoimmunity to insulin receptor and hypoglycaemia in patient with Hodgkin's disease. Lancet 1987;1:237-40.
4. Walters EG, Tavaré JM, Denton RM, Walters G. Hypoglycaemia due to an insulin-receptor antibody in Hodgkin's disease. Lancet 1987;1:241-3.
5. Boden G, Fujita-Yamaguchi Y, Shimoyama R, et al. Nonbinding inhibitory antiinsulin receptor antibodies. J Clin Invest 1988;81:1971-8.
6. Dean BM, McNally JM, Bonifacio E, et al. Comparison of insulin autoantibodies in diabetes-related and healthy populations by precise displacement ELISA. Diabetes 1989;38:1275-81.
7. Ziegler AG, Ziegler R, Vardi P, et al. Life-table analysis of progression to diabetes of anti-insulin autoantibody-positive relatives of individuals with type 1 diabetes. Diabetes 1989;38:1320-5.

INTEGRINS

Integrins are non-covalent heterodimeric cell-surface receptors for certain heterodimeric cell adhesion molecules (CAMs) which belong to a superfamily of proteins present in blood, on white cells and in extracellular matrices. CAMs are characterized by tripeptide arginine-glycine-aspartic acid (RGD) group(s) present in the recognition site(s) by which they are bound to the integrins. The cell adhesion molecules and their receptors include fibronectin and its receptor, vitronectin and its receptor (cf. 1) fibrinogen and gpIIb/IIIa, ICAM-1 and LFA-1 (CD11a), as well as C3bi and Mac-1 (CD11b). For review, cf. 2 and 3. See also **LEUKOCYTE ADHESION MOLECULES** and **CLUSTERS OF DIFFERENTIATION**.

REFERENCES:
1. Suzuki S, Huang Z-S, Tanihara H. Cloning of an integrin β subunit exhibiting high homology with integrin β_3 subunit. Proc Natl Acad Sci USA 1990;87:5354-8.
2. Ruoslahti E, Pierschbacher MD. New perspectives in cell adhesion: RGD and integrins. Science 1987;238:491-7.
3. Hogg N. The leukocyte integrins. Immunol Today 1989;10:111-4.

INTERCALATED CELL ANTIBODIES

Antibodies to intercalated cell antibodies of the renal collecting tubules were reported in a patient with three spontaneous abortions.[1] These antibodies to cells responsible for HCO3-/Cl-exchange and those containing a proton pump should be sought in patients with autoimmune disease and relevant acid-base problems.

REFERENCES:
1. Raghunath M, Gilbert P, Miedaner-Maier I, et al. Detection of a human autoantibody against intercalated cells of kidney-collecting tubule. J Autoimmunity 1989;2:889-94.

INTERCELLULAR ADHESION MOLECULE 1

Intercellular adhesion molecule 1 (ICAM-1) is a member of the immunoglobulin gene super-family, one of the large family of cell adhesion molecules.[1] It is found at the surface of cells, including endothelial cells for which it acts as a ligand for leukocyte function antigen 1 (LFA-1). Interaction of ICAM-1 and LFA-1 is one of the steps by which lymphocytes bind to and traverse endothelial cells.[2-5] Known to be upregulated (possibly by inflammatory cytokines) in the mesangium and proximal tubules in murine lupus nephritis,[6] ICAM-1 expression is also upregulated on inflamed bronchial endothelium; airway eosinophilia and hyper-responsiveness are attenuated by a monoclonal antibody to ICAM-1 in experimental asthma.[7] ICAM-1 is the cellular receptor for a subgroup of rhinoviruses (cf. 8); a soluble form of

ICAM-1 inhibits infection of cells by rhinoviruses,[8] which cause 50% of common colds. See also **LEUKOCYTE ADHESION MOLECULES.**

REFERENCES:
1. Edelman GM. Topobiology. Sci Am 1989;260(5):76-88.
2. Hale LP, Martin ME, McCollum DE, et al. Immunohistologic analysis of the distribution of cell adhesion molecules within the inflammatory synovial microenvironment. Arthritis Rheum 1989;32:22-30.
3. Smith CW, Rothlein R, Hughes BJ, et al. Recognition of an endothelial determinant for CD18-dependent human neutrophil adherence and transendothelial migration. J Clin Invest 1988;82:1746-56.
4. Mentzer SJ, Rothlein R, Springer TA, Faller DV. Intercellular adhesion molecule-1 (ICAM-1) is involved in the cytolytic T lymphocyte interaction with a human synovial cell line. J Cell Physiol 1988;137:137-73.
5. Makgoba MW, Sanders ME, Shaw S. The CD2-LFA-3 and LFA-1-ICAM pathways: relevance to T-cell recognition. Immunol Today 1989;10:417-22.
6. Wuthrich RP, Jevnikar AM, Takei F, et al. Intercellular adhesion molecule-1 (ICAM-1) expression is upregulated in autoimmune murine lupus nephritis. Am J Pathol 1990;136:441-50.
7. Wegner CD, Gundel RH, Reilly P, et al. Intercellular adhesion molecule-1 (ICAM-1) in the pathogenesis of asthma. Science 1990;247:456-9.
8. Marlin SD, Staunton DE, Springer TA, et al. A soluble form of intercellular adhesion molecule-1 inhibits rhinovirus infection. Nature 1990;334:70-2.

INTERFERONS

IFN-α (leukocyte) and IFN-γ ("immune") are produced by lymphocytes and macrophages, and T lymphocytes, respectively, whereas IFNβ is produced by fibroblasts (cf. 1 for review). These cytokines are widely exploited for their induction of antiviral activities and for their roles as regulators of growth, differentiation and development.[2] Of three additional IFNs, the acid-labile IFNs found in patients with SLE or AIDS are best characterized.[3,4] Increased levels of IFN-α are found in CSF of many patients with viral meningitis[5,6] and in sera of patients with ARC and AIDS; persistence of serum IFN-α is thought to predict development of AIDS in HIV-infected individuals.[7,8] Immunoreactive IFN-α is said to be decreased in plasma of patients with rheumatoid arthritis,[9] but mitogen-induced IFN-γ production is impaired in rheumatoid arthritis and related diseases.[10] Although elevated levels of IFN-α in serum or CSF are seen in a variety of viral and mycoplasma infections (e.g., in sera of patients with *Mycoplasma pneumoniae* infection),[11] the test does not function well in a setting of acute infectious disease.[12] Bioassays and immunoassays for IFN-α and IFN-γ are available. Inhibitors of interferon activity are found by bioassay in some patients with AIDS, advanced cancer and SLE.[13] Natural, non-neutralizing IgG antibodies to IFN-γ found in serum of normal individuals of all ages are greatly increased in a wide variety of viral infections,[14] but the clinical utility of this observation is as yet unproved. In chronic carriers of HBV, clearance of serum HBsAg during IFN-α therapy correlates with increased spontaneous in vitro production of TNF-α and IL-1Bβ by PBMC.15 See 16 for recent review.

REFERENCES:
1. Greenberg SB. Human interferon in viral diseases. Antiviral Chemotherapy 1987;891:383-423.
2. Romeo G, Fiorucci G, Rossi GB. Interferons *in* cell growth *and* development. Trends in Genetics 1989;5:19-24.
3. Preble OT, Black RJ, Friedman RM, Klippel JH, Vilcek J. Systemic lupus erythematosus: presence in human serum of an unusual acid-labile leukocyte interferon. Science 1982;216:429-31.
4. Preble OT, Rook AH, Steis R, et al. Interferon-induced 2'-5' oligoadenylate synthetase during interferon-α therapy in homosexual men with Kaposi's sarcoma: marked deficiency in biochemical response to interferon in patients with acquired immunodeficiency syndrome. J Infect Dis 1985;152:457-65.
5. Ho-Yen D, Carrington D. Alpha-interferon responses in cerebrospinal fluid of patients with suspected meningitis. J Clin Pathol 1987;40:83-6.

6. Burke DS, Morrill JC. Levels of interferon in the plasma and cerebrospinal fluid of patients with acute Japanese encephalitis. J Infect Dis 1987;155:797-9.
7. Skidmore SJ, Mawson SJ. α-Interferon in anti-HIV positive patients [Letter]. Lancet 1987;2:520.
8. Abb J. Interferon-alpha in sera of HIV-infected patients [Letter]. Lancet 1987;2:1092-3.
9. Shiozawa S, Chihara K, Shiozawa K, et al. A sensitive radioimmunoassay for alpha-interferon: circulating α-interferon-like substance in the plasma of healthy individuals and rheumatoid arthritis patients. Clin Exp Immunol 1986;66:77-87.
10. Stolzenburg T, Binz R, Fontana A, Felder NA, Wagenhauser FJ. Impaired mitogen-induced interferon gamma production in rheumatoid arthritis and related diseases. Scand J Immunol 1988;27:73-82.
11. Nakayama T, Urano T, Osano M, Maehara N, Makino S. α-Interferon in the sera of patients infected with Mycoplasma pneumoniae. J Infect Dis 1986;154:904-6.
12. Flowers D, Scott GM. How useful are serum and CSF interferon levels as a rapid diagnostic aid in virus infections? J Med Virol 1985;15:35-47.
13. Ambrus JL, Poiesz BJ, Lillie MA, et al. Interferon and interferon inhibitor levels in patients infected with varicella-zoster virus, acquired immunodeficiency syndrome, acquired immunodeficiency syndrome-related complex, or Kaposi's sarcoma, and in normal individuals. Am J Med 1989;87:405-7.
14. Caruso A, Bonfanti C, Colombrita D, et al. Natural antibodies to IFN-γ in man and their increase during viral infection. J Immunol 1990;144:685-90.
15. Daniels HM, Meager A, Eddleston ALW, et al. Spontaneous production of tumour necrosis factor α and interleukin-1β during interferon-α treatment of chronic HBV infection. Lancet 1990;1:875-7.
16. Balkwill FR. Interferons. Lancet 1989;1:1060-3.

INTERLEUKIN-1 (IL-1)

Produced by many nucleated cells in response to a huge variety of stimuli, IL-1 (like IL-2) increases IL-2R expression and increases production of a variety of lymphokines and cytokines.[1,2] IL-1 is an endogenous pyrogen.[3] Plasma levels of IL-1β, which are increased in RA, correlate with disease activity.[4] Synovial fluids levels of IL-1 are increased in RA and OA.[5,6] Serum levels of IL-1 are increased during the acute phase of Kawasaki disease[7] and are increased (with TNF-α) in children with severe infectious purpura.[8] IL-1β and TNF are often increased in cerebrospinal fluid in neonatal Gram-negative enteric bacillary meningitis, and IL-1 is usually increased in aseptic meningitis.[9] High levels of CSF IL-1β correlate with poor prognosis.[10] Plasma IL-1 (EDTA/aprotinin) is probably more appropriate for study than serum.[11] Antibodies to IL-1α are reported in normal serum.[12] Blockade of the IL-1 receptor is expected to be an important approach to the treatment of several diseases. Plasma levels of IL-1β, but not IL-1. which is largely cell-associated for several hours afters endotoxin administration, are elevated twofold after endotoxin-infusion and are three to fourfold elevated in septic shock, where higher levels are found in surviving patients.[13] IL-1 functions as an autocrine inhibitor of endothelial growth, probably by decreasing expression of binding sites for fibroblast growth factor.[14] See also **IL-1 INHIBITOR** and **TUMOR NECROSIS FACTOR**.

REFERENCES:
1. Malkovský M, Sondel PM, Strober W, Dagleish AG. The interleukins in acquired disease. Clin Exp Immunol 1988;74:151-61.
2. Dinarello CA, Mier JW. Lymphokines. N Engl J Med 1987;317:940-5.
3. Duff GW, Durum SK. The pyrogenic and mitogenic actions of interleukin-1 are related. Nature 1983;304:449-51.
4. Eastgate JA, Symons JA, Wood NC, Grinlinton FM, DiGiovine FS, Duff GW. Correlation of plasma interleukin 1 levels with disease activity in rheumatoid arthritis. Lancet 1988;2:706-9.
5. Miyasaka N, Sato K, et al. Augmented interleukin-1 production and HLA-DR expression in the synovium of rheumatoid arthritis patients. Arthritis Rheum 1988;31:480-5.
6. Buchan G, Barrett K, Turner M, Chantry D, Maini RN, Feldmann M. Interleukin-1 and tumour necrosis factor mRNA expression in rheumatoid arthritis: prolonged production of IL-1α. Clin Exp Immunol 1988;73:449-55.
7. Maury CPJ, Salo E, Pelkonen P. Circulating interleukin-1β in patients with Kawasaki disease [Letter]. N Engl J Med 1988;319:1670-1.

8. Girardin E, Grau GE, Dayer J-M, Roux-Lombard P, The Study Group, Lambert P-H. Tumor necrosis factor and interleukin-1 in the serum of children with severe infectious purpura. N Engl J Med 1988;319:397-400.

9. Ramilo O, Mustafa MM, Sáez-Llorens X, et al. Role of interleukin 1-beta in meningeal inflammation. Pediatr Infect Dis J 1989;8:909-10.

10. McCracken GH Jr, Mustafa MM, Ramilo O, Olsen KD, Risser RC. Cerebrospinal fluid interleukin 1-beta and tumor necrosis factor concentrations and outcome from neonatal Gram-negative enteric bacillary meningitis. Pediatr Infect Dis J 1989;8:155-9.

11. Cannon JG, van der Meer JWM, Kwiatkowski D, et al. Interleukin-1β in human plasma: optimization of blood collection, plasma extraction, and radioimmunoassay methods. Lymphokine Res 1988;7:457-67.

12. Svenson M, Poulsen LK, Fomsgaard A, Bendtzen K. IgG autoantibodies against interleukin 1. in sera of normal individuals. Scand J Immunol 1989;29:489-92.

13. Cannon JG, Tompkins RG, Gelfand JA, et al. Circulating interleukin-1 and tumor necrosis factor in septic shock and experimental endotoxin fever. J Infect Dis 1990;161:79-84.

14. Cozzolino F, Torcia M, Aldinucci D, et al. Interleukin 1 is an autocrine regulator of human endothelial cell growth. Proc Natl Acad Sci USA 1990;87:6487-91.

INTERLEUKIN-1 RECEPTOR ANTAGONISTS [INTERLEUKIN-1 INHIBITORS (IL-1INHs)]

Natural inhibitors of IL-1 are found in urine of patients with monocytic leukemia,[1] in urine of some febrile patients,[2] in serum and urine of febrile patients with systemic type of juvenile chronic arthritis (S-JCA),[3] in serum of some patients with rheumatoid arthritis,[4] and in culture supernatants of mononuclear cells from patients with systemic sclerosis.[5] Some IL-1 INH(s) interfere with the IL-1/MCF (mononuclear-cell factor) activity which stimulates production of collagenase and PGE_2 by synovial cells.[6] IL-1 INH(s) probably inhibit by competition for binding to the IL-1 receptor.[7] TNF also stimulates production of PGE_2 by synovial cells.[8] Serum from patients with S-JCA also inhibits normal erythropoiesis *in vitro*.[9] Uromodulin, an immunosuppressive glycoprotein found in human pregnancy urine, inhibits IL-1 activity by direct binding to IL-1.[10] Recently cloned IL-1R antagonists might be therapeutically useful[11-13] (cf. 14 for discussion). Blockage of IL-1R with MAbs inhibits weight loss, induction of IL-6 and acute-phase protein synthesis during inflammation.[15] A soluble form of the IL-1R inhibits in vivo development alloreactivity and prolongs survival of murine heterotopic heart allografts; these effects are overcome by IL-1 administration.[16] See also **TUMOR NECROSIS FACTOR.**

REFERENCES:

1. Balavoine J-F, de Rochemonteix B, Williamson K, et al. Prostaglandin E_2 and collagenase production by fibroblasts and synovial cells is regulated by urine-derived human interleukin 1 and inhibitor(s). J Clin Invest 1986;78:1120-4.

2. Seckinger P, Dayer J-M. Interleukin-1 inhibitors. Ann Inst Pasteur Immunol 1987;138:486-8.

3. Prieur A-M, Kaufmann M-T, Griscelli C, Dayer J-M. Specific interleukin-1 inhibitor in serum and urine of children with systemic juvenile chronic arthritis. Lancet 1987;2:1240-2.

4. Suzuki H, Akama T, Okane M, et al. Interleukin-1-inhibitory IgG in sera from some patients with rheumatoid arthritis. Arthritis Rheum 1989;32:1528-38.

5. Westacott CI, Whicher JT, Hutton CW, Dieppe PA. Increased spontaneous production of interleukin-1 together with inhibitory activity in systemic sclerosis. Clin Sci 1988;75:561-7.

6. Dayer J-M, Demczuk S. Cytokines and other mediators in rheumatoid arthritis. Springer Semin Immunopathol 1984;7:387-413.

7. Seckinger P, Lowenthal JW, Williamson K, et al. A urine inhibitor of interleukin 1 activity that blocks ligand binding. J Immunol 1987;139:1546-9.

8. Dayer J-M, Beutler B, Cerami A. Cachectin/tumor necrosis factor stimulates collagenase and prostaglandin E2 production by human synovial cells and dermal fibroblasts. J Exp Med 1985;162:2163-8.

9. Prouse PJ, Harvey AR, Bonner B, et al. Anaemia in juvenile chronic arthritis: serum inhibition of normal erythropoiesis in vitro. Ann Rheum Dis 1987;46:127-34.

10. Muchmore AV, Shifrin S, Decker JM. In vitro evidence that carbohydrate moieties derived from uromodulin, an 85,000 dalton immunosuppressive glycoprotein isolated from human pregnancy urine, are immunosuppressive in the absence of intact protein. J Immunol 1987;138:2547-53.
11. Hannum CH, Wilcox CJ, Arend WP, et al. Interleukin-1 receptor antagonist activity of a human interleukin-1 inhibitor. Nature 1990;343:336-40.
12. Eisenberg SP, Evans RJ, Arend WP, et al. Primary structure and functional expression from complementary DNA of a human interleukin-1 receptor antagonist. Nature 1990;343:341-6.
13. Carter DB, Deibel MR Jr, Dunn CJ, et al. Purification, cloning, expression and biological characterization of an interleukin-1 receptor antagonist protein. Nature 1990;344:633-8.
14. Whicher J. Control of receptor appetite. Nature 1990;344:584.
15. Gershenwald JE, Fong Y, Fahey TJ III, et al. Interleukin 1 receptor blockade attenuates the host inflammatory response. Proc Natl Acad Sci USA 1990;87:4966-70.
16. Fanslow WC, Sims JE, Sassenfeld H, et al. Regulation of alloreactivity in vivo by a soluble form of the interleukin-1 receptor. Science 1990;248:739-42.

INTERLEUKIN-2 (IL-2)

IL-2 production is impaired in a variety of immunodeficiency diseases (e.g., AIDS, Nezelof's syndrome and SCID) and in autoimmune diseases, including SLE and insulin-dependent diabetes mellitus (cf. 1 and 2 for review). Other data suggest overproduction of IL-2 in SLE.[3] Striking increases of IL-2 in serum and/or CSF[4-7] and IL-2R in serum and CSF5 are found in few patients with multiple sclerosis. IL-2 and IL-2R are increased in the serum in diffuse and limited scleroderma;[8,9] serum IL-2 is increased in pre-eclampsia.[10] Plasma and urine IL-2 and plasma IL-2R levels are greatly increased during renal allograft rejection or CMV infection in patients with renal allografts.[11,12] As well as increasing their survival, decreasing autoantibody and RF titers and decreasing kidney and synovial pathology, infection of MRL/lpr mice with recombinant IL-2/vaccinia virus is said to cause decreases in the increased numbers of CD3[+] CD4[-] CD8[-] ("double negative") T cells which characterize these mice and patients with SLE and RA.[13] See also **INTERLEUKIN-2 RECEPTOR.**

REFERENCES:
1. Malkovský M, Sondel PM, Strober W, Dalgleish AG. The interleukins in acquired disease. Clin Exp Immunol 1988;74:151-61.
2. Dinarello CA, Mier JW. Lymphokines. N Engl J Med 1987;317:940-5.
3. Warrington RJ. Interleukin-2 abnormalities in systemic lupus erythematosus and rheumatoid arthritis: a role for overproduction of interleukin-2 in human autoimmunity? J Rheumatol 1988;15:616-20.
4. Gallo P, Piccinno M, Pagni S, Tavolato B. Interleukin-2 levels in serum and cerebrospinal fluid of multiple sclerosis patients. Ann Neurol 1988; 24:795-7.
5. Trotter JL, Clifford DB, Anderson CB, et al. Elevated serum interleukin-2 levels in chronic progressive multiple sclerosis [Letter]. N Engl J Med 1988;318:1206.
6. Boctor FN, Peter JB, Barka NE, Tourtellotte WW. Lymphokines in multiple sclerosis (MS): concordance of the abnormal levels in serum [Abstract]. Neurology 1989;39:331.
7. Adachi K, Kumamoto T, Araki S. Interleukin-2 receptor levels indicating relapse in multiple sclerosis. Lancet 1989;1:559-60.
8. Kahaleh MB, LeRoy EC. Interleukin-2 in scleroderma: correlation of serum level with extent of skin involvement and disease duration. Ann Intern Med 1989;110:446-50.
9. Peter JB, Agopian MS, Clements PJ, Telian NS, Furst DE. Elevated serum levels of interleukin-2 receptor (IL-2R) and IL-2 in diffuse (DS) and limited scleroderma (LS) [Abstract]. Arthritis Rheum 1989;32(Suppl 4):S77.
10. Sunder-Plassmann G, Derfler K, Wagner L, et al. Increased serum activity of interleukin-2 in patients with pre-eclampsia. J Autoimmunity 1989;2:203-5.
11. Cornaby A, Simpson MA, Vann Rice R, Dempsey RA, Madras PN, Monaco AP. Interleukin-2 production in plasma and urine, plasma interleukin-2 receptor levels, and urine cytology as a means of monitoring renal allograft recipients. Transplant Proc 1988;20:108-10.
12. Colvin RB, Fuller TC, Mackeen L, Kung PC, Ip SH, Cosimi AB. Plasma interleukin 2 receptor levels in renal allograft recipients. Clin Immunol Immunopathol 1987;43:273-6.
13. Gutierrez-Ramos JC, Andreu JL, Revilla Y, et al. Recovery from autoimmunity of MRL/lpr mice after infection with an interleukin-2/vaccinia recombinant virus. Nature 1990;346:271-4.

INTERLEUKIN-2 RECEPTOR (IL-2R)

Soluble IL-2R (sIL-2R; also known as Tac), the 55 kd low-affinity IL-2 binding component of IL-2R (a high-affinity IL-2R composed of the p75 and Tac proteins), is released by activated cells (probably including T cells, B cells and macrophages) during a variety of immune responses.[1] These include autoimmune disease [rheumatoid arthritis,[2,3] SLE,[4] scleroderma,[5-8] polymyositis,[9] host versus graft reaction,[10,11] lymphoreticular malignancies,[12] systemic parasitic diseases,[13] AIDS[14] and chronic progressive multiple sclerosis[15-17] (cf. also 18 and 19). High serum levels of IL-2 and sIL-2R in patients with RA and SLE probably correlate with disease activity;[20] elevated levels of sIL-2R are found in bile and in lower concentrations in serum of liver transplant patients before and during acute rejection episodes.[21] Release of IL-2 and sIL-2R by PHA-stimulated peripheral blood mononuclear cells is decreased[22] in type I diabetes mellitus. Serum levels of sIL-2R are increased progressively from stages I and II to stages III and IV of IgA nephropathy,[23] but the significance of this is uncertain because serum sIL-2R increases in patients with chronic renal failure.[24] Although of pathogenetic interest, none of these increases have been shown to be clinically useful for evaluation of disease activity or therapeutic monitoring.

REFERENCES:
1. Rubin LA. The soluble interleukin-2 receptor in rheumatic disease [Editorial]. Arthritis Rheum 1990;33:1145-8.
2. Campen DH, Horwitz DA, Quismorio FP Jr, Ehresmann GR, Martin J. Serum levels of interleukin-2 receptor and activity of rheumatic diseases characterized by immune system activation. Arthritis Rheum 1988;31:1358-64.
3. Keystone EC, Snow KM, Bombardier C, et al. Elevated soluble interleukin-2 receptor levels in the sera and synovial fluids of patients with rheumatoid arthritis. Arthritis Rheum 1988;31:844-9.
4. Wolf RE, Brelsford WG. Soluble interleukin-2 receptors in systemic lupus erythematosus. Arthritis Rheum 1988;31:729-35.
5. Engel EE, Charley MR, Steen VD, Medsger TA Jr. Soluble interleukin 2 receptors in systemic sclerosis (scleroderma) [Abstract]. Arthritis Rheum 1989;32(Suppl 1):R39.
6. Peter JB, Agopian MS, Clements PJ, Telian NS, Furst DE. Elevated serum levels of interleukin-2 receptor (IL-2R) and IL-2 in diffuse (DS) and limited scleroderma (LS) [Abstract]. J Rheumatol 1990;17:908-10.
7. Degiannis D, Seibold JR, Czarnecki M, et al. Soluble interleukin-2 receptors in patients with systemic sclerosis. Arthritis Rheum 1990;33:375-80.
8. Famularo G, Procopio A, Giacomelli R, et al. Soluble interleukin-2 receptor, interleukin-2 and interleukin-4 in sera and supernatants from patients with progressive systemic sclerosis. Clin Exp Immunol 1990;81:368-72.
9. Wolf RE, Baethge BA. Interleukin-1., interleukin-2, and soluble interleukin-2 receptors in polymyositis. Arthritis Rheum 1990;33:1007-14.
10. Colvin RB, Fuller TC, MacKeen L, Kung PC, Ip SH, Cosimi AB. Plasma interleukin 2 receptor levels in renal allograft recipients. Clin Immunol Immunopathol 1987;43:273-6.
11. Cornaby A, Simpson MA, Vann Rice R, Dempsey RA, Madras PN, Monaco AP. Interleukin-2 production in plasma and urine, plasma interleukin-2 receptor levels, and urine cytology as a means of monitoring renal allograft recipients. Transplant Proc 1988;20:108-10.
12. Marcon L, Rubin LA, Kurman CC, et al. Elevated serum levels of soluble tac peptide in adult T-cell leukemia: correlation with clinical status during chemotherapy. Ann Intern Med 1988;109:274-9.
13. Josimovic-Alasevic O, Feldmeier H, Zwingenberger K, et al. Interleukin 2 receptor in patients with localized and systemic parasitic diseases. Clin Exp Immunol 1988;72:249-54.
14. Sethi KK, Näher H. Elevated titers of cell-free interleukin-2 receptor in serum and cerebrospinal fluid specimens of patients with acquired immunodeficiency syndrome. Immunol Lett 1986;13:179-84.
15. Greenberg SJ, Marcon L, Hurwitz BJ, Waldmann T, Nelson DL. Elevated levels of soluble interleukin-2 receptors in multiple sclerosis [Letter]. N Engl J Med 1988;319:1019-20.
16. Adachi K, Kumamoto T, Araki S. Interleukin-2 receptor levels indicating relapse in multiple sclerosis. Lancet 1989;1:559-60.
17. Hartung H-P, Hughes RAC, Taylor WA, et al. T cell activation in Guillain-Barré syndrome and in MS: elevated serum levels of soluble IL-2 receptors. Neurology 1990;40:215-8.

18. Boctor FN, Peter JB, Barka NE, Tourtellotte WW. Lymphokines in multiple sclerosis (MS): concordance of the abnormal levels in serum [Abstract]. Neurology 1989;39:331.
19. Trotter JL, Clifford DB, Andersen CB, van der Veen RC, Hicks BC, Banks G. Elevated serum interleukin-2 levels in chronic progressive multiple sclerosis [Letter]. N Engl J Med 1988;318:1206.
20. Manoussakis MN, Papadopoulos GK, Drosos AA, Moutsopoulos HM. Soluble interleukin 2 receptor molecules in the serum of patients with autoimmune diseases. Clin Immunol Immunopathol 1989;50:321-32.
21. Adams DH, Wang L, Hubscher SG, Elias E, Neuberger JM. Soluble interleukin-2 receptors in serum and bile of liver transplant recipients. Lancet 1989;1:469-71.
22. Giordano C, PantJ F, Caruso C, et al. Interleukin 2 and soluble interleukin 2-receptor secretion defect in vitro in newly diagnosed type I diabetic patients. Diabetes 1989;38:310-15.
23. Tomino Y, Ozaki T, Koide H, et al. Serum levels of interleukin-2 receptor and disease activity in patients with IgA nephropathy. J Clin Lab Analysis 1989;3:355-9.
24. Takamatsu T, Yasuda N, Ohno T, et al. Soluble interleukin-2 receptors in the serum of patients with chronic renal failure. Tohoku J Exp Med 1988;155:343-7.

INTERLEUKIN-3 (IL-3)

Levels of IL-3, a regulator of growth and differentiation of hematopoietic and lymphoid progenitors, have not yet been defined in human diseases,[1] but an important role in chronic allergic diseases and perhaps in hematological diseases is a good possibility.[2] IL-3R was cloned,[3] as was a homologous gene for which the ligand is not yet known.[4]

REFERENCES:
1. Malkovský M, Sondel PM, Strober W, Dalgleish AG. The interleukins in acquired disease. Clin Exp Immunol 1988;74:151-61.
2. Schrader JW. The panspecific hemopoietin of activated lymphocytes (interleukin-3). Annu Rev Immunol 1986;4:205-30.
3. Itoh N, Yonehara S, Schreurs J, et al. Cloning of an interleukin-3 receptor gene: a member of a distinct receptor gene family. Science 1990;247:324-327.
4. Gorman DM, Itoh N, Kitamura T, et al. Cloning and expression of a gene encoding an interleukin 3 receptor-like protein: identification of another member of the cytokine receptor gene family. Proc Natl Acad Sci USA 1990;87:5459-63.

INTERLEUKIN-4 (IL-4)

IL-4, a T cell, mast cell and B cell product which affects activation, differentiation and proliferation of hematopoietic and lymphoid cells, has not yet been studied in health and disease.[1,2] IL-4 influences production of IgE *in vivo*.[3] Studies in patients with allergic diseases will be of great interest (cf. 4 for review). As with other T cell lymphokines, IL-4 is not increased in RA synovial fluid.[5] A soluble IL-4-binding protein, the free (unoccupied) form of which is low in SCID mouse serum,[6] could be another example of a soluble receptor (in this case, IL-4R)[7] of possible importance in immunoregulation, as may also be the case with soluble forms of IL-2R,[8] IL-6R,[9] Fc IgE,[10] IFN-γ-R,[11] as well as TNFR, IL-1R and others.

REFERENCES:
1. Malkovský M, Sondel PM, Strober W, Dalgleish AG. The interleukins in acquired disease. Clin Exp Immunol 1988;74:151-61.
2. Dinarello CA, Mier JW. Lymphokines. N Engl J Med 1987;317:940-5.
3. Vercelli D, Jabara HH, Arai K-I, Geha RS. Induction of human IgE synthesis requires interleukin 4 and T/B cell interactions involving the T cell receptor/CD3 complex and MHC class II antigens. J Exp Med 1989;169:1295-307.
4. Paul WE, Ohara J. B-cell stimulatory factor-1/interleukin 4. Annu Rev Immunol 1987;5:429-59.
5. Miossec P, Naviliat M, D'Angeac AD, Sany J, Banchereau J. Low levels of interleukin-4 and high levels of transforming growth factor β in rheumatoid arthritis. Arthritis Rheum 1990;33:1180-8.
6. Fernandez-Botran R, Vitetta ES. A soluble, high-affinity, interleukin-4-binding protein is present in the biological fluids of mice. Proc Natl Acad Sci USA 1990;87:4202-6.

7. Harada N, Castle BE, Gorman DM, et al. Expression cloning of a cDNA encoding the murine interleukin 4 receptor based on ligand binding. Proc Natl Acad Sci USA 1990;87:857-61.
8. Baran D, Korner M, Theze J. Characterization of the soluble murine IL-2R and estimation of its affinity for IL-2. J Immunol 1988;141:539-46.
9. Hirano T, Taga T, Matsuda T, et al. Interleukin 6 and its receptor in the immune response and hematopoiesis. Int J Cell Cloning 1990;8(Suppl 8):155-66.
10. Ikuta K, Takami M, Kim CW, et al. Human lymphocyte Fc receptor for IgE: sequence homology of its cloned cDNA with animal lectins. Proc Natl Acad Sci USA 1987;84:819-23.
11. Novick D, Engelman H, Wallach D, Rubinstein M. Soluble cytokine receptors are present in normal human urine. J Exp Med 1989;170:1409-14.

INTERLEUKIN-5 (IL-5)

Clinical conditions have not yet been associated with excess or deficient production of IL-5, which is important in differentiation and proliferation of eosinophils and B cells and perhaps in isotype differentiation as an IgA-specific switch factor.[1-3] There may, however, be species differences. In mice, IL-5 (like IL-4 which stimulates IgE responses) is produced by the TH2 subset of CD4+ T-cell lines; treatment with MAb to IL-5 inhibits helminth-induced eosinophilia in bone marrow and peripheral blood and in the egg granulomas of acute schistosomiasis.[4] Extension of IL-5 studies to helminth-related and other eosinophilias in humans is awaited.

REFERENCES:
1. Malkovský M, Sondel PM, Strober W, Dalgleish AG. The interleukins in acquired disease. Clin Exp Immunol 1988;74:151-61.
2. Dinarello CA, Mier JW. Lymphokines. N Engl J Med 1987;317:940-5.
3. Harriman GR, Strober W. Interleukin 5, a mucosal lymphokine? J Immunol 1987;139:3553-5.
4. Sher A, Coffman RL, Hieny S, et al. Interleukin 5 is required for the blood and tissue eosinophilia but not granuloma formation induced by infection with *Schistosoma mansoni*. Proc Natl Acad Sci USA 1990;87:61-5.

INTERLEUKIN-6 (IL-6)

IL-6 is involved in terminal differentiation of stimulated B cells into immunoglobulin-secreting plasma cells and is associated with hyperglobulinemia and autoantibody production when secreted by cardiac myxomas or cervical carcinomas[1-4] (cf. 5 and 6 for review). IL-6 is also elevated in infection/endotoxemia[7,8] and in alcoholic liver cirrhosis.[9] IL-6, which is bound to alpha 2-macroglobulin in serum,[10] is increased in serum of children with Still disease,[11] in synovial fluid and sometimes in serum in rheumatoid arthritis[12, 13] and in CSF of patients with CNS-LE.[14] The fact that serum levels of IL-6 correlate with and precede increases in acute phase reactants in serum probably reflects the identity of hepatocyte-stimulating factor (HSF) activity and IL-6.[15-17] IL-6 is a co-stimulus for con A activation of purified T cells.[18] IL-1, TNF-α and IL-6 regulate several cellular functions involved in connective tissue destruction.[19] Release of all three of these monokines is induced by the neuropeptides substance P and substance K.[20] Release of IL-6 by normal and neoplastic B cells and by cells derived from AIDS Kaposi sarcomas[21] is expected to have important effects on cells in their microenvironment;[22] serum levels of IL-6 correlate with disease severity in plasma cell dyscrasias.[23] Plasma (EDTA and aprotinin at least for IL-1) is probably more appropriate for study than serum.[24] IL-6 is increased in plasma and on dermal and epidermal cells in lesional skin of psoriasis.[25] Note that increased transforming growth factor α[26,27] and decreased IL-1 bioactivity[28] are also characteristic of hyperplastic psoriatic lesions. Increases of serum IL-6 are found in Castleman disease,[29] in which inappropriate synthesis of IL-6 probably has a primary role in pathogenesis.[30] IL-6 mRNA is increased in synoviocytes and endothelial cells in RA;[31] cytokines produced by macrophages and fibroblasts (including IL-1β, TNF; CSF) are present in the next highest concentrations, and IFN-γ and IL-2 (which are produced by T cells) show the smallest increases.[31,32]

REFERENCES:

1. Hirano T, Taga T, Yasukawa K, et al. Human B-cell differentiation factor defined by an anti-peptide antibody and its possible role in autoantibody production. Proc Natl Acad Sci USA 1987;84:228-31.

2. St. John Sutton MG, Mercier L-A, Giuliani ER, Lie JT. Atrial myxomas. A review of clinical experience in 40 patients. Mayo Clin Proc 1980;55:371-6.

3. Hirano T, Yasukawa K, Harada H, et al. Complementary DNA for a novel human interleukin (BSF-2) that induces B lymphocytes to produce immunoglobulin. Nature 1986;324:73-6.

4. Jourdan M, Bataille R, Seguin J, et al. Constitutive production of interleukin-6 and immunologic features in cardiac myxomas. Arthritis Rheum 1990;33:398-402.

5. Malkovský M, Sondel PM, Strober W, Dalgleish AG. The interleukins in acquired disease. Clin Exp Immunol 1988;74:151-61.

6. O'Garra A. Interleukins and the immune system 1. Lancet 1989;1:943-4.

7. Helfgott DC, Tatter SB, Santhanam U, et al. Multiple forms of IFN-β_2/IL-6 in serum and body fluids during acute bacterial infection. J Immunol 1989;142:948-53.

8. Fong Y, Moldawer LL, Marano M, et al. Endotoxemia elicits increased circulating β_2-IFN/IL-6 in man. J Immunol 1989;142:2321-4.

9. Deviere J, Content J, Denys C, et al. High interleukin-6 serum levels and increased production by leucocytes in alcoholic liver cirrhosis. Correlation with IgA serum levels and lymphokines production. Clin Exp Immunol 1989;77:221-5.

10. Matsuda T, Hirano T, Nagasawa S, Kishimoto T. Identification of $\alpha 2$-macroglobulin as a carrier protein for IL-6. J Immunol 1989;142:148-52.

11. Kishimoto T. Factors affecting B-cell growth and differentiation. Annu Rev Immunol 1985;3:133-57.

12. Houssiau F, Devogelaer J-P, Van Damme J, de Deuxchaisnes CN, Van Snick J. Interleukin-6 in synovial fluid and serum of patients with rheumatoid arthritis and other inflammatory arthritides. Arthritis Rheum 1988;31:784-8.

13. Waage A, Kaufmann C, Espevik T, Husby G. Interleukin-6 in synovial fluid from patients with arthritis. Clin Immunol Immunopathol 1989;50:394-8.

14. Hirohata S, Miyamoto T. Elevated levels of Interleukin-6 in cerebrospinal fluid from patients with systemic lupus erythematosus and central nervous system involvement. Arthritis Rheum 1990;33:644-9.

15. Gauldie J, Richards C, Harnish D, Lansdorp P, Baumann H. Interferon β_2/B-cell stimulating factor type 2 shares identity with monocyte-derived hepatocyte-stimulating factor and regulates the major acute phase protein response in liver cells. Proc Natl Acad Sci USA 1987;84:7251-5.

16. Nijsten MWN, de Groot ER, ten Duis HJ, Klasen HJ, Hack CE, Aarden LA. Serum levels of interleukin-6 and acute phase responses. Lancet 1987;2:921.

17. Nishimoto N, Yoshizaki K, Tagoh H, et al. Elevation of serum interleukin 6 prior to acute phase proteins on the inflammation by surgical operation. Clin Immunol Immunopathol 1989;50:399-401.

18. Garman RD, Jacobs KA, Clark SC, Raulet DH. B-cell stimulatory factor 2 (β_2 interferon) functions as a second signal for interleukin 2 production by mature murine T cells. Proc Natl Acad Sci USA 1987;84:7629-33.

19. Le J, Vilcek J. Biology of disease. Tumor necrosis factor and interleukin 1: cytokines with multiple overlapping biological activities. Lab Invest 1987;56:234-48.

20. Lotz M, Vaughan JH, Carson DA. Effect of neuropeptides on production of inflammatory cytokines by human monocytes. Science 1988;241:1218-20.

21. Miles SA, Rezai AR, Salazar-González JF, et al. AIDS Kaposi sarcoma-derived cells produce and respond to interleukin 6. Proc Natl Acad Sci USA 1990;87:4068-72.

22. Freeman GJ, Freedman AS, Rabinowe SN, et al. Interleukin 6 gene expression in normal and neoplastic B cells. J Clin Invest 1989;83:1512-8.

23. Bataille R, Jourdan M, Zhang X-G, Klein B. Serum levels of interleukin 6, a potent myeloma cell growth factor, as reflect of disease severity in plasma cell dyscrasias. J Clin Invest 1989;84:2008-11.

24. Cannon JG, van der Meer JWM, Kwiatkowski D, et al. Interleukin-1β in human plasma: optimization of blood collection, plasma extraction, and radioimmunoassay methods. Lymphokine Res 1988;7:457-67.

72

25. Grossman RM, Krueger J, Yourish D, et al. Interleukin 6 is expressed in high levels in psoriatic skin and stimulates proliferation of cultured human keratinocytes. Proc Natl Acad Sci USA 1989;86:6367-71.
26. Gottlieb AB, Chang CK, Posnett DN, et al. Detection of transforming growth factor α in normal, malignant, and hyperproliferative human keratinocytes. J Exp Med 1988;167:670-5.
27. Elder JT, Fisher GJ, Lindquist PB, et al. Overexpression of transforming growth factor α in psoriatic epidermis. Science 1989;813:811-4.
28. Cooper KD, Baadsgaard O, Elder JT, et al. Increased levels of an interleukin-1 inhibitor block interleukin-1 activity but not immunoreactivity or RNA expression of interleukin-1 beta in psoriasis skin [Abstract]. J Invest Dermatol 1988;90:552.
29. Yoshizaki K, Matsuda T, Nishimoto N, et al. Pathogenic significance of interleukin-6 (IL-6/BSF-2) in Castleman's disease. Blood 1989;74:1360-7.
30. Brandt SJ, Bodine DM, Dunbar CE, Nienhus AW. Dysregulated interleukin 6 expression produces a syndrome resembling Castleman's disease in mice. J Clin Invest 1990;86:592-9.
31. Firestein GS, Xu W-D, Townsend K, et al. Cytokines in chronic inflammatory arthritis. I. Failure to detect T cell lymphokines (interleukin 2 and interleukin 3) and presence of macrophage colony stimulating factor (CSF-1) and a novel mast cell growth factor in rheumatoid synovitis. J Exp Med 1988;168:1573-86.
32. Guerne P-A, Zuraw BL, Vaughan JH, et al. Synovium as a source of interleukin 6 in vitro: contribution to local and systemic manifestations of arthritis. J Clin Invest 1989;83:585-92.

INTERLEUKIN-7 (IL-7)

IL-7, a potent growth stimulus for pre-B cells, is also co-stimulus for Con A activation of T cells. This activation is independent of IL-6 induced activation of Con A-stimulated T cells.[1] IL-7 also induces proliferation and expression of IL-2R and transferrin receptor on memory T cells (CD45R), indicating an important role for IL-7 in the normal physiology of human T cells.[2] Studies of IL-7 in human disease are not yet available. Unlike other interleukins described to date, IL-7 seems not to induce differentiation (cf. 3 for review).

REFERENCES:
1. Morrissey PJ, Goodwin RG, Nordan RP, et al. Recombinant interleukin-7, pre-B cell growth factor, has costimulatory activity on purified mature T cells. J Exp Med 1989;169:707-16.
2. Welch PA, Namen AE, Goodwin RG, et al. Human IL-7: a novel T cell growth factor. J Immunol 1989;143:3562-7.
3. Henney CS. Interleukin 7: effects on early events in lymphopoiesis. Immunol Today 1989;10:170-3.

INTERLEUKIN-8 (IL-8)

IL-8, a 4q12-q21 monocyte-derived factor which was formerly known as neutrophil-activating protein (NAP-1) and T cell chemotactic factor, causes T cell and neutrophil activation, chemotaxis and edema formation.[1-4] IL-8 can down regulate expression of its own receptor[5] on human neutrophils.[6] Through its capacity to inhibit neutrophil adhesion to cytokine-activated endothelial cells, IL-8 may attenuate neutrophil-mediated damage of endothelial cells at sites of inflammation.[7] Studies of IL-8 in clinical conditions are expected to be very useful.

REFERENCES:
1. Larsen CG, Anderson AO, Appella E, Oppenheim JJ, Matsushima K. The neutrophil-activating protein (NAP-1) is also chemotactic for T lymphocytes. Science 1989;243:1464-6.
2. Westwick J, Li SW, Camp RD. Novel neutrophil-stimulating peptides. Immunol Today 1989;10:146-7.
3. Rampart M, Van Damme J, Zonnekeyn L, Herman AG. Granulocyte chemotactic protein/interleukin-8 induces plasma leakage and neutrophil accumulation in rabbit skin. Am J Pathol 1989;135:21-5.

4. Modi WS, Dean M, Seuanez HN, et al. Monocyte-derived neutrophil chemotactic factor (MDNCF/IL-8) resides in a gene cluster along with several other members of the platelet factor 4 gene superfamily. Hum Genet 1990;84:185-7.
5. Grob PM, David E, Warren TC, et al. Characterization of a receptor for human monocyte-derived neutrophil chemotactic factor/interleukin-8. J Biol Chem 1990;265:8311-6.
6. Samanta AK, Oppenheim JJ, Matsushima K. Interleukin 8 (monocyte-derived neutrophil chemotactic factor) dynamically regulates its own receptor expression on human neutrophils. J Biol Chem 1990;265:183-9.
7. Gimbrone MA Jr, Obin MS, Brock AF, et al. Endothelial interleukin-8: a novel inhibitor of leukocyte-endothelial interactions. Science 1989;246:1601-3.

INTERLEUKIN-10 (IL-10)

The mechanisms which determine whether antibody-mediated immunity or delayed type hypersensitivity (DTH) will dominate the response to antigens are largely unknown,[1,2] but may reflect documented differences in function of cloned T cell subtypes including T_H1 cells which secrete IL-2 and IFN-γ, activate macrophages and preferentially induce DTH, and T_H2 cells which produce IL-4 and IL-5 and provide B cell help.[3,4] Part of this mutual inhibition may be due to products of these cells[5] including IL-10 (cytokine synthesis inhibitory factor produced by T_H2 cells) which inhibits synthesis of IFN-γ and other cytokines by stimulated T_H1 cells[6] and by IFN-γ which inhibits proliferation of T_H2 clones in vitro.[7] See also **CYTOKINES** and reference 8 for discussion of T_H1 and T_H2 T cell clones.

REFERENCES:

1. Katsura Y. Cell-mediated and humoral immune responses in mice. III. Dynamic balance between delayed-type hypersensitivity and antibody response. Immunology 1977;32:227-35.
2. Howard JG, Hale C, Liew FY. Genetically determined susceptibility to Leishmania tropica infection is expressed by haematopoietic donor cells in mouse radiation chimaeras. Nature 1980;288:161-2.
3. Boom WH, Liano D, Abbas AK. Heterogeneity of helper/inducer T lymphocytes. II. Effects of interleukin 4- and interleukin 2-producing T cell clones on resting B lymphocytes. J Exp Med 1988;167:1350-63.
4. Stout RD, Bottomly K. Antigen-specific activation of effector macrophages by IFN-γ producing (T_H1) T cell clones. Failure of IL-4 producing (T_H2) T cell clones to activate effector function in macrophages. J Immunol 1989;142:760-5.
5. Moore KW, Vieira P, Fiorentino DF, et al. Homology of cytokine synthesis inhibitory factor (IL-10) to the Epstein-Barr virus gene BCRFI. Science 1990;248:1230-4.
6. Fiorentino DF, Bond MW, Mosmann TR. Two types of mouse T helper cell. IV. Th2 clones secrete a factor that inhibits cytokine production by Th1 clones. J Exp Med 1989;170:2081-95.
7. Gajewski TF, Fitch FW. Anti-proliferative effect of IFN-γ in immune regulation. I. IFN-γ inhibits the proliferation of Th2 but not Th1 murine helper T lymphocyte clones. J Immunol 1990;140:4245-52.
8. Fernandez-Botran R, Sanders VM, Mosmann TR, Vitetta ES. Lymphokine-mediated regulation of the proliferative response of clones of T helper 1 and T helper 2 cells. J Exp Med 1988;168:543-58.

INTERLEUKINS

Interleukins (and interferons) are polypeptide members of the family of cytokines which affect functions of specific cell types.[1-4] They are produced by lymphocytes, monocytes, and various other cell types and are released by cells in response to antigenic and non-antigenic stimuli. The interleukins, of which there were 8 well defined members in 1989, modulate inflammation and immunity by regulating growth, mobility, and differentiation of lymphoid and other cells. Included among the cytokines are cachectin and lymphotoxin which are now known as tumor necrosis factor-α and TNF-β, respectively.[2] IL-1 inhibitors are the first well described proteins involved in the feedback regulation of interleukin activities.[5] A synopsis of recent research on lymphokine receptor interactions is available.[6] Assays for interleukins are expected to become important in autoimmune, infectious and neoplastic diseases (cf. 7 for review of early studies in RA, reference 8 for early studies of the role of interleukins in T and B cell-mediated immunity, and references 9 and 10 for recent review). Other seemingly distinct cytokines, including natural killer cell stimulatory factor,[11] are not yet officially recognized by assignation of a specific number in the interleukin series. The cells of origin and the diverse activities of IL-1 through IL-7 on cell growth, differentiation and activation were recently reviewed.[12] See also **CYTOKINES, IL-1** through **IL-8, IL-1 INHIBITOR, LYMPHOKINES** and **PEPTIDE REGULATORY FACTORS.**

REFERENCES:
1. Malkovský M, Sondel PM, Strober W, Dalgleish AG. The interleukins in acquired disease. Clin Exp Immunol 1988;74:151-61.
2. Dinarello CA, Mier JW. Lymphokines. N Engl J Med 1987;317:940-5.
3. Smith EM. Hormonal activities of lymphokines, monokines, and other cytokines. Prog Allergy 1988;43:121-39.
4. Romeo G, Fiorucci G, Rossi GB. Interferons *in* cell growth *and* development. Trends in Genetics 1989;5:19-24.
5. Prieur A-M, Kaufmann M-T, Griscelli C, Dayer J-M. Specific interleukin-1 inhibitor in serum and urine of children with systemic juvenile chronic arthritis. Lancet 1987;2:1240-2.
6. Banchereau J. Lymphokine receptor interactions. Immunol Today 1989;10:73-6.
7. Dayer J-M, Demczuk S. Cytokines and other mediators in rheumatoid arthritis. Springer Semin Immunopathol 1984;7:387-413.
8. Gately MK, Jenson JC, Benjamin WR. Role of cytokines in T and B cell mediated immmunity. Concepts Immmunopathol 1986;3:74-108.
9. O'Garra A. Interleukins and the immune system 1. Lancet 1989;1:943-4.
10. O'Garra A. Interleukins and the immune system 2. Lancet 1989;1:1003-5.
11. Kobayashi M, Fitz L, Ryan M, et al. Identification and purification of natural killer cell stimulatory factor (NKSF), a cytokine with multiple biologic effects on human lymphocytes. J Exp Med 1989;170:827-45.
12. Mizel SB. The interleukins. FASEB J 1989;3:2379-88.

INTRINSIC FACTOR ANTIBODIES

Anti-intrinsic factor antibodies (AIFA) exhibit very high specificity[1,2] and are found in approximately 75% of patients with pernicious anemia (PA). High serum levels of vitamin B12 (cobalamin) cause false positive results for AIFA. Assays are now available for type I AIFA (reactive with B12 binding site of IF), type II AIFA [reactive with site(s) on IF other than the B12 binding site] and total antibodies, but the combined method which detects total AIFA (types I and II) provides only a modest increase in diagnostic sensitivity.[2] Levels of pepsinogen (PG) I and II, and the PGI/PGII ratio, are decreased in most (∿90%) patients with pernicious anemia.[3] Increasing data indicate that detection of elevated levels of methylmalonic acid and total homocysteine in serum and/or urine is the most reliable assay for cobalamin deficiency in patients with decreased levels of serum cobalamin (4-7; see also 8-9). See also **PEPSINOGEN I** and **II.**

REFERENCES:
1. Nimo RE, Carmel R. Increased sensitivity of detection of the blocking (type I) anti-intrinsic factor antibody. Am J Clin Pathol 1987;88:729-33.
2. Waters HM, Smith C, Howarth JE, Dawson DW, Delamore IW. New enzyme immunoassay for detecting total, type I, and type II intrinsic factor antibodies. J Clin Pathol 1989;42:307-12.
3. Carmel R. Pepsinogens and other serum markers in pernicious anemia. Am J Clin Pathol 1988;90:442-5.
4. Norman EJ, Logan D, Terrell P. Falsely high serum B_{12} levels [Letter]. Am J Clin Pathol 1986;86:692.
5. Matchar DB, Feussner JR, Millington DS, Wilkinson RH Jr, Watson DJ, Gale D. Isotope-dilution assay for urinary methylmalonic acid in the diagnosis of vitamin B_{12} deficiency: a prospective clinical evaluation. Ann Intern Med 1987;106:707-10.
6. Stabler SP, Marcell PD, Podell ER, Allen RH, Savage DG, Lindenbaum J. Elevation of total homocysteine in the serum of patients with cobalamin or folate deficiency detected by capillary gas chromatography-mass spectrometry. J Clin Invest 1988;81:466-74.

7. Chu RC, Hall CA. The total serum homocysteine as an indicator of vitamin B_{12} and folate status. Am J Clin Pathol 1988;90:446-9.
8. Lindenbaum J, Healton EB, Savage DG, et al. Neuropsychiatric disorders caused by cobalamin deficiency in the absence of anemia or macrocytosis. N Engl J Med 1988;318:1720-8.
9. Herbert V, Norman EJ, Alston TA, Lindenbaum J. Cobalamin deficiency and neuropsychiatric disorders [Letters]. N Engl J Med 1988;319:1733-5.

ISLET CELL ANTIBODIES

In first-degree relatives of probands with insulin-dependent diabetes mellitus (IDDM) the presence of high titer ICA of the IgG cytoplasmic variety (IgG-ICA) and ICA of the complement-fixing subgroup (CF-ICA) confer a relative risk of 75 for development of IDDM.[1] The presence of ICA combined with a decrease in the first-phase of insulin secretion (less than 25 microU/ml) is predictive with a 95% likelihood of the development of IDDM within 12 months.[2] Reproducible results among laboratories are possible with careful attention to selection of the human pancreas as substrate as well as to the use of dilutions to generate standard curves and to the conversion of results to units.[3,4] The prozone phenomena described elsewhere[5] are not common in our experience. 50% of relatives with a single positive ICA test will develop IDDM within 10 years,[6] and 60-80% of relatives with both ICA and insulin autoantibodies IAA will develop IDDM within 10 years.[7,8] The predictive value for health of negative results for ICA and IAA is almost 99%.[8] Strong, persistently positive ICA (i.e., ≥ 40 JDF U), especially if accompanied by markedly decreased insulin secretion, are the best predictors of subsequent development of IDDM.[9-12] The 64 kd β-cell autoantigen long thought to be an important target for ICA is not yet available from expression cloning despite efforts by several groups.[13] ICA positivity correlates with rapid loss of C-peptide secretory capacity in newly diagnosed ICA-positive IDDM.[14] The predictive values of ICA for development of IDDM within 10 years in first-degree relatives of patients with IDDM increase from 40% at low levels of ICA to 100% at high levels, whereas the sensitivity is 88% at low levels and 31% at high levels.[15]

Prediabetics positive for ICA and IAA have increased suppressor-inducer (CD45R) and decreased helper-inducer (CDw29) peripheral blood lymphocytes.[16] In two randomized, prospective, placebo-controlled studies of recent-onset IDDM, cyclosporine immunosuppression increased the rate of non-insulin-requiring remissions as well as β-cell function during drug treatment.[17,18] Although 12 months of cyclosporine therapy decreases titers of ICA and insulin antibodies (IA) and increases glucagon-stimulated levels of serum C-peptide, the determination of ICA and IA and HLA-DR type are of no predictive value in selecting recent-onset IDDM patients for cyclosporine immunointervention.[19] See 20 for discussion of genetic control of autoimmunity in IDDM. EIA for autoantibodies to a 64 kd islet-cell protein is promising for prediction of IDDM, but sensitivity and specificity are still suboptimal.[21] See also **INSULIN ANTIBODIES.**

REFERENCES:
1. Tarn AC, Thomas JM, Dean BM, et al. Predicting insulin-dependent diabetes. Lancet 1988;1:845-50.
2. Chase HP, Voss MA, Butler-Simon N, Hoops S, O'Brien D, Dobersen MJ. Diagnosis of pre-type I diabetes. J Pediatr 1987;111:807-12.
3. Bonifacio E, Lernmark A, Dawkins RL, Peter JB, et al. Serum exchange and use of dilutions have improved precision of measurement of islet cell antibodies. J Immunol Methods 1988;106:83-8.
4. Landin-Olsson M. Precision of the islet-cell antibody assay depends on the pancreas. J Clin Lab Analysis 1990;4:289-94.
5. Colman PG, DiMario U, Rabizadeh A, Dotta F, Anastasi E, Eisenbarth GS. A prozone phenomenon interferes in islet cell antibody detection: direct comparison of two methods in subjects at risk of diabetes and in insulin dependent diabetics at onset. J Autoimmunity 1988;1:109-17.
6. Bruining GJ, Molenaar JL, Grobbee DE, et al. Ten-year follow-up study of islet-cell antibodies and childhood diabetes mellitus. Lancet 1989;1:1100-3.
7. Ziegler AG, Ziegler R, Vardi P, et al. Life-table analysis of progression to diabetes of anti-insulin autoantibody-positive relatives of individuals with type 1 diabetes. Diabetes 1989;38:1320-5.

8. Dean BM, McNally JM, Bonifacio E, et al. Comparison of insulin autoantibodies in diabetes-related and healthy populations by precise displacement ELISA. Diabetes 1989;38:1275-81.
9. Sachs JA, Cudworth AG, Jaraquemade D, et al. Type I diabetes and the HLA locus. Diabetologia 1980;18:41-3.
10. McCulloch DK, Klaff LJ, Kahn SE, et al. Nonprogression of subclinical β-cell dysfunction among first-degree relatives of IDDM patients. 5-yr follow-up of the Seattle Family study. Diabetes 1990;39:549-56.
11. Tarn AC, Thomas JM, Dean BM, et al. Predicting insulin dependent diabetes. Lancet 1988;1:845-50.
12. Srikanta S, Ganda OP, Jackson RA, et al. Type I diabetes in monozygotic twins: chronic progressive beta cell dysfunction. Ann Intern Med 1983;99:320-6.
13. Atkinson MA, Maclaren NK, Holmes NK, et al. The natural history and predictive value of $M_r64,000$ autoantibodies for insulin-dependent diabetes mellitus. J Autoimmunity 1990;3:41-5.
14. Peig M, Gomis R, Ercilla G, et al. Correlation between residual β-cell function and islet cell antibodies in newly diagnosed type 1 diabetes. Follow-up study. Diabetes 1989;38:1396-1401.
15. Bonifacio E, Bingley P, Shattock M, et al. Quantification of islet-cell antibodies and prediction of insulin-dependent diabetes. Lancet 1990;1:147-9.
16. Faustman D, Eisenbarth G, Daley J, Breitmeyer J. Abnormal T-lymphocyte subsets in type 1 diabetes. Diabetes 1989;38:1462-8.
17. Feutren G, Papoz L, Assan R, et al. Cyclosporin increases the rate and length of remissions in insulin-dependent diabetics of recent onset: results of a multicentre double-blind trial. Lancet 1986;2:119-23.
18. The Canadian-European Randomized Control Trial Group. Cyclosporin-induced remission of IDDM after early intervention: association of 1 year of cyclosporin treatment with enhanced insulin secretion. Diabetes 1988;37:1574-82.
19. Mandrup-Poulsen T, Molvig J, Andersen HU, et al. Lack of predictive value of islet cell antibodies, insulin antibodies, and HLA-DR phenotype for remission in cyclosporin-treated IDDM patients. Diabetes 1990;39:204-10.
20. Todd JA. Genetic control of autoimmunity in type 1 diabetes. Immunology Today 1990;11:122-9.
21. Atkinson MA, Maclaren NK, Scharp DW, et al. 64,000 M_r autoantibodies as predictors of insulin-dependent diabetes. Lancet 1990;1:1357-60.

Jo-1 (HISTIDYL-TRANSFERASE RNA SYNTHETASE) ANTIBODIES

Antibodies to the Jo-1 antigen (histidyl-tRNA synthetase)[1,2] are found in approximately 25% of adult patients with myositis (including polymyositis, dermatomyositis; overlap syndromes) and are particularly common (~68%) in patients with both myositis and cryptogenic fibrosing alveolitis (pulmonary interstitial fibrosis)[1-4] (cf. 5 for review of early literature). A negative result for nuclear and cytoplasmic fluorescence (e.g., by IFA on HEp-2 cells) does not rule out the presence of anti-Jo-1 antibodies, which should be tested by DD or preferably by EIA.[4,6-9] This antibody, which is apparently highly specific for myositis, was detected by EIA in 35-48% of polymyositis sera, i.e., double the frequency by commercial thymus extract.[9] Antibodies to 56 kd protein are found in sera of 85% of patients with myositis; antibody levels might reflect disease activity in adults.[10]

REFERENCES:
1. Rosa MD, Hendrick JP Jr, Lerner MR, et al. A mammalian tRNA [His]-containing antigen is recognized by the polymyositis-specific antibody anti-Jo-1. Nucleic Acids Res 1983;11:853-70.
2. Hochberg MC, Feldman D, Stevens MB, Arnett FC, Reichlin M. Antibody to Jo-1 in polymyositis/dermatomyositis: association with interstitial pulmonary disease. J Rheumatol 1984;11:663-5.
3. Bernstein RM, Morgan SH, Chapman J, et al. Anti-Jo-1 antibody: a marker for myositis with interstitial lung disease. Br Med J 1984;289:151-2.
4. Targoff IN, Reichlin M. Measurement of antibody to Jo-1 by ELISA and comparison to enzyme inhibitory activity. J Immunol 1987;138:2874-82.

5. Fudman EJ, Schnitzer TJ. Clinical and biochemical characteristics of autoantibody systems in polymyositis and dermatomyositis. Semin Arthritis Rheum 1986;15:255-60.
6. Biswas T, Miller FW, Takagaki Y, Plotz PH. An enzyme-linked immunosorbent assay for the detection and quantitation of anti-Jo-1 antibody in human serum. J Immunol Methods 1987;98:243-8.
7. Reichlin M, Arnett FC Jr. Multiplicity of antibodies in myositis sera. Arthritis Rheum 1984;27:1150-6.
8. Biswas T, Miller FW, Plotz PH. Stimulation and partial stabilization of human histidyl-tRNA synthetase by hemoglobin. FEBS Lett 1988;229:203-5.
9. Walker EJ, Tymms KE, Webb J, Jeffrey PD. Improved detection of anti-Jo-1 antibody, a marker for myositis, using purified histidyl-tRNA synthetase. J Immunol Methods 1987;96:149-56.
10. Arad-Dann H, Isenberg D, Ovadia E, et al. Autoantibodies against a nuclear 56 kDa protein: a marker for inflammatory muscle disease. J Autoimmunity 1989;2:877-88.

Ki ANTIBODIES

These antibodies to a 32 kd protein component of rabbit thymus are found in about 21% and 8% of patients with SLE by ELISA and DID respectively and in smaller proportions in MCTD, systemic sclerosis and RA.[1] Although, perhaps more common in CNS lupus, anti-Ki antibodies and anti-SL antibodies,[2] with which they are identical, are not clinically useful at this time.

REFERENCES:
1. Sakamoto M, Takasaki Y, Yamanaka K, et al. Purification and characterization of Ki antigen and detection of anti-Ki antibody by enzyme-linked immunosorbent assay in patients with systemic lupus erythematosus. Arthritis Rheum 1989;32:1554-62.
2. Bernstein RM, Morgan SH, Bunn CC, et al. The SL autoantibody-antigen system: clinical and biochemical studies. Ann Rheum Dis 1986;45:353-8.

KINETOCHORE ANTIBODIES

Usually referred to as anti-centromere, these antibodies stain the mitotic spindle apparatus in broad peripolar patterns.[1,2] See also **CENTROMERE ANTIBODIES.**

REFERENCES:
1. Powell FC, Winkelmann RK, Venencie-Lemarchand F, Spurbeck JL, Schroeter AL. The anticentromere antibody: disease specificity and clinical significance. Mayo Clin Proc 1984;59:700-6.
2. Moroi Y, Peebles C, Fritzler MJ, Steigerwald J, Tan EM. Autoantibody to centromere (kinetochore) in scleroderma sera. Proc Natl Acad Sci USA 1980;77:1627-31.

Ku ANTIBODIES

Anti-Ku antibodies are found in approximately 30-50% of patients with SLE, mixed connective tissue disease and scleroderma,[1,2] in about 5% of patients with myositis in the US and in a larger proportion in Japan (cf. 3 for review). Availability of the cloned Ku antigen (Ku is now known to be identical to Ki antigen, p70/p80 antigen, and p86-70 kd protein complex) may help clarify the clinical utility, if any, of assays for anti-Ku antibodies (cf. 4 for review).

REFERENCES:
1. Reeves WH. Use of monoclonal antibodies for the characterization of novel DNA-binding proteins recognized by human autoimmune sera. J Exp Med 1985;161:18-39.
2. Reeves WH. Antinuclear antibodies as probes to explore the structural organization of the genome. J Rheumatol 1987;14(Suppl 13):97-105.
3. Fudman EJ, Schnitzer TJ. Clinical and biochemical characteristics of autoantibody systems in polymyositis and dermatomyositis. Semin Arthritis Rheum 1986;15:255-60.
4. Reeves WH, Sthoeger ZM. Molecular cloning of cDNA encoding the p70 (Ku) lupus autoantigen. J Biol Chem 1989;264:5047-52.

LAMIN ANTIBODIES

Displaying a ring- or rim-type ANA pattern by IFA assay, these antibodies are found in a few patients with SLE and more commonly in patients with chronic autoimmune disease with an unusual triad of conditions including hepatitis; cytopenia(s) with a circulating anti-coagulant or anti-cardiolipin antibodies; and cutaneous luekocytoclastic angiitis or probable brain vasculitis.[1-4]

REFERENCES:
1. Lassoued K, Guilly M-N, Danon F, et al. Antinuclear autoantibodies specific for lamins. Ann Intern Med 1988;108:829-33.
2. Tan EM. Autoantibodies to nuclear lamins. Ann Intern Med 1988;108:897-8.
3. Reeves WH, Chaudhary N, Salerno A, Blobel G. Lamin B autoantibodies in sera of certain patients with systemic lupus erythematosus. J Exp Med 1987;165:750-62.
4. Guilly M-N, Danon F, Brouet J-C, Bornens M, Courvalin J-C. Autoantibodies to nuclear lamin B in a patient with thrombopenia. Eur J Cell Biol 1987;43:266-72.

LEUKOCYTE ADHESION MOLECULES

Leukocyte adhesion (which among other vital functions, is essential for adhesion to vascular endothelium, aggregation, binding of iC3B-coated particles, chemotaxis, cytotoxicity, lymphocyte proliferation and phagocytosis) is mediated by binding of Leu-CAMs composed of heterodimer molecules [3 α subunits known as CD11a-c and a common β subunit (CD18)] on leukocytes to CD54(ICAM-1) on epithelial cells, fibroblasts, mononuclear leukocytes, vascular endothelial cells and by the binding of CD2 on T cells to CD58, which is found on a wide variety of cells. Leu-CAMs are members of the integrin family of adhesion receptors among which the β subfamilies are composed of $\alpha\beta$ glycoprotein heterodimers including the 3 members of the $\beta2$ Leu-CAMs subfamily which are composed of a common β subunit [i.e., $\beta2$(CD18)] and 3 different α subunits. The $\beta1$ subfamily (receptors for fibronectin and late-activation antigens) and the $\beta3$ subfamily (receptors for fibrinogen, vibronectin, platelet IIb/IIIa) are each composed of unique β subunits common to their respective families and several α subunits (cf. 1 for review of Leu-CAMs); the $\beta1$ and $\beta3$ integrins, which recognize the arg-gly-asp (RGD) tripeptide, are involved in a wide variety of functions ranging from matrix assembly to morphogenesis and wound healing. Leu-CAM deficiencies, also known as leukocyte adhesion deficiencies (LADs), are partial or complete inherited deficiencies of cell surface expression of CD18 and CD11a-c which result in recurrent infection, inability of granulocytes to reach extravascular sites of inflammation, and death before age 2 in severely deficient patients.[2-4] See also **CLUSTERS OF DIFFERENTIATION, INTEGRINS** and **INTERCELLULAR ADHESION MOLECULE 1.**

REFERENCES:
1. Patarroyo M, Makgoba MW. Leucocyte adhesion to cells in immune and inflammatory responses. Lancet 1989;2:1139-42.
2. Anderson DC, Springer TA. Leukocyte adhesion deficiency: an inherited defect in the Mac-1, LFA-1, and p150,95 glycoproteins. Ann Rev Med 1987;38:175-94.
3. Patarroyo M, Makgoba MW. Leukocyte adhesion to cells. Molecular basis, physiological relevance and abnormalities [Editorial]. Scand J Immunol 1989;30:129-64.
4. Arnaout MA, Dana N, Gupta SK, et al. Point mutations impairing cell surface expression of the common β subunit (CD18) in a patient with leukocyte adhesion molecule (Leu-CAM) deficiency. J Clin Invest 1990;85:977-81.

LEUKOTRIENES C$_4$, D$_4$ and E$_4$ (LTC$_4$, LTD$_4$ and LTE$_4$)

LTD$_4$, an arachidonic acid metabolite which is several hundredfold more potent as a bronchoconstrictor than histamine, is rapidly metabolized to LTE$_4$ (cf. 1 for review). Urinary excretion of LTE$_4$ (ng/mmol creatinine) is increased approximately fivefold after antigen challenge of atopic patients.[2] Large increases of LTD$_4$ and LTC$_4$ in bronchoalveolar lavage fluids induced by antigen challenge are associated with increases of histamine and prostaglandin D$_2$; the immediate response to antigen challenge is inhibited approximately ⅓ by LTD$_4$ antagonists.[3] Although local challenge increases LTD$_4$ in nasal washes[4] and tear fluid,[5] urinary LTE$_4$ is not increased in allergic rhinitis, perhaps because the number of relevant cells is smaller than with pulmonary challenge.[2] Leukotrienes are now recognized as mediators in liver[6] and cardiovascular diseases[7] as well as hypersensitivity (8; cf. 1, 9 and 10 for reviews of the early literature and references 11-13 for reviews of the recent literature). Analytical methods now available[2] promise incisive studies of the clinical utility of leukotriene quantitation in a variety of conditions.

REFERENCES:
1. Zipser RD, Laffi G. Prostaglandins, thromboxanes and leukotrienes in clinical medicine. West J Med 1985;143:485-97.
2. Taylor GW, Taylor I, Black P, et al. Urinary leukotriene E_4 after antigen challenge and in acute asthma and allergic rhinitis. Lancet 1989;1:584-8.
3. Britton JR, Hanley SP, Tattersfield AE. The effect of an oral leukotriene D_4 antagonist, L-649,923, on the response to inhaled antigen in asthma. J Allergy Clin Immunol 1987;79:811-16.
4. Creticos PS, Peters SP, Adkinson NF Jr, et al. Peptide leukotriene release after antigen challenge in patients sensitive to ragweed. N Engl J Med 1984;310:1626-30.
5. Bisgaard H, Ford-Hutchinson AW, Charleson S, Taudorf E. Detection of leukotriene C_4-like immunoreactivity in tear fluid from subjects challenged with specific allergen. Prostaglandins 1984;27:369-74.
6. Keppler D, Huber M, Baumert T. Leukotrienes as mediators in diseases of the liver. Semin Liver Dis 1988;8:357-66.
7. Piper PJ, Stanton AW, Yaacob HB, Antoniw J. Leukotrienes in the cardiovascular system. Biochem Soc Trans 1988;16:482-3.
8. Marone G, Casolaro V, Cirillo R, et al. Pathophysiology of human basophils and mast cells in allergic disorders. Clin Immunol Immunopathol 1989;50:S24-40.
9. Samuelsson B. Leukotrienes: mediators of immediate hypersensitivity reactions and inflammation. Science 1983;220:568-75.
10. Goetzl EJ, Payan DG, Goldman DW. Immunopathogenetic roles of leukotrienes in human diseases. J Clin Immunol 1984;4:79-84.
11. Feuerstein G, Hallenbeck JM. Leukotrines in health and disease. FASEB J 1987;1:186-92.
12. Salmon JA, Higgs GA. Prostaglandins and leukotrienes as inflammatory mediators. Br Med Bull 1987;43:285-96.
13. Piper PJ, Samhoun MN. Leukotrienes. Br Med Bull 1987;43:297-311.

LIPOMODULIN ANTIBODIES

IgM antibodies to lipomodulin, a phospholipase A_2 inhibitory protein, were reported in some patients with RA and SLE.[1] Further studies have not appeared.

REFERENCES:
1. Hirata F, del Carmine R, Nelson CA, et al. Presence of autoantibody for phospholipase inhibitory protein, lipomodulin in patients with rheumatic diseases. Proc Natl Acad Sci USA 1981;78:3190-4.

LIVER-KIDNEY MICROSOMAL ANTIBODIES

These antibodies, which stain the cytoplasm of hepatocytes and proximal renal tubules (and hence are often difficult to distinguish from anti-mitochondrial antibody by IFA assay) are found in a subgroup of patients with ANA-negative autoimmune chronic active hepatitis (CAH) (which is by definition HBsAg negative); anti-LKM antibodies are not found in CAH non-A, non-B.[1,2] Liver-kidney microsomal (LKM1)-antibody-positive CAH (i.e., autoimmune chronic active hepatitis type 2),[3] which represents less than 10% of HBsAg-negative CAH, is the most common autoimmune liver disease of childhood and has a relatively unfavorable prognosis.[4] Anti-LKM1 antibodies are unlikely to be of pathogenic significance in childhood autoimmune CAH because they do not bind to hepatocyte membrane antigens.[5] Other antibodies to endoplasmic reticulin include anti-LKM2 antibodies found in tienilic acid (ticrynafen)-induced hepatitis[6,7] and anti-LKM3 found in approximately 10% of chronic delta virus hepatitis.[8] The delta-associated LKM3 antibodies in chronic delta hepatitis are organ (liver)- and species (human)-specific in contrast to typical anti-LKM antibodies.[8,9] Reaction of LKM-positive CAH sera with a species-nonspecific 50-57 kd polypeptide may reflect quantitative increases of a naturally occurring antibody.[10] The LKM1 and 2 antigens are now known to be cytochromes P-450IID6 and P-450IIC8/9/10, respectively (cf. 11). Dihydralazine-induced hepatitis is characterized by anti-liver-microsome (anti-LM) antibodies which are directed to cytochrome P-450IA1.[11] Organ-specific antibodies to liver cytosol (anti-LC1) were recently described in chronic active hepatitis type 2. These antibodies were not found in classic chronic active hepatitis type 1 which is associated with anti-actin antibodies.[12] Antibodies to hepatitis C virus (HCV) in ANA/smooth muscle antibody-positive CAH[13] and in LKM-antibody-positive type 2 AI-CAH patients[14,15] may be false positives[16] but whether the "stickiness" of some of these sera is due to immune complexes,[17] anti-idiotypic antibodies or other factors is not known. The disputed relationship of HCV to AI-CAH is, of course, important because interferon causes development of autoantibodies in CAH type 2[18-20] and can cause exacerbations of disease.[19,20] See also **LIVER-SPECIFIC LIPOPROTEIN, LIVER MEMBRANE ANTIGEN** and **SOLUBLE LIVER ANTIGEN**.

REFERENCES:
1. Manns M, Gerken G, Kyriatsoulis A, Meyer zum Büschenfelde K-H. Significant autoimmune markers of autoimmune liver disorders: current status. J Clin Lab Analysis 1987;1:363-70.
2 Zanger UM, Hauri H-P, Loeper J, Homberg J-C, Meyer UA. Antibodies against human cytochrome P-450db1 in autoimmune hepatitis type II. Proc Natl Acad Sci USA 1988;85:8256-60.
3. Homberg J-C, Abuaf N, Bernard O, et al. Chronic active hepatitis associated with antiliver/kidney microsome antibody type 1: a second type of "autoimmune" hepatitis. Hepatology 1987;7:1333-9.
4. Maggiore G, Bernard O, Homberg J-C, et al. Liver disease associated with anti-liver-kidney microsome antibody in children. J Pediatr 1986;108:399-404.
5. Peakman M, Lobo-Yeo A, Mieli-Vergani G, Davies ET, Mowat AP, Vergani D. Characterization of anti-liver kidney microsomal antibody in childhood autoimmune chronic active hepatitis: evidence for IgG1 subclass restriction, polyclonality and non cross-reactivity with hepatocyte surface antigens. Clin Exp Immunol 1987;69:543-9.
6. Homberg JC, Andre C, Abuaf N. A new anti-liver-kidney microsome antibody (anti-LKM2) in tienilic acid-induced hepatitis. Clin Exp Immunol 1984;55:561-70.
7. Beaune P, Dansette PM, Mansuy D, et al. Human anti-endoplasmic reticulum auto-antibodies appearing in a drug-induced hepatitis are directed against a human liver cytochrome P-450 that hydroxylates the drug. Proc Natl Acad Sci USA 1987;84:551-5.
8. Crivelli O, Lavarini C, Chiaberge E, et al. Microsomal autoantibodies in chronic infection with the HBsAg associated delta (δ) agent. Clin Exp Immunol 1983;54:232-8.
9. Caredda F, de Bartolo G, Zampini L, et al. Detection and further characterization of a newly described microsomal autoantibody associated with chronic delta infection. Digestion 1986;33:181-8.
10. Kyriatsoulis A, Manns M, Gerken G, et al. Distinction between natural and pathological autoantibodies by immunoblotting and densitometric subtraction: liver-kidney microsomal antibody (LKM) positive sera identify multiple antigens in human liver tissue. Clin Exp Immunol 1987;70:53-60.
11 Bourdi M, Larrey D, Nataf J, et al. Anti-liver endoplasmic reticulum autoantibodies are directed against human cytochrome P-450IA2. A specific marker of dihydralazine-induced hepatitis. J Clin Invest 1990;85:1967-73.
12. Maddrey WC. Subdivisions of idiopathic autoimmune chronic active hepatitis. Hepatology 1987;7:1372-5.
13. Esteban JI, Esteban R, Viladomiu L, et al. Hepatitis C virus antibodies among risk groups in Spain. Lancet 1989;2:294-6.
14. Lenzi M, Ballardini G, Fusconi M, et al. Type 2 autoimmune hepatitis and hepatitis C virus infection. Lancet 1990;1:258-9.
15. Dussaix E, Maggiore G, De Giacomo C, et al. Autoimmune hepatitis in children and hepatitis C virus testing [Letter]. Lancet 1990;335:1160-1.
16. McFarlane IG, Smith HM, Johnson PJ, et al. Hepatitis C virus antibodies in chronic active hepatitis: pathogenetic factor or false-positive result? Lancet 1990;335:754-7.
17. McFarlane IG, Tolley P, Major G, et al. Development of a micro enzyme-linked immunosorbent assay for antibodies against the liver-specific membrane lipoprotein. J Immunol Methods 1983;64:215-25.

18. Mayet W-J, Hess G, Gerken G, et al. Treatment of chronic type B hepatitis with recombinant α-interferon induces autoantibodies not specific for autoimmune chronic hepatitis. Hepatology 1989;10:24-8.
19. Vento S, Di Perri G, Garofano T, et al. Hazards of interferon therapy for HBV-seronegative chronic hepatitis [Letter]. Lancet 1989;2:926.
20. Vento S, Di Perri G, Luzzati R, et al. Type 2 autoimmune hepatitis and hepatitis C virus infection [Letter]. Lancet 1990;1:921-2.

LIVER MEMBRANE ANTIGEN ANTIBODIES

Antibodies to LMA, which react with surface membranes of rabbit hepatocytes, are found in approximately 70% of patients with HBsAg-negative autoimmune chronic active hepatitis. As expected in the so-called "lupoid" variety of autoimmune chronic active hepatitis, anti-LMA antibodies are commonly accompanied by positive tests for ANA and for anti-smooth muscle antibodies. As with other antibodies involved in chronic liver diseases (ANA, anti-LSP; anti-LKM antibodies), the presence of anti-LMA antibodies is not in itself of diagnostic or prognostic value (1-3, see 4 and 5 for review of early and recent literature). See also **LIVER-KIDNEY MICROSOME ANTIBODIES** and **LIVER-SPECIFIC LIPOPROTEIN ANTIBODIES**.

REFERENCES:
1. Hopf U, Meyer zum Büschenfelde K-H, Arnold W. Detection of a liver-membrane autoantibody in HB_s Ag-negative chronic active hepatitis. N Engl J Med 1976;294:578-82.
2. Manns M, Meyer zum Büschenfelde K-H, Hess G. Autoantibodies against liver-specific membrane lipoprotein in acute and chronic liver diseases: studies on organ-, species-, and disease-specificity. Gut 1980;21:955-61.
3. Gerken G, Manns M, Ramadori G, et al. Liver membrane autoantibodies in chronic active hepatitis. Studies on mechanically and enzymatically isolated rabbit hepatocytes. J Hepatol 1987;5:65-74.
4. Meyer zum Büschenfelde K-H, Hütteroth TH, Manns M, Möller B. The role of liver membrane antigens as targets in autoimmune type liver disease. Springer Semin Immunopathol 1980;3:297-315.
5. Meyer zum Büschenfelde K-H. Immunologie der lebererkrankungen. Schweiz Med Wochenschr 1987;117:1065-75.

LIVER-SPECIFIC MEMBRANE LIPOPROTEIN ANTIBODIES

Sera from most patients with acute viral hepatitis A and B and from a few patients with non-A, non-B hepatitis react with a liver-specific membrane lipoprotein fraction known as LSMP. Anti-LSMP antibodies are initially high and decline during recovery from acute viral hepatitis A and B. The LSMP complex contains liver cell membranes, including plasma membrane (1-5; cf. 6 for review of early literature). Antibodies to the galactose-specific asialoglycoprotein receptor (also known as hepatic lectin, HL) are detected by the assay for anti-LSMP antibodies in acute viral hepatitis A and B and, like anti-LSMP antibodies, are found to a much lesser extent in acute non-A, non-B viral hepatitis. Persistence or reappearance of anti-LSP antibodies in patients in remission of autoimmune chronic active hepatitis during withdrawal of treatment (prednisone/azathioprine) are associated with the reactivation of disease,[7] but confirmation of these observations is not yet available. Autoantibodies to LSMP are found not only in acute viral hepatitis and chronic active hepatitis of adults and children, but also in primary biliary cirrhosis,[8] alcoholic liver disease,[9] and to a lesser extent in liver disease due to α_1 antitrypsin deficiency.[10] See also **SOLUBLE LIVER ANTIGEN** and **LIVER MEMBRANE ANTIGEN**.

REFERENCES:
1. Jensen DM, McFarlane IG, Portmann BS, Eddleston ALWF, Williams R. Detection of antibodies directed against a liver-specific membrane lipoprotein in patients with acute and chronic active hepatitis. N Engl J Med 1978;299:1-7.
2. Kakumu S, Arakawa Y, Goji H, Kashio T, Yata K. Occurrence and significance of antibody to liver-specific membrane lipoprotein by double-antibody immunoprecipitation method in sera of patients with acute and chronic liver diseases. Gastroenterology 1979;76:665-72.

3. Manns M, Meyer zum Büschenfelde KH, Hess G. Autoantibodies against liver-specific membrane lipoprotein in acute and chronic liver diseases: studies on organ-, species- and disease-specificity. Gut 1980;21:955-61.
4. Meliconi R, Baraldini M, Stefanini GF, et al. Antibodies against human liver-specific protein (LSP) in acute and chronic viral hepatitis types A, B and non-A, non-B. Clin Exp Immunol 1981;46:382-90.
5. Vento S, McFarlane BM, McSorley CG. Liver autoreactivity in acute virus A, B and non-A, non-B hepatitis. J Clin Lab Immunol 1988;25:1-7.
6. Meyer zum Büschenfelde KH, Hütteroth TH, Manns M, Möller B. The role of liver membrane antigens as targets in autoimmune type liver disease. Springer Semin Immunopathol 1980;3:297-315.
7. McFarlane IG, Hegarty JE, McSorley CG, McFarlane BM, Williams R. Antibodies to liver-specific protein predict outcome of treatment withdrawal in autoimmune chronic active hepatitis. Lancet 1984;2:954-6.
8. Tsantoulas D, Perperas A, Portmann B, Eddleston ALWF, Williams R. Antibodies to a human liver membrane lipoprotein (LSP) in primary biliary cirrhosis. Gut 1980;21:557-60.
9. Perperas A, Tsantoulas D, Portmann B, Eddleston ALWF, Williams R. Autoimmunity to a liver membrane lipoprotein and liver damage in alcoholic liver disease. Gut 1981;2:149-52.
10. Larcher VF, MacDonald A, Vegnente A, Mowat AP, Eddleston AL, Williams R. Antibodies to liver-specific lipoprotein in children with chronic liver disease due to "autoimmune" chronic active hepatitis, cystic fibrosis and α_1-antitripsin deficiency. J Pediatr Gastroenterol Nutr 1984;3:728-33.

LUNG ANTIBODIES

Reported to be present in sera of patients with farmer's lung disease, the specificity of anti-lung antibodies is not yet well defined.[1,2] Likewise, cytotoxic antibodies to lung in sarcoidosis and in extrinsic asthma have not been well characterized.[3]

REFERENCES:
1. Braun SR, Flaherty DK, Burrell R, Rankin J. Importance of anti-lung antibody in farmer's lung disease. Am J Med 1983;74:535-9.
2. Dewair M, Baur X, Fruhmann G. Lung-reactive antibodies in sera of patients with farmer's lung disease. Respiration 1987;51:146-54.
3. Ende N, Grizzanti JN, Orsi EV, et al. Sarcoid and cytotoxic lung antibodies. Life Sci 1986;39:2435-40.

LUPUS ANTICOAGULANTS

Lupus anticoagulants (LAC) are a common cause of a prolonged activated partial thromboplastin (APTT) which is corrected by addition of platelet-rich plasma (or phospholipids) and not by platelet-poor plasma (cf. 1-3 for review). The method of choice for detection of LAC is the kaolin clotting time using the rabbit brain neutralization procedure.[4] Current data suggest that LAC and antibodies to negatively charged phospholipids (cardiolipin, phosphatidylserine, phosphatidic acid and phosphatidylinositol) are risk factors for arterial and venous thrombosis and for recurrent abortions in populations of patients which àre distinct but overlapping.[1,5-7] Drug-induced LAC are also associated with increased risk of thrombosis.[2,8] Current testing for LAC and anti-phospholipid antibodies (cardiolipin plus phosphatidylserine or cardiolipin plus phosphatidylglycerol) may be useful for assessing risk in patients with SLE.[1,9,10] Some data indicate that LAC assays are more reliable predictors of thrombosis, fetal loss and thrombocytopenia than are ACA assays.[11] Although the technology is in many ways more reliable, the rush to describe associations of LACs with various disorders has been much less scientifically unseemly than has been that of ACAs with their bewildering variety of clinical associations. The contribution of one serious study[12] must, it seems, render tolerable the excess of trivia recently published in this area. See also **CARDIOLIPIN ANTIBODIES** and **PHOSPHOLIPID ANTIBODIES.**

REFERENCES:
1. Triplett DA, Brandt JT, Musgrave KA, Orr CA. The relationship between lupus anticoagulants and antibodies to phospholipid. JAMA 1988;259;550-4.

2. Tobelem G, Cariou R, Camez A. The lupus anticoagulant and its role in thrombosis. Blood Rev 1987;1:21-4.
3. Petri M, Golbus M, Anderson R, Whiting-O'Keefe Q, Corash L, Hellmann D. Antinuclear antibody, lupus anticoagulant, and anticardiolipin antibody in women with idiopathic habitual abortion. A controlled, prospective study of forty-four women. Arthritis Rheum 1987;30:601-6.
4. Rosove MH, Ismail M, Kozoil BJ, et al. Lupus anticoagulants: improved diagnosis with a kaolin clotting time using rabbit brain phospholipid in standard and high concentrations. Blood 1986;68:472-8.
5. Howard MA, Firkin BG, Healy DL, Choong S-CC. Lupus anticoagulant in women with multiple spontaneous miscarriage. Am J Hematol 1987;26:175-8.
6. Carreras LO, Perez GN, Vega HR, Casavilla F. Lupus anticoagulant and recurrent fetal loss: successful treatment with gammaglobulin. Lancet 1988;i:393-4.
7. Li GC, Greenberg CS, Currie MS. Procainamide-induced lupus anticoagulants and thrombosis. South Med J 1988;81:262-4.
8. Fisher M, McGehee W. Cerebral infarct, TIA, and lupus inhibitor. Neurology 1986;36:1234-7.
9. Rosove MH, Brewer PM, Runge A, Hirji K. Simultaneous lupus anticoagulant and anticardiolipin assays and clinical detection of antiphospholipids. Am J Hematol 1989;32:148-9.
10. Alving BM, Barr CF, Tang DB. Correlation between lupus anticoagulants and anticardiolipin antibodies in patients with prolonged activated partial thromboplastin times. Am J Med 1990;88:112-6.
11. Derksen RHWM, Hasselaar P, Blokziji L, et al. Coagulation screen is more specific than the anticardiolipin antibody ELISA in defining a thrombotic subset of lupus patients. Ann Rheum Dis 1988;47:364-71.
12. Thiagarajan P, Shapiro SS, De Marco L. Monoclonal immunoglobulin Mλ coagulation inhibitor with phospholipid specificity. J Clin Invest 1980;66:397-405.

Ly-6

Products of the Ly-6 multigene family, long known to be expressed on murine T and B lymphocytes (cf. 1 for review) are also present on several non-lymphoid organs. Homologues of Ly-6 are also apparently present in man, but as in mice their function is unknown.[2]

REFERENCES:
1. Shevach EM, Korty PE. Ly-6: a multigene family in search of a function. Immunol Today 1989;10:195-200.
2. Stefanová I, Hilgert I, Kristofová H, et al. Characterization of a broadly expressed human leucocyte surface antigen MEM-43 anchored in membrane through phosphatidylinositol. Mol Immunol 1989;26:153-61.

LYMPHOCYTE ANTIBODIES

Two separate categories of anti-lymphocyte antibodies are well recognized.

Anti-lymphocyte autoantibodies:

In several autoimmune diseases (including RA, SLE and PSS), anti-lymphocyte autoantibodies are frequently found.[1,2] Classically, these are IgM in isotype and best detected in the cold. Although the amount may relate to disease activity,[1] the precise indications for this investigation are not established. MHC genes control the titer to some degree.[3,4] IgG autoantibodies may also be found in SLE.[5,6] Lymphocyte autoantibodies, which are detected in HIV infection, may play a role in the development of immunodeficiency.[7-9]

Anti-lymphocyte alloantibodies:

Following transfusion, transplantation and pregnancy, IgG alloantibodies (which react with lymphocytes of a particular subject) are often demonstrable at room temperature or 37 °C. Recently, flow cytometry has been shown to be useful.[10] The demonstration of these antibodies is critical in renal transplantation and possibly helpful in the assessment of spontaneous abortion.[11]

To distinguish between these two classes of antibody, the test can be performed at 4° to 37 °C in addition to screening at room temperature.

REFERENCES:
1. Dawkins RL, Witt C, Richmond J, et al. Lymphocytotoxic antibodies in disease. Aust N Z J Med 1978;2:81-6.
2. Herrmann K, Schaller J, Haustein U-F, Baldauf Ch, Kiessig S. Lymphocytotoxic auto-antibodies in progressive systemic sclerosis. Arch Dermatol Res 1988;280:399-404.
3. Zilko PJ, Dawkins RL, Holmes K, Witt C. Genetic control of suppressor lymphocyte function in myasthenia gravis: relationship of impaired suppressor function to HLA-B8/DRW3 and cold reactive lymphocytotoxic antibodies. Clin Immunol Immunopathol 1979;14:222-30.
4. Donaldson PT, Hussain MJ, Mieli-Vergani G, Mowat AP, Vergani D. Anti-lymphocytic antibodies in autoimmune chronic active hepatitis starting in childhood. Clin Exp Immunol 1989;75:41-6.
5. Edwards BS, Searles RP, Brozek CM, et al. Isotype and cytotoxicity spectra of anti-lymphocyte antibodies in patients with systemic lupus erythematosus. Clin Immunol Immunopathol 1987;45:333-47.
6. Minota S, Winfield JB. Nature of IgG anti-lymphocyte autoantibody-reactive molecules shed from activated T cells in systemic lupus erythematosus. Rheumatol Int 1988;8:165-70.
7. Stricker RB, McHugh TM, Moody DJ, et al. An AIDS-related cytotoxic autoantibody reacts with a specific antigen on stimulated CD4+ T cells. Nature 1987;327:710-3.
8. Ozturk GE, Kohler PF, Horsburgh CR Jr, Kirkpatrick CH. The significance of antilym-phocyte antibodies in patients with acquired immune deficiency syndrome (AIDS) and their sexual partners. J Clin Immunol 1987;7:130-9.
9. Peković DD, Gornitsky M, Garzon S, et al. Mechanisms of HIV-associated immunosuppression. Cancer Detect Prev 1988;12:195-203.
10. Wormsley SB. Applications of monoclonal antibodies in organ transplantation. In: Moulds JE, Masouredis SP, eds. Monoclonal antibodies. Arlington, Virginia, American Association of Blood Banks 1989. In press.
11. Smith JB, Cowchock FS. Immunological studies in recurrent spontaneous abortion: ef-fects of immunization of women with paternal mononuclear cells on lymphocytotoxic and mixed lymphocyte reaction blocking antibodies and correlation with sharing of HLA and pregnancy outcome. J Reprod Immunol 1988;14:99-113.

LYMPHOCYTE ANTIGEN STIMULATION

Antigen-specific lymphocyte stimulation is used to assess cell-mediated immunity in acquired and inherited immunodeficiencies, in the response to immunotherapies, and in detection of previous exposure to a variety of antigens, allergens and pathogens.[1-3] Previously sensitized lymphocytes will proliferate and produce measurable amounts of lymphokines when stimulated *in vitro* with the specific antigen. Defects in the ability of lymphocytes to proliferate and produce IL-2 in response to sensitizing antigen are found in immunodeficient states, par-ticularly AIDS.[4,5] Lymphocyte proliferation is measured by incorporation of ^{3}H-thymidine into newly synthesized DNA. Supernatants from the same antigen-stimulated cultures can be assessed for cytokine production by ELISA. The lymphocyte response to antigen *in vitro* cor-relates with the existence of delayed-type hypersensitivity *in vivo*.[1] The variability in T cell responses to common antigens in normal individuals makes the clinical utility of measuring cell mediated immunity *in vitro* somewhat dubious as compared to DTH skin testing using the Multitest system.[6,7] However, the usefulness of *in vitro* assays is apparent when testing previous exposure to infrequently encountered infectious agents. For example, T cell blastogenic responses to *Borrelia burgdorferi* can be used as evidence of infection in seronegative individuals in whom Lyme disease is suspected.[8]

REFERENCES:
1. Räsänen L. Skin test reactivity and *in vitro* response to microbes and microbial antigens. Clin Exp Immunol 1980;40:566-72.
2. Maluish AE, Strong DM. Lymphocyte proliferation. In: Rose NR, Friedman H, Fahey JL, eds. Clinical Laboratory Immunology. Am Society Microbiol, 1986;274-81.
3. Oppenheim JJ, Dougherty S, Chan SP, Baker J. Use of lymphocyte transformation to assess clinical disorders. In: Vyas GN, ed. Laboratory diagnosis of immunologic disorders. New York: Grune & Stratton, 1975:87-109.

4. Antonen J, Krohn K. Interleukin 2 production in HTLV-III/LAV infection: evidence of defective antigen-induced, but normal mitogen-induced IL-2 production. Clin Exp Immunol 1986;65:489-96.
5. Lane HC, Depper JM, Greene WC, Whalen G, Waldmann TA, Fauci AS. Qualitative analysis of immune function in patients with the acquired immunodeficiency syndrome. N Engl J Med 1985;313:79-84.
6. Kniker WT, Anderson CT, McBryde JL, Roumiantzeff M, Lesourd B. Multitest CMI for standardized measurement of delayed cutaneous hypersensitivity and cell-mediated immunity. Normal values and proposed scoring system for healthy adults in the U.S.A. Ann Allergy 1984;52:75-81.
7. Grimsley G. The significance of tests of cell-mediated immunity: an evaluation of the utility of tests used for the assessment of cell-mediated immunity [Thesis]. Western Australia: The University of Western Australia, 1987. 7 p.
8. Dattwyler RJ, Volkman DJ, Luft BJ, Halperin JJ, Thomas J, Golightly MG. Seronegative Lyme disease. Dissociation of specific T- and B-lymphocyte responses to *Borrelia burgdorferi*. N Engl J Med 1988;319:1441-6.

LYMPHOCYTE FUNCTION-ASSOCIATED ANTIGEN 1 (LFA-1)

LFA-1 (CD11A), a heterodimer expressed on the surface of cell lymphocytes, is a member of the family of leukocyte adhesion molecules which includes Mac-1 [CD11B, complement receptor 3 (CR3)] and p150/95 (CD11C). In leukocyte adhesion deficiency,[1] the β subunit is genetically deficient and normal interaction of T and B cells is impaired due to deficient LFA-1 expression on T cells.[2]

REFERENCES:
1. Springer TA, Thompson WS, Miller LJ, Schmalstieg F, Anderson DC. Inherited deficiency of the Mac-1, LFA-1, p150,95 glycoprotein family and its molecular basis. J Exp Med 1984;160:1901-18.
2. Mazerolles F, Lumbroso C, Lecomte O, Le Deist F, Fischer A. The role of lymphocyte function-associated antigen 1 (LFA-1) in the adherence of T lymphocytes to B lymphocytes. Eur J Immunol 1988;18:1229-34.

LYMPHOCYTE MITOGEN STIMULATION

In vitro lymphocyte stimulation by mitogens is a common method of measuring cell-mediated immunity. In humans, the plant lectin concanavalin A stimulates CD4 and CD8 lymphocyte subsets.[1] Pokeweed mitogen and phytohemagglutinin stimulate both T and B cells[2-4] and the protein A component of *Staphylococcus aureus* Cowan strain I is a potent B cell stimulator.[5] Lymphocyte stimulation is measured by ^{3}H-thymidine incorporation into newly synthesized DNA. Supernatants from mitogen-stimulated lymphocyte cultures often contain measurable amounts of lymphokines, most notably IL-2.[6] B cells can be induced to produce immunoglobulin under the appropriate conditions.[5] Inability of lymphocytes to proliferate and/or produce lymphokines or immunoglobulin upon mitogen stimulation is a sign of impaired cell-mediated immunity[7] as is found in acquired or genetic immunodeficiencies.[7-9] Recent data suggest that a decrease in PWM response is an early indicator for development of AIDS in HIV-seropositive individuals.[10] Cell-mediated immune responses are also impaired in a variety of other conditions, including bacterial or viral infections,[7] chemotherapy,[7,11] autoimmune diseases such as Sjögren syndrome and SLE,[7,12] motor neurone disease,[13] surgery and anesthesia, stress, aging, malnutrition, cancer, uremia and major burns.[7,14,15] Despite all these reports, the extremely large ranges of normal and the relatively poor reproducibility of mitogen stimulation (even in the same individual) strongly suggest that lymphocyte mitogen stimulation is overused and of poor cost-effectiveness compared to DTH skin tests using the Multitest system.[16,17]

REFERENCES:
1. Stobo J, Paul W. Functional heterogeneity of murine lymphoid cells. III. Differential responsiveness of T cells to phytohemagglutinin and concanavalin A as a probe for T cell subsets. J Immunol 1973;110:362-75.
2. Keightley RG, Cooper MD, Lawton AR. The T cell dependence of B cell differentiation induced by pokeweed mitogen. J Immunol 1976;117:1538-44.

3. Fitzgerald MG. The establishment of a normal human population dose-response curve for lymphocytes cultured with PHA (phytohaemagglutinin). Clin Exp Immunol 1971;8:421-5.
4. Phillips B, Roitt IM. Evidence for transformation of human B lymphocytes by PHA. Nature New Biol 1973;241:254-6.
5. Banck G. *Staphylococcus aureus* Cowan I and *Branhamella catarrhalis* as B lymphocyte mitogens. Culture conditions for optimal DNA synthesis and selective stimulation of human B lymphocytes. J Immunol Methods 1982;51:279-86.
6. Rocklin RE, MacDermott RP, Chess L, Schlossman SF, David JR. Studies on mediator production by highly purified human T and B lymphocytes. J Exp Med 1974;140:1303-16.
7. Oppenheim JJ, Dougherty S, Chan SP, Baker J. Use of lymphocyte transformation to assess clinical disorders. In: Vyas GN, ed. Laboratory diagnosis of immunologic disorders. New York: Grune & Stratton, 1975:87-109.
8. Reuben JM, Hersh EM, Murray JL, Munn CG, Mehta SR, Mansell PWA. IL-2 production and response *in vitro* by the leukocytes of patients with acquired immune deficiency syndrome. Lymphokine Res 1985;4:103-6.
9. Bowen DL, Lane HC, Fauci AS. Immunopathogenesis of the acquired immunodeficiency syndrome. Ann Intern Med 1985;103:704-9.
10. Hofmann BO, Lindhardt BO, Gerstoft J, et al. Lymphocyte transformation response to pokeweed mitogen as a predictive marker for development of AIDS and AIDS related symptoms in homosexual men with HIV antibodies. Br Med J 1987;295:293-7.
11. Thomas JW, Coy P, Lewis HS, Yuen A. Effect of therapeutic irradiation on lymphocyte transformation in lung cancer. Cancer 1971;27:1046-50.
12. Alcocer-Varela J, Alarcon-Segovia D. Decreased production of and response to interleukin 2 by cultured lymphocytes from patients with systemic lupus erythematosus. J Clin Invest 1982;69:1388-92.
13. Aspin J, Harrison R, Jehanli A, Lunt G, Campbell M. Stimulation by mitogens and neuronal membranes of lymphocytes from patients with motor neurone disease. J Neuroimmunol 1986;11:31-40.
14. Eilber FR, Morton DL. Impaired immunologic reactivity and recurrence following cancer surgery. Cancer 1970;25:362-7.
15. Lamb D, Pilney F, Kelly WD, Good RA. A comparative study of the incidence of anergy in patients with carcinoma, leukemia, Hodgkin's disease and other lymphomas. J Immunol 1962;89:555-8.
16. Kniker WT, Anderson CT, McBryde JL, Roumiantzeff M, Lesourd B. Multitest CMI for standardized measurement of delayed cutaneous hypersensitivity and cell-mediated immunity. Normal values and proposed scoring system for healthy adults in the U.S.A. Ann Allergy 1984;52:75-81.
17. Grimsley G. The significance of tests of cell-mediated immunity: an evaluation of the utility of tests used for the assessment of cell-mediated immunity [Thesis]. Western Australia: The University of Western Australia, 1987:1-194.

LYMPHOKINES

The effects of helper/induced T cells are mediated by a set of polypeptides known as lymphokines, each of which seems to have multiple functions (pleiotropy) and some of which mediate the same or very similar function in a very redundant fashion (cf. 1 for review). T cell lines (T_{H1} and T_{H2}) that produce distinctive populations of lymphokines include T_{H1} cells that produce IL-2, IFN γ and lymphotoxin as well as T_{H2} cells which produce IL-4, IL-5 and IL-6. Both T_{H1} and T_{H2} produce IL-3 and GM-CSF. Whether T_{H1} and T_{H2} cells exist among normal populations of T cells is not established for mouse cells, much less for human cells. Nevertheless, the putative distinction is helpful in identifying products which are probably important in allergic and anti-parasite inflammatory responses (e.g., IL-3, IL-4 and IL-5) and T_{H1}-like products (IL-2 and IFNγ) which may be protective against obligatory intracellular organisms. See also **COLONY STIMULATING FACTORS, INTERFERONS, INTERLEUKINS** and **PEPTIDE REGULATORY FACTORS.**

REFERENCES:
1. Paul WE. Pleiotropy and redundancy: T cell-derived lymphokines in the immune response. Cell 1989;57:521-4.

MACROPHAGE INFLAMMATORY PROTEINS (MIPs)

MIP-1 and MIP-2 are prototypic members of two families of structurally related cytokines.[1] The effects of MIP-1, which is produced by macrophages after stimulation with endotoxin as well as by activated T cells and fibroblasts, are largely unknown, except that MIP-1 is probably an important negative regulator [i.e., a chalone (cf. 2)] of hematopoietic stem cell proliferation.[3-5] MIP-2, which is also produced by endotoxin-stimulated macrophages, is a member of the platelet factor 4 (PF4) family which includes PF4 and β-thromboglobulin and perhaps neutrophil activating factor/peptide (IL-8). Members of the MIP-2 family have effects on fibroblasts, hematopoietic cells, neutrophils and melanoma cells.[1] See also **CYTOKINES, IL-8** and **PEPTIDE REGULATORY FACTORS.**

REFERENCES:
1. Wolpe SD, Cerami A. Macrophage inflammatory proteins 1 and 2: members of a novel superfamily of cytokines. FASEB J 1989;3:2565-73.
2. Iversen OH. The chalones. In: Baserga R, ed. Tissue growth factors. New York: Springer-Verlag, 1981:491-550.
3. Wright EG, Sheridan P, Moore MA. An inhibitor of murine stem cell proliferation produced by normal human bone marrow. Leuk Res 1980;4:309-14.
4. Graham GJ, Wright EG, Hewick R, et al. Identification and characterization of an inhibitor of haemopoietic stem cell proliferation. Nature 1990;344:442-4.
5. Dexter TM, White H. Growth without inflation. Nature 1990;344:380-1.

MAJOR HISTOCOMPATIBILITY COMPLEX

The major histocompability complex (MHC), which occupies about 1% of human chromosome 6 on its short arm, includes about 3000 kb of DNA within which are the class I genes (including the highly polymorphic, classical genes, the products of which bind peptides for presentation to T cells as well as the E, F and G genes and their products which are not T cell restricting), class II genes (*HLA-DR, DQ, DP, DN* and *DO*) and class III genes (*Bf, C2, C4, TNF, HSP70* and *BAT2&3*), among others. Class II genes are centromeric to and class I genes are telomeric to a central interval of about 1000 kb (the MHC class III region). Examples of the approved nomenclature for HLA genes, their molecular characteristics, alleles and specificity are given below (cf. 1-3 for details of nomenclature).

NAME OF GENE	MOLECULAR CHARACTERISTICS	HLA ALLELES	HLA SPECIFICITY
HLA-A	Class I α chain	A*0101	A1
HLA-B	Class I α chain	B*2701 to B*2706	B27
HLA-DRA	DR α chain		
HLA-DRB1	DR β1 chain (DR1, DR3, DR4, DR5, etc.)	DR B1*0101	
HLA-DQA1	DQ α chain	DQA1*0101	
HLA-DQB1	DQ β chain	DQB1*0501	

The major function of the MHC gene products (class I are composed of a glycoprotein chain complexed with β_2-microglobulin, and class II are glycoprotein α/β heterodimers) is to bind and display peptides from foreign antigens to enable their recognition by T cells. Complexes of a specific peptide (e.g., viral peptides derived from cytoplasmic proteins of the infected cells) with class I molecules are recognized by specific receptors on CD8+ cytotoxic T cells with resultant death of cells presenting such complexes. Complexes of specific peptides (which are processed from internalized exogenous proteins) with class II molecules presented by B-cells, macrophages and other cells are recognized by and cause proliferation of CD4+ helper T cells. Only cells of similar MHC type can interact with each other, i.e., the processes are MHC restricted.[1-4] Current evidence,[5] however, points up the oversimplification of grouping antigens into two discrete categories,[4] i.e., the grouping of antigens as 1) non-replicating, exogenous entities that after endosomal processing are presented at the cell surface in association with class II molecules in preparation for CD4+ T cell activation (as required for antibody production or CD4+ class II-restricted cytotoxic T cells) or 2) as endogenously synthesized and processed proteins (e.g. viral peptides) that are presented with class I molecules as primers for CD8+ cytotoxic T cells (cf. 6 for review). Peptides are bound with high affinity not only by the complete class II α/β heterodimers, but also by monomers of the α and β chains.[7] Mice deficient in β_2-microglobulin lack CD4-8+ T cells.[8] The absence of the non-polymorphic invariant chain currently referred to as Ii causes altered expression of class II at the cell surface but does not greatly influence processing or presentation of intact antigen.[9]

Despite a prodigious amount of work relating the amino acid sequences of certain class II molecules to susceptibility to certain autoimmune diseases (e.g., non-aspartate at position 57 in the DQβ chain with susceptibility to IDDM in caucasians[10] but not Japanese[11] [cf. 12 for review]; HLA-DQw1.2 [one of the polymorphic forms of the DQβ molecule] with protection against IDDM;[13] DRβI [DR4-associated] and DQB1.3 [DRw6-associated] with pemphigus vulgaris;[14] a DPB2.1 allele with pauciarticular juvenile rheumatoid arthritis but not adult rheumatoid arthritis;[15] and DRB1 with adult rheumatoid arthritis),[16] the clinical utility of such associations has not been enhanced over the past ten years. In addition to alleles at one locus shown to be of importance to susceptibility (or resistance), alleles at other linked loci may have important roles.[17] The association of HLA-B27 with ankylosing spondylitis[18] and HLA-DR3/4 with IDDM[19] remains to be explained. The relationships of failure of tolerance to the trimolecular complex (MHC-Ag-TCR) were recently reviewed[20] and critiqued.[12] See also **BETA$_2$-MICROGLOBULIN** and **Mls (MINOR LYMPHOCYTE STIMULATING) ANTIGENS**.

REFERENCES:
1. WHO - HLA Nomenclature Committee. Nomenclature for factors of the HLA system, 1987. Vox Sang 1988;55:119-26.
2. Bodmer WF, Albert E, Bodmer JG, et al. Immunobiology of HLA. In: Dupont B, ed. Histocompatibility testing. New York: Springer Verlag, 1987:72-9.
3. Bodmer JG, Marsh SGE, Albert E. Nomenclature for factors of the HLA system, 1989. Immunol Today 1990;11:3-10.
4. Germain RN. The ins and outs of antigen processing and presentation. Nature 1986;322:687-9.
5. Takahashi H, Takeshita T, Morein B, et al. Induction of CD8+ cytotoxic T cells by immunization with purified HIV-1 envelope protein in ISCOMs. Nature 1990;344:873-5.
6. Bolognesi DP. Fresh pathways to follow. Nature 1990;344:818-9.
7. Rothenhäusler B, Dornmair K, McConnell HM. Specific binding of antigenic peptides to separate α and β chains of class II molecules of the major histocompatibility complex. Proc Natl Acad Sci USA 1990;87:352-4.
8. Zijlstra M, Bix M, Simister NE, et al. β2-microglobulin deficient mice lack CD4-8+ cytolytic T cells. Nature 1990;344:742-6.
9. Peterson M, Miller J. Invariant chain influences the immunological recognition of MHC class II molecules. Nature 1990;345:172-4.
10. Sinha AA, Brautbar C, Szafer F, et al. A newly characterized HLA DQ$_\beta$ allele associated with pemphigus vulgaris. Science 1988;239:1026-9.
11. Ikegami H, Tahara Y, Cha T, et al. Aspartic acid at position 57 of the HLA-DQβ chain is not protective against insulin-dependent diabetes mellitus in Japanese people. J Autoimmunity 1990;3:167-74.
12. Parham P. A diversity of diabetes. Nature 1990;345:662-4.
13. Baisch JM, Weeks T, Giles R, et al. Analysis of HLA-DQ genotypes and susceptibility in insulin-dependent diabetes mellitus. N Engl J Med 1990;322:1836-41.
14. Scharf SJ, Friedmann A, Brautbar C, et al. HLA class II allelic variation and susceptibility to pemphigus vulgaris. Proc Natl Acad Sci USA 1988;;85:3504-8.
15. Begovich AB, Bugawan TL, Nepom BS, et al. A specific HLA-DPβ allele is associated with pauci articular juvenile rheumatoid arthritis but not adult rheumatoid arthritis. Proc Natl Acad Sci USA 1989;86:9489-93.
16. Wordsworth BP, Lanchbury SS, Sakkas LI, et al. HLA-DR4 subtype frequencies in rheumatoid arthritis indicate that DRB1 is the major susceptibility locus within the HLA class II region. Proc Natl Acad Sci USA 1989;86:10049-53.
17. Segall M, Bach FH. HLA and disease. The perils of simplification [Editorial]. N Engl J Med 1990;322:1879-81.
18. Benjamin R, Parham P. Guilt by association: HLA-B27 and ankylosing spondylitis. Immunol Today 1990;11:137-42.
19. Tait BD. Genetic susceptibility to type I diabetes: a review. J Autoimmunity 1990;3:3-11.
20 Sinha AA, Lopez MT, McDevitt HO. Autoimmune diseases: the failure of self tolerance. Science 1990;248:1380-7.

MALIGNIN ANTIBODIES

Malignin is a 10 kd protein of 89 amino acids of which thirteen are glutamic acids and nine are aspartic acids. Anti-malignin antibodies are said to be elevated in cancer regardless of cell type, and the concentration of antibody is said to relate quantitatively to survival (cf. 1 for review). These studies by one group have not yet been independently confirmed.

REFERENCES:
1. Bogoch S, Bogoch ES, Iliescu VM. In vitro production of the general transformation antibody related to survival in human cancer patients: antimalignin antibody. Cancer Detect Prev 1988;12:313-20.

MANNAN-BINDING PROTEIN

Deficiency of mannan-binding protein (Man-BP) is associated with failure to opsonize bakers' yeast (*Saccharomyces cerevisiae*), but the high frequency (∿5-7%) of impaired opsonic function in normal populations shows that the putative relationship of Man-BP deficiency to recurrent infections, chronic diarrhea, otitis media or allergies will not be straightforward. Perhaps Man-BP will prove to be a risk factor for infection in infants ages 6-24 months (cf. 1 for review).

REFERENCES:
1. Super M, Thiel S, Lu J, et al. Association of low levels of Mannan-binding protein with a common defect of opsonisation. Lancet 1989;2:1236-9.

MEMBRANE ATTACK COMPLEX (SC5b-9)

Increased levels of serum SC5b-9 reflect accelerated production of the C5b-9 complex which binds to S-protein, an important inhibitor of the C5b-9 complex. Serum levels of SC5b-9 are a more sensitive measure of activity of SLE than are C4, C3 or CH50 (1; cf. 2 for review). Three distinctive concentration patterns of the terminal complement components are seen in idiopathic membranoproliferative glomerulonephritis (MPGN), and in acute postinfectious glomerulonephritis (APGN).[3] 1) Depression of C5 and all of the late complement components as well as C3 is seen in patients with MPGN type I (4, see 5 for diagnostic criteria for MPGN types I, II and III). 2) In acute postinfectious glomerulonephritis C3 and C5 are decreased but C6-C9 are within reference range. 3) In MPGN II C5-C9 are normal but C3 is decreased. In MPGN I the complement levels fall into pattern 1 or 3.[5] Plasma SC5b-9 and factor Ba may be better indices of activity of SLE than are C3 or C4.[6] Glomerular deposition of MAC and S-protein are found in about 75% of lupus membranous nephropathy (MN) and 50% of idiopathic MN.[7]

REFERENCES:
1. Falk RJ, Dalmasso AP, Kim Y, et al. Radioimmunoassay of the attack complex of complement in serum from patients with systemic lupus erythematosus. N Engl J Med 1985;312:1594-9.
2. Dalmasso AP. Complement in the pathophysiology and diagnosis of human diseases. CRC Crit Rev Clin Lab Sci 1986;24:123-83.
3. Tucker ES. Complement activation in autoimmune disease. J Clin Immunoassay 1984;7:310-20.
4. Clardy CW, Forristal J, Strife CF, West CD. Serum terminal complement component levels in hypocomplementemic glomerulonephritides. Clin Immunol Immunopathol 1989;50:307-20.
5. West CD, McAdams AJ. The chronic glomerulonephritides of childhood. Part II. J Pediatr 1978;93:167-76.
6. Petri M, Kolb W, Morrow P, Tamerius J. Association of complement activation tests with clinical measurement of lupus activity [Abstract]. Clin Res 1989;37(2):510A.
7. Lai KN, Lo STH, Mac-Moune Lai F. Immunohistochemical study of the membrane attack complex of complement and S-protein in idiopathic and secondary membranous nephropathy. Am J Pathol 1989;135:469-76.

MINOR LYMPHOCYTE STIMULATING (Mls) ANTIGENS

Mls antigens, which have been detected to date only in mice, can stimulate up to 10% of the murine T cell repertoire. The large range of the response, which resembles that seen with certain bacterial toxins, contrasts with the response of well less than 1% of all T cells to ordinary immunological stimuli.[1] The Mls "superantigens," like bacterial toxins, interact only with the β chain of the T cell receptor after binding to specific non-groove regions of MHC molecules. Presumably, the combination of bacterial toxin with MHC protein or Mls with MHC protein causes T cell activation, but how this might in turn cause immune suppression is unknown. Experiments employing Mls-mismatched mice are providing insight into mechanisms of anergy.[2]

REFERENCES:
1. Marrack P, Kappler J. The staphylococcal enterotoxins and their relatives. Science 1990;248:705-11.
2. Mueller DL. Do tolerant T cells exist? Nature 1989;339:513-6.

MITOCHONDRIAL ANTIBODIES

Anti-mitochondrial antibodies are found in 90-95% of patients with primary biliary cirrhosis (PBC). These IgG antibodies are directed against the E2 component (lipoate acetyltransferase) of the pyruvate dehydrogenase enzyme complex located at the inner mitochondrial membrane (M2) as well as against another protein present in E2 preparations (1-2; cf. 3 for review). AMA which do not react with M2 are found in other situations, including anti-M1 in syphilis, anti-M3 in pseudolupus, anti-M5 in undefined collagen diseases, anti-M6 in iproniazid-induced hepatitis, anti-M7 in cardiomyopathy and myocarditis, anti-M8 which may be a prognostic marker, and anti-M9 which is a marker for early PBC which also occurs in healthy family members (cf. 4 for review). The titer of AMA in PBC tends to correlate with disease progression.[5] AMA with titers of 1:40 or greater suggest PBC even in the absence of symptoms and the presence of a normal alkaline phosphatase.[6] AMA in low titers are common in chronic active hepatitis and their presence does not preclude response to corticosteroids.[7] AMA disappear in about 1 month after orthotopic liver transplantation[8] and decrease with cyclosporine treatment which may be useful in PBC.[9]

Approximately 3% of patients with PBC have scleroderma, usually of the CREST syndrome variety.[10] In addition, AMA reactive with M2 complex are found in some patients with CREST or diffuse scleroderma,[11] sometimes in the absence of overt liver disease. Scleroderma typically precedes PBC in those patients with both diseases.[11]

Four patients with mitochondrial antibodies, hepatic granulomas (4/4), lung granulomas (3/4), pulmonary signs and symptoms, some features of Sjögren syndrome, coeliac disease and mixed connective tissue disease (MCTD) suggest these problems sometimes form a continuum.[12]

Anti-nuclear antibodies specific for nuclear membrane are found in a subset of patients with PBC, including a few who are AMA-negative.[13,14] AMA are found in less than 1% of apparently healthy caucasoid adults.[15,16] AMA-positive sera react with antigens from mutants of gram-negative bacteria which are defective in polysaccharide synthesis;[17] enterobacterial antigens are found in CIC of patients with PBC.[18] Immunoblotting reveals PBC-specific AMA-reactive proteins in *E. coli* R-forms isolated from patients' stools.[19] See also **CENTROMERE ANTIBODIES.**

REFERENCES:
1. Yeaman SJ, Fussey SPM, Danner DJ, James OFW, Mutimer DJ, Bassendine MF. Primary biliary cirrhosis: identification of two major M2 mitochondrial autoantigens. Lancet 1988;1:1067-70.
2. Gershwin ME, Mackay IR, Sturgess A, Coppel RL. Identification and specificity of a cDNA encoding the 70 kd mitochondrial antigen recognized in primary biliary cirrhosis. J Immunol 1987;138:3525-31.
3. Kaplan MM. Primary biliary cirrhosis. N Engl J Med 1987;316:521-8.
4. Berg PA, Klein R. Immunology of primary biliary cirrhosis. Ballieres Clin Gastroenterol 1987;1:675-706.

5. Christensen E, Crowe J, Doniach D, et al. Clinical pattern and course of disease in primary biliary cirrhosis based on an analysis of 236 patients. Gastroenterology 1980;78:236-46.
6. Mitchison HC, Bassendine MF, Hendrick A, et al. Positive antimitochondrial antibody but normal alkaline phosphatase: is this primary biliary cirrhosis? Hepatology 1986;6:1279-84.
7. Kenny RP, Czaja AJ, Ludwig J, Dickson ER. Frequency and significance of antimitochondrial antibodies in severe chronic active hepatitis. Dig Dis Sci 1986;31:705-11.
8. Haagsma EB, Manns M, Klein R, et al. Subtypes of antimitochondrial antibodies in primary biliary cirrhosis before and after orthotopic liver transplantation. Hepatology 1987;7:129-33.
9. Wiesner RH, Ludwig J, Lindor KD, et al. A controlled trial of cyclosporine in the treatment of primary biliary cirrhosis. N Engl J Med 1990;322:1419-24.
10. van Venrooij WJ, Stapel SO, Houben H, et al. Scl-86, a marker antigen for diffuse scleroderma. J Clin Invest 1985;75:1053-60.
11. Fregeau DR, Leung PSC, Coppel RL, McNeilage LJ, Medsger TA Jr, Gershwin ME. Autoantibodies to mitochondria in systemic sclerosis. Arthritis Rheum 1988;31:386-92.
12. Fagan EA, Moore-Gillon JC, Turner-Warwick M. Multiorgan granulomas and mitochondrial antibodies. N Engl J Med 1983;308:572-75.
13. Ruffatti A, Arslan P, Floreani A, et al. Nuclear membrane-staining antinuclear antibody in patients with primary biliary cirrhosis. J Clin Immunol 1985;5:357-61.
14. Lassoued K, Guilly MN, Andre C, et al. Autoantibodies to 200 kd polypeptide(s) of the nuclear envelope: a new serologic marker of primary biliary cirrhosis. Clin Exp Immunol 1988;74:283-8.
15. Triger DR, Charlton CAC, Ward AM. What does the antimitochondrial antibody mean? Gut 1982;23:814-18.
16. Hawkins BR, O'Conner KJ, Dawkins RL, Dawkins B, Rodger B. Autoantibodies in an Australian population: I. Prevalence and persistence. J Clin Lab Immunol 1979;2:211-5.
17. Stemerowicz R, Hopf U, Möller B, et al. Are antimitochondrial antibodies in primary biliary cirrhosis induced by R (rough)-mutants of enterobacteriaceae? Lancet 1988;2:1166-70.
18. Stemerowicz R, Möller B, Küther D, et al. Are antigenic components of circulating immune complexes (CIC) in primary biliary cirrhosis (PBC) of enterobacterial origin? J Hepatol 1989;8(Suppl 1):S231.
19. Hopf U, Möller B, Stemerowicz R, et al. Relation between Escherichia coli R(rough)-forms in gut, lipid in liver, and primary biliary cirrhosis. Lancet 1989;2:1419-22.

MOLECULAR MIMICRY

That amino acid sequences common to a microbial (or other non-self) molecule and a host protein result in an immunologic response with subsequent cross-reaction with self determinants is the basis of the molecular mimicry hypothesis (cf. 1 and 2 for review). Examples of such cross-reactions of potential importance to human diseases include adenovirus 12 Elb protein and coeliac disease,[3] components of certain streptococci and rheumatic heart disease,[4,5] a nitrogenase of *Klebsiella pneumoniae* and ankylosing spondylitis[6] and a peptide common to herpes simplex virus and the acetylcholine receptor in patients with myasthenia gravis of whom a small proportion have antibodies to this peptide.[7]

REFERENCES:
1. Oldstone MBA. Molecular mimicry and autoimmune disease. Cell 1987;50:819-20.
2. Dyrberg T, Oldstone MBA. Peptides as probes to study molecular mimicry and virus induced autoimmunity. Curr Top Microbiol Immunol 1986;130:25-37.
3. Kagnoff MF, Austin RK, Hubert JJ, et al. Possible role for a human adenovirus in the pathogenesis of celiac disease. J Exp Med 1984;160:1544-7.
4. Dale JB, Beachey EH. Epitopes of streptococcal M proteins shared with cardiac myosin. J Exp Med 1985;162:583-91.
5. Krisher K, Cunningham M. Myosin: a link between streptococci and heart. Science 1985;227:413-5.

6. Schwimmbeck PL, Yu DTY, Oldstone MBA. Autoantibodies to HLA B27 in the sera of HLA B27 patients with ankylosing spondylitis and Reiter's syndrome: molecular mimicry with *Klebsiella pneumoniae* as potential mechanism of autoimmune disease. J Exp Med 1987;166:173-81.
7. Schwimmbeck PL, Dyrberg T, Drachman DB, Oldstone MBA. Molecular mimicry and myasthenia gravis. an autoantigenic site of the acetylcholine receptor α-subunit that has biologic activity and reacts immunochemically with herpes simplex virus. J Clin Invest 1989;84:1174-80.

MONOCLONAL IMMUNOGLOBULIN DEPOSITION DISEASE

Mononuclear immunoglobulin deposition diseases, characterized by deposits of monotypic light or heavy chains, can be fibrillar and Congo Red binding, as in light chain amyloidosis, or nonfibrillar as in light or light and heavy chain deposition diseases, which lack amyloid P component. Patients with MIDD usually present with albuminuria, hypogammaglobulinemia, azotemia, nephropathy or cardiomyopathy whether accompanied by multiple myeloma or other neoplastic plasma cell proliferation or not. Mononuclear serum or urine proteins or marrow plasmacytosis of restricted clonality occur in 80% or more of such patients (cf. 1 for review). See also **AMYLOID.**

REFERENCES:
1. Buxbaum JN, Chuba JV, Hellman GC, et al. Monoclonal immunoglobulin deposition disease: light chain and light and heavy chain deposition diseases and their relation to light chain amyloidosis. Clinical features, immunopathology, and molecular analysis. Ann Intern Med 1990;112:455-64.

MOUSE IMMUNOGLOBULIN ANTIBODIES

Human antibodies to mouse immunoglobulins can cause falsely elevated results in immunoassays that employ mouse antibodies.[1,2] AMIA, sometimes with anti-Id-like activities, are produced in response to repeated infusions of mouse monoclonal antibodies to CD2 or CD4 for immune suppression.[3] Monitoring for anti-mouse Ig antibodies is increasingly used in transplantation medicine.[4]

REFERENCES:
1. McCarthy RC, Ryan FJ, McKenzie CM. Interference in immunoenzymometric assays caused by IgM anti-mouse IgG antibodies. Arch Pathol Lab Med 1988;112:901-7.
2. Csako G, Weintraub BD, Zweig MH. The potency of immunoglobulin G fragments for inhibition of interference caused by anti-immunoglobulin antibodies in a monoclonal immunoradiometric assay for thyrotropin. Clin Chem 1988;34:1481-3.
3. Hafler DA, Ritz J, Schlossman SF, Weiner HL. Anti-CD4 and anti-CD2 monoclonal antibody infusions in subjects with multiple sclerosis: immunosuppressive effects and human anti-mouse responses. J Immunol 1988;141:131-8.
4. Shawler DL, McCallister TJ, Sobol RE, Dillman RO. Serologic and cellular assays to monitor therapy with murine monoclonal antibodies. J Clin Lab Analysis 1987;1:184-90.

MYELIN ANTIBODIES

The measurement of AMyA which are reactive with peripheral nerve myelin is of no clinical utility, because their frequency (17%) in patients with peripheral neuropathy, in the absence of a monoclonal immunoglobulin, is essentially identical (16%) to that found in normals.[1] Antibodies to myelin basic protein may or may not be elevated in CSF of patients with multiple sclerosis.[2,3] Anti-peripheral nerve myelin antibodies are said to occur early in Guillain-Barré syndrome;[4] the correlation of complement fixing antibodies to peripheral nerve myelin (PNM) and tissue-damaging C5b-9 complex suggests that PNM might serve as the target for antibody-mediated complement damage in Guillain-Barré syndrome.[5]

REFERENCES:
1. Cruz M, Ernerudh J, Olsson T, HNjeberg B, Link H. Occurrence and isotype of antibodies against peripheral nerve myelin in serum from patients with peripheral neuropathy and healthy controls. J Neurol Neurosurg Psychiatry 1988;51:820-5.

2. Matsiota P, Blancher A, Doyon B, et al. Comparative study of natural autoantibodies in the serum and cerebrospinal fluid of normal individuals and patients with multiple sclerosis and other neurological diseases. Ann Inst Pasteur Immunol 1988;139:99-108.
3. Warren KG, Catz I, Bauer C. Cerebrospinal fluid antibodies to myelin basic protein in acute idiopathic optic neuritis. Ann Neurol 1988;23:297-9.
4. Koski CL, Gratz E, Sutherland J, Mayer RF. Clinical correlation with anti-peripheral-nerve myelin antibodies in Guillain-Barré syndrome. Ann Neurol 1986;19:573-7.
5. Koski CL, Sanders ME, Swoveland PT, et al. Activation of terminal components of complement in patients with Guillain-Barré syndrome and other demyelinating neuropathies. J Clin Invest 1987;80:1492-7.

MYELIN-ASSOCIATED GLYCOPROTEIN (MAG)

Myelin-associated glycoprotein (MAG), a glycoprotein component of the myelin of central and peripheral nervous systems, is present in the periaxonal region, Schmidt-Lantermann incisures, lateral loops and outer mesaxon of the myelin sheath.[1] Due to the difficulties in obtaining sufficient pure MAG from human nerve tissue, a cross-reacting antigen SGPG (sulfate-3-glucoronyl paragloboside) is commonly used as a substitute for MAG in an immunoassay system.[2]

IgM anti-MAG antibodies are detected in some patients with inflammatory neuropathies such as Guillain-Barré syndrome, chronic inflammatory neuropathy,[2,3] IgM paraproteinemias with peripheral neuropathy,[2,4] multiple sclerosis, myasthenia gravis and systemic lupus erythematosus.[3,5] Low titers of anti-MAG antibodies are also detected in some normal individuals.[5] The clinical utility of anti-MAG antibodies assay is undefined.

REFERENCES:
1. Latov N. Neuropathic syndromes associated with autoreactive IgM antibodies. Neurology 1989;I:2-4.
2. Quarles RH, Ilyas AA, Willison HJ. Antibodies to glycolipids in demyelinating diseases of the human peripheral nervous system. Ann Neurol 1990;27:S48-52.
3. Sato S, Baba H, Inuzuka T, Miyatake T. Anti-myelin-associated glycoprptein antibody in sera from patients with demyelinating diseases. Acta Neurol Scand 1986;74:115-20.
4. Murray N, Page N, Steck AJ. The human anti-myelin-associated glycoprotein IgM system. Ann Neurol 1986;19:473-8.
5. McGinnis S, Kohriyama T, Yu RK, et al. Antibodies to sulfated glucoronic acid containing glycosphingolipids in neuropathy associated with anti-MAG antibodies and in normal subjects. J Neuroimmunol 1988;17:119-26.

MYELIN BASIC PROTEIN

Myelin basic protein (MBP) and proteolytic fragments of MBP are found in the CSF and urine of patients with MS.[1,2] The test is not entirely specific for MS but may be positive in some degree in any disease with major demyelination. This would include transverse myelitis, optic neuritis and other diseases where there is major destruction of myelin but in which demyelination is not the primary process, e.g., radiation or chemotherapy of neoplasms in or near the CNS.[3,4] The presence of activated T cells responsive to MBP in the CSF of MS patients is now recognized as an important concomitant of demyelination. Whether MBP-reactive T cells contribute to demyelination or arise as a secondary phenomenon in response to myelin breakdown products is yet to be determined.[5] Careful studies showed only minor increases in MBP-induced lymphoproliferation in vitro in patients with MS compared with controls[6] (see 5 and 7 for review). A decapeptide within the 69-89 aa sequence is the relevant antigenic epitope of human MBP.[8] Use of antisera capable of recognizing epitopes present in the carboxyl half of a MBP peptide (69-89 aa) in a competitive inhibition immunoassay provides high sensitivity (upper limits of normal = 0.16 ng/ml) for detection of MBP-like fragments in CSF of about 80% of patients with acute MS and 40% of chronic progressive MS but very few patients with stable MS.[8] Due to normal protein turnover, MBP-like peptides are detected at a low level in unconcentrated urine of nondiseased individuals. However, the concentration of MBP-like peptides is much higher in the urine of MS patients, but further chemical characterization of the MBP-like material in urine is needed before clinical utility can be evaluated. Detection of MBP and MBP fragments is appropriate for following the course of demyelinating diseases because values fluctuate with disease activity[1,4,9] and therapy.[10] High values indicate active demyelination as seen in MS, SSPE and radiation damage. A result greater than 4 ng/ml of CSF is highly suggestive of a rapid rate of myelin degradation as in a recent exacerbation of MS. Results of 1-3 ng/ml are consistent with a slower rate of myelin degradation or with recovery from an acute flare of demyelination. Levels of 1-3 ng/ml are seen in patients with MS whose acute attack is greater than one week old and in some patients with chronic, active MS. Less than 5% of patients with inactive MS will have values in the greater than 1 ng/ml range. Results less than 1 ng/ml indicate a lack of rapid demyelination[11] (see 7, 12, 13 for review). Turbidity of CSF may cause spurious elevation of MBP but not in the second generation assay developed at SLI. New diagnostic criteria for MS, including laboratory features (oligoclonal immunoglobulins or increased synthesis of IgG) are available.[14] Treatment of animals with peptide analogues of MBP or with peptides from shared epitopes of the relevant T cell receptors prevents experimental allergic encephalomyelitis, an animal model of multiple sclerosis (cf. 15 and 16 for review). Some clones of somatically mutated T cells isolated from peripheral blood of patients with chronic progressive MS (but not relapsing remitting MS) react with MBP[17] (cf. 18 for review of method for monitoring humans for somatic cell mutations that occur spontaneously or after exposure to environmental mitogens); DR2+ patients with relapsing-remitting MS have increased numbers of T cells reactive with an immunodominant peptide (amino acids 84-102) of MBP.[19] The shared usage of TCR V_β genes for recognition of immunodominant regions of MBP by T cells from MS patients promises insights into the mechanisms of and possible therapies for MS.[20] See also GENE REARRANGEMENTS.

REFERENCES:
1. Whitaker JN. Myelin encephalitogenic protein fragments in cerebrospinal fluid of persons with multiple sclerosis. Neurology 1977;27:911-20.
2. Whitaker JN. The antigenic reactivity of small fragments derived from human myelin basic protein peptide 43-88. J Immunol 1982;129:2729-33.
3. Gerson B, Cohen SR, Gerson IM, Guest GH. Myelin basic protein, oligoclonal bands, and IgG in cerebrospinal fluid as indicators of multiple sclerosis. Clin Chem 1981;27:1974-7.
4. Cohen SR, Brooks BR, Herndon RM, McKhann GM. A diagnostic index of active demyelination: myelin basic protein in cerebrospinal fluid. Ann Neurol 1980;8:25-31.
5. Calder V, Owen S, Watson C, et al. MS: a localized immune disease of the central nervous system. Immunol Today 1989;10:99-103.
6. Johnson D, Hafler DA, Fallis RJ, et al. Cell-mediated immunity to myelin-associated glycoprotein, proteolipid protein, and myelin basic protein in multiple sclerosis. J Neuroimmunol 1986;13:99-108.
7. Hafler DA, Weiner HL. MS: a CNS and systemic autoimmune disease. Immunology Today 1989;10:104-8.
8. Whitaker JN, Herman PK. Human myelin basic protein peptide 69-89: immunochemical features and use in immunoassays of cerebrospinal fluid. J Neuroimmunol 1988;19:47-57.
9. Whitaker JN. The presence of immunoreactive myelin basic protein peptide in urine of persons with multiple sclerosis. Ann Neurol 1987;22:648-55.
10. Lamers KJB, Uitdehaag BMJ, Hommes OR, et al. The short-term effect of an immunosuppressive treatment on CSF myelin basic protein in chronic progressive multiple sclerosis. J Neurol Neurosurg Psychiatry 1988;51:1334-7.
11. Thompson AJ, Brazil J, Feighery C, et al. CSF myelin basic protein in multiple sclerosis. Acta Neurol Scand 1985;72:577-83.
12. Thompson AJ, Brazil J, Hutchinson M, Feighery C. Three possible laboratory indexes of disease activity in multiple sclerosis. Neurology 1987;37:515-9.
13. McFarland HF, Dhib-Jalbut S. Multiple sclerosis: possible immunological mechanisms. Clin Immunol Immunopathol 1989;50:S96-S105.
14. Poser CM, Paty DW, Scheinberg L, et al. New diagnostic criteria for multiple sclerosis: guidelines for research protocols. Ann Neurol 1983;13:227-31.
15. Janeway CA. Immunotherapy by peptides? Nature 1989;341:482-3.
16. Wraith DC, McDevitt HO, Steinman L, Acha-Orbea H. T cell recognition as the target for immune intervention in autoimmune disease. Cell 1989;57:709-15.
17. Allegretta M, Nicklas JA, Sriram S, Albertini RJ. T cells responsive to myelin basic protein in patients with multiple sclerosis. Science 1990;247:718-21.
18. O'Neill JP, Sullivan LM, Booker JK, et al. Longitudal study of the in vivo hprt mutant frequency in human T-lymphocytes as determined by a cell cloning assay. Environ Mol Mutagen 1989;13:289-93.

19. Ota K, Matsui M, Milford EL, et al. T-cell recognition of an immunodominant myelin basic protein epitope in multiple sclerosis. Nature 1990;346:183-7.
20. Wucherpfennig KW, Ota K, Endo N, et al. Shared human T cell receptor V_β usage to immunodominant regions of myelin basic protein. Science 1990;248:1016-9.

MYOCARDIAL ANTIBODIES

Anti-myocardial antibodies (AMyA) are found in a variety of patterns in a number of clinical conditions,[1] including Dressler syndrome.[2,3] The titer of these antibodies also rises in approximately 66% of patients with coronary artery bypass and need not be related to postcardiotomy syndrome.[2] AMyA, largely with sarcolemmal, intermyofibrillar or myofibrillar patterns, are found in most patients with acute rheumatic fever (4,5; cf. 6 for review). See also **ENDOTHELIAL CELL ANTIBODIES.**

REFERENCES:
1. Nicholson GC, Dawkins RL, McDonald BL, Wetherall JD. A classification of anti-heart antibodies: differentiation between heart-specific and heterophile antibodies. Clin Immunol Immunopathol 1977;7:349-63.
2. Baker JR Jr, Cohen DJ, Head HD, DeShong JL, Graeber GM. Development of circulating antiheart antibodies as a result of coronary bypass surgery. Ann Thorac Surg 1986;41:507-10.
3. Engle MA. Humoral immunity and heart disease: postpericardiotomy syndrome. Clin Immunol Newsletter 1982;3:155-8.
4. Kaplan MH, Meyeresian M, Kushner I. Immunologic studies of heart tissue: IV. serologic reactions with human heart tissue as revealed by immunofluorescent methods: isoimmune, Wassermann, and autoimmune reactions. J Exp Med 1961;113:17-35.
5. Kaplan MH, Frengley JD. Autoimmunity to the heart in cardiac disease: current concepts of the relation of autoimmunity to rheumatic fever, postcardiotomy and postinfarction syndromes and cardiomyopathies. Am J Cardiol 1969;24:459-73.
6. Zabriskie JB, Friedman JE. The role of heart binding antibodies in rheumatic fever. Adv Exp Med Biol 1983;161:457-70.

NATURAL AUTOANTIBODIES

These antibodies, also known as "polyreactive antibodies", are usually low-affinity IgM and are produced by $CD5^+B$ cells, which represent 10-25% of circulating B lymphocytes in normals, 27-52% in RA and less than 25% in SLE (cf. 1 and 2 for review). Assay conditions which favor detection of low-affinity antibodies are expected to show an enormous number of cross-reactions between decavalent IgM antibodies and seemingly unrelated antigens, but such cross-reactions are likely irrelevant to *in vivo* conditions under which antigens bind to bivalent IgM on surfaces of B cells (cf. 3). Natural autoantibodies, although sometimes reactive with the same antigens, differ from autoantibodies produced by $CD5^-$ B cells, which are usually monoreactive and high affinity and are typically detectable only in autoimmune individuals.[1-3]

In general, monoreactive high-affinity IgG or IgA antibodies use a restricted number of VH gene segments and are not derived from the same $CD5^+$ cells as are polyreactive low-affinity IgM antibodies which use an assortment of VH gene segments.[4]

REFERENCES:
1. Casali P, Notkins AL. CD^+ B lymphocytes, polyreactive antibodies and the human B-cell repertoire. Immunol Today 1989;10:364-8.
2. van Rooijen N. Are bacterial endotoxins involved in autoimmunity by $CD5^+$ (Ly-1^+) B cells? Immunol Today 1989;10:334-6.
3. Nossal GJV. Immunologic tolerance: collaboration between antigen and lymphokines. Science 1989;245:147-53.
4. Ueki Y, Goldfard IS, Harindranath N, et al. Clonal analysis of a human antibody response. J Exper Med 1990;171:19-34.

NATURAL KILLER CELLS

These $CD3^-NKH1^+CD16^+$ large granular lymphocytes, which constitute about 15% of total circulating lymphocytes, mediate natural immunity, are not MHC restricted and can kill tumor cells and virus-infected cells, including those lacking MHC glycoproteins. Abnormalities of activity and/or absolute numbers of natural killer (NK) cells are reported in AIDS and several other viral infections, autoimmune diseases, cancer, chronic fatigue syndrome, depression and certain immunodeficiencies (cf. 1 for review). In no case, however, can measurement of NK numbers or function be considered clinically useful at this time; this includes evaluation of the chronic fatigue syndrome.

REFERENCES:
1. Whiteside TL, Herberman RB. Short analytical review. The role of natural killer cells in human disease. Clin Immunol Immunopathol 1989;53:1-23.

NEOPTERINS

Increased concentrations of neopterins in urine are found in hyperphenylalaninemia and in conditions with activated cellular immunity.[1-3] Among these conditions are a variety of bacterial, viral and protozoal infections (including AIDS,[4] tuberculosis,[5] and malaria[6]), tumors,[7] graft-versus-host disease,[8] inflammatory bowel disease[9,10] and autoimmune disease.[11-14] Levels of neopterins can be measured in plasma, CSF, synovial fluid and urine. The exact clinical utility of quantitation of neopterins is not yet clearly defined,[13] but urinary neopterin may be of use in monitoring HIV infection.[15]

REFERENCES:
1. Anonymous. Neopterins in clinical medicine [Editorial]. Lancet 1988;1:509-11.
2. Rokos H, Frisius H, Kunze R. Neopterin and dihydroneopterin in serum of control and patients with various diseases. Circadian rhythms of neopterin. Influence of cortisol? In: Cooper BA, Whitehead VM, eds. Chemistry and biology of pteridines. Berlin: Walter de Gruyter, 1986:411-4.
3. Bagasra O, Fitzharris JW, Bagasra TR. Neopterin: an early marker of development of pre-AIDS conditions in HIV-seropositive individuals. Clin Immunol Newsletter 1988;9:197-9.
4. Wachter H, Fuchs D, Hausen A, Reibnegger G, Werner ER, Dierich MP. Who will get AIDS? [Letter]. Lancet 1986;2:1216-7.
5. Fuchs D, Hausen A, Kofler M, Kosanowski H, Reibnegger G, Wachter H. Neopterin as an index of immune response in patients with tuberculosis. Lung 1984;162:337-46.
6. Schutzhard E, Fuchs D, Hausen A, Reibnegger G, Wachter H. Neopterin ein neuer parameter in der malariadiagnostik? Mit Oster Tropenmed Parasitol 1985;72:63-70.
7. Reibnegger GJ, Bichler AH, Dapunt O, et al. Neopterin as a prognostic indicator in patients with carcinoma of the uterine cervix. Cancer Res 1986;46:950-5.
8. Niederwieser D, Huber C, Gratwohl A, et al. Neopterin as a new biochemical marker in the clinical monitoring of bone marrow transplant recipients. Transplantation 1984;38:497-500.
9. Prior Ch, Bollbach R, Fuchs D, et al. Urinary neopterin, a marker of clinical activity in patients with Crohn's disease. Clin Chim Acta 1986;155:11-22.
10. Niederwieser D, Fuchs D, Hausen A, et al. Neopterin as a new biochemical marker in the clinical assessment of ulcerative colitis. Immunobiology 1985;170:320-6.
11. Fuchs D, Granditsch G, Hausen A, Reibnegger G, Wachter H. Urinary neopterin excretion in coeliac disease [Letter]. Lancet 1983;2:463-4.
12. Reibnegger G, Egg D, Fuchs D, et al. Urinary neopterin reflects clinical activity in patients with rheumatoid arthritis. Arthritis Rheum 1986;29:1063-70.
13. Peter JB, Agopian MS, Clements PJ, Telian NS, Furst DE. Elevated serum levels of interleukin-2 receptor (IL-2R) and IL-2 in diffuse (DS) and limited scleroderma (LS) [Abstract]. Arthritis Rheum 1989;32(Suppl 4):S77.
14. Krause A, Protz H, Goebel KM. Correlation between synovial neopterin and inflammatory activity in rheumatoid arthritis. Ann Rhem Dis 1989;48:636-40.
15. Fuchs D, Banekovich M, Hausen A, et al. Neopterin estimation compared with the ratio of T-cell subpopulations in persons infected with human immunodeficiency virus-1. Clin Chem 1988;34:2415-7.

NEURONAL ANTIBODIES

Anti-neuronal antibodies, which react with human neuroblastoma cell lines, were increased in the CSF of approximately 74% of the patients with neuropsychiatric SLE (NP-SLE) and in approximately 11% of SLE patients without NP manifestations, but serum levels in these two groups were similar in some studies,[1] but were elevated in serum of NP-SLE in other studies.[2,3] There is agreement that anti-neuronal antibodies are especially common (up to 90%) in SLE patients with cognitive impairment or non-focal NP-SLE.[3-5] As expected, sera containing these antibodies react with a variety of proteins.[6] Anti-neuronal antibodies in CSF of patients with NP-SLE are found only in the presence of serum anti-neuronal antibodies and probably reflect, at least in part, an increased permeability of the blood-brain barrier in CNS lupus.[3,7,8] At a minimum, studies showing increased intra-blood-brain-barrier synthesis of anti-neuronal antibodies are critical for evaluation of the potential pathogenetic significance of these antibodies for neuropsychiatric for NP-SLE, but these are not yet available. See also **RIBOSOMAL P PROTEIN ANTIBODIES.**

REFERENCES:
1. Bluestein HG, Williams GW, Steinberg AD. Cerebrospinal fluid antibodies to neuronal cells: association with neuropsychiatric manifestations of systemic lupus erythematosus. Am J Med 1981;70:240-6.
2. How A, Dent PB, Liao S-K, Denburg JA. Antineuronal antibodies in neuropsychiatric systemic lupus erythematosus. Arthritis Rheum 1985;28:789-95.
3. Nai-Zheng Z, Zheng CW. Antineuronal antibodies in Chinese patients with neuropsychiatric systemic lupus erythematosus (NP-SLE). Proceedings of the second international conference on systemic lupus erythematosus. Singapore: Professional Postgraduate Services, K.K., 1989;109-11.
4. Denburg JA, Carbotte RM, Denburg SD. Neuronal antibodies and cognitive function in systemic lupus erythematosus. Neurology 1987;37:464-7.
5. Bluestein HG. Neuropsychiatric manifestations of systemic lupus erythematosus. N Engl J Med 1987;317:309-11.
6. Hanly JG, Rajaraman S, Behmann S, Denburg JA. A novel neuronal antigen identified by sera from patients with systemic lupus erythematosus. Arthritis Rheum 1988;31:1492-9.
7. Kelly MC, Denburg JA. Cerebrospinal fluid immunoglobulins and neuronal antibodies in neuropsychiatric systemic lupus erythematosus and related conditions. J Rheumatol 1987;14:740-4.
8. Winfield JB, Shaw M, Silverman LM, Eisenberg RA, Wilson HA III. Intrathecal IgG synthesis and blood-brain barrier impairment in patients with systemic lupus erythematosus and central nervous system dysfunction. Am J Med 1983;74:837-44.

NEUROPEPTIDES

With the exceptions of angiotensins and bradykinin which are liberated extracellularly, neuropeptides (unlike peptide regulatory factors) are processed intracellularly from larger precursors and are stored in specialized neuronal vesicles. In addition, neuropeptides activate intracellular second messages via G-protein-coupled receptors with 7 transmembrane segments in contrast to the single-transmembrane-segment growth factor receptors which activate tyrosine kinases, among other probable mechanisms.[1] Neuropeptide Y, a 36-amino acid peptide with a sequence similar to pancreatic polypeptide and peptide YY,[2] is readily measured in serum and CSF[3] and is known to be increased in plasma of some patients with pheochromocytoma and neuroblastoma (cf. 3). Although a potent vasoconstrictor, NPY levels are not abnormal in hypertension. A member of the mammalian tachykinin family[4] which includes neurokinins A and B and neuropeptides K and γ, substance P (SP) is an 11-amino acid transmitter of nociception with excitatory effects on central and peripheral neurones (cf. 5). SP also affects chemotaxis and phagocytosis by neutrophils, histamine release by mast cells, T-cell activation as well as B-cell maturation (cf. 6) and is increased in RA, OA and Reiter syndrome in synovial fluid and especially in posttrauma effusions.[7] Conditions modulating the expression of the recently cloned SP receptor[5] will be of clinical interest. Although SP is reported to be increased in CSF, but not plasma in fibromyalgia,[8,9] the differences are small and the clinical relevance is suspect, as is also the case with reported elevations of plasma dopamine and PGE.[10] Beta-endorphin and calcitonin gene-related peptides (which are both pain-modulatory neuropeptides) are normal in CSF in fibrositis.[11,12] Assays for a wide variety of neuropeptides are now available for research, but at present none answer clinically important questions. See also **PEPTIDE REGULATORY FACTORS** and **SUBSTANCE P.**

REFERENCES:
1. Hanley MR. Peptide regulatory factors in the nervous system. Lancet 1989;2:1373-6.
2. Tatemotor K. Neuropeptide Y: complete amino acid sequence of the brain peptide. Proc Natl Acad Sci USA 1982;79:5485-9.
3. Stridsberg M, Lundquist G. Radioimmunoassay of neuropeptide Y (NPY) in biological fluids. Circulating NPY levels depend on renal function. Clin Chim Acta 1989;185:61-72.
4. Erspamer V. The tachykinin peptide family. Trends Neurosci 1981;4:267-9.
5. Hershey AD, Krause JE. Molecular characterization of a functional cDNA encoding the rat substance P receptor. Science 1990;247:958-62.
6. Lotz N, Carson DA, Vaughan JH. Effect of neuropeptides on production of inflammatory cytokines by human monocytes. Science 1988;241:1218-21.
7. Marshall KW, Chiu B, Inman RD. Substance P and arthritis: analysis of plasma and synovial fluid levels. Arthritis Rheum 1990;33:87-90.
8. Reynolds WJ, Chiu B, Inman RD. Plasma substance P levels in fibrositis. J Rheumatol 1988;15:1802-3.
9. Vaeroy H, Helle R, Ferre O, et al. Elevated CSF levels of substance P and high incidence of Raynaud phenomenon in patients with fibromyalgia: new features for diagnosis. Pain 1988;32:21-6.
10. Hamaty D, Valentine JL, Howard R, et al. The plasma endorphin, prostaglandin and catecholamine profile of patients with fibrositis treated with cyclobenzaprine and placebo: a 5-month study. J Rheumatol 1989;19:164-8.
11. Vaeroy H, Helle R, Ferre O, et al. Cerebrospinal fluid levels of beta-endorphin in patients with fibromyalgia (fibrositis syndrome). J Rheumatol 1988;15:1804-6.
12. Vaeroy H, Sakurada T, Ferre O, et al. Modulation of pain in fibromyalgia (fibrositis syndrome): cerebrospinal fluid (CSF) investigation of pain related neuropeptides with special reference to calcitonin gene related peptide (CGRP). J Rheumatol 1989;19:94-7.

NEUROTROPHIC FACTORS

Neurotrophic factors, including ciliary neurotrophic factor (CNTF), nerve growth factor (NGF), brain-derived neurotrophic factor and neurotrophin-3 are in early stages of characterization.[1-4] NGF induces growth and differentiation of human B lymphocytes and IgM secretion.[5] Assays have not been applied to clinical materials. See also **NEUROPEPTIDES.**

REFERENCES:
1. Davies AM. The emerging generality of the neurotrophic hypothesis. Trends Neurosci 1988;11:234-4.
2. Hanley MR. Peptide regulatory factors in the nervous system. Lancet 1989;1:1373-6.
3. Lin L-FH, Mismer D, Lile JD, et al. Purification, cloning, and expression of ciliary neurotrophic factor (CNTF). Science 1989;246:1023-5.
4. Maisonpierre PC, Belluscio L, Squinto S, et al. Neurotrophin-3: a neurotrophic factor related to NGF and BDNF. Science 1990;247-1446-51.
5. Otten U, Ehrhard P, Peck R. Nerve growth factor induces growth and differentiation of human B lymphocytes. Proc Natl Acad Sci USA 1989;86:10059-63.

NEUTROPHIL CYTOPLASM ANTIBODIES

Detectable by their reaction with fixed neutrophils, anti-neutrophil cytoplasm antibodies (ANCA), which are also known as anti-cytoplasmic antibodies (ACPA), are present in 84-100% of patients with generalized active Wegener granulomatosis.[1-6] Positive results are also obtained in patients with microscopic polyarteritis, which may or may not be a variant of WG (cf. 7 for review of this problem). The amount of serum ANCA can best be quantified by flow cytometry (which allows accuracy and precision based on a standard curve and a working international standard)[8] combined with indirect fluorescent antibody (IFA) microscopy. This allows precise localization of the antibody reactivity in cytoplasm.[4] The amount of antibody parallels disease activity.[4-6] Antibody levels often decline to a nadir somewhat above the upper limits of normal in asymptomatic patients after treatment.[4,5] Anti-myeloperoxidase antibodies, which are a variety of ANCA giving a perinuclear staining pattern [P-ANCA as opposed to the diffuse cytoplasmic pattern (C-ANCA)] are associated not with classical Wegener granulomatosis but with pauci-immune glomerulonephritis.[6,9] P-ANCA must be carefully differentiated from granulocyte-specific ANAs which are largely associated with rheumatoid arthritis and autoimmune neutropenia.[9] Antibodies to proteinase 3[10] are one component of C-ANCA. Antibodies to elastase (a lysosomal protease of granulocytes) are found by ELISA in same patients with SLE (especially with neurological disease) but do not give a C-ANCA pattern by IFA;[11] confirmation of these results is awaited. False-positive ANCA results can occur in HIV infection.[12,13] Antibodies to myeloperoxidase or to the 29 kd serine proteinase are highly sensitive and specific for vasculitis-associated and idiopathic crescentic glomerulonephritis, classical polyarteritis, Churg-Strauss syndrome and polyangiitis overlap syndrome without renal manifestations of vasculitis.[14] See also **GRANULOCYTE ANTIBODIES** and **GRANULOCYTE-SPECIFIC ANTINUCLEAR ANTIBODIES.**

REFERENCES:
1. van der Woude FJ, Rasmussen N, Lobatto S, et al. Autoantibodies against neutrophils and monocytes: tool for diagnosis and marker of disease activity in Wegener's granulomatosis. Lancet 1985;2:425-9.
2. Savage COS, Winearls CG, Jones S, Marshall PD, Lockwood CM. Prospective study of radioimmunoassay for antibodies against neutrophil cytoplasm in diagnosis of systemic vasculitis. Lancet 1987;1:1389-93.
3. Lüdemann G, Gross WL. Autoantibodies against cytoplasmic structures of neutrophil granulocytes in Wegener's granulomatosis. Clin Immunol 1987;69:350-7.
4. Wormsley SB, Leavitt RJ, Peter JB, Boctor FN, Fauci AS. Antineutrophil cytoplasm antibodies (ANCA) in systemic vasculitis: clinical utility of quantitation by flow cytometry. Arthritis Rheum 1988;31(Suppl 4):S34.
5. Specks U, Wheatley CL, McDonald TJ, Rohrbach MS, DeRemee RA. Anticytoplasmic autoantibodies in the diagnosis and follow-up of Wegener's granulomatosis. Mayo Clin Proc 1989;64:28-36.
6. Falk RJ, Jennette JC. Anti-neutrophil cytoplasmic autoantibodies with specificity for myeloperoxidase in patients with systemic vasculitis and idiopathic necrotizing and crescentic glomerulonephritis. N Engl J Med 1988;318:1651-7.
7. Savage COS, Winearls CG, Evans DJ, Rees AJ, Lockwood CM. Microscopic polyarteritis: presentation, pathology and prognosis. Q J Med 1985;56:467-83.
8. Rasmussen N, Wiik A, Hoier-Madsen M, Borregaard N, van der Woude F. Antineutrophil cytoplasm antibodies 1988 [Letter]. Lancet 1988;1:706-7.
9. Wiik A. Granulocyte-specific antinuclear antibodies. Allergy 1980;35:263-89.
10. Jenne DE, Tschopp J, Lodemann J, et al. Wegener's autoantigen decoded [Letter]. Nature 1990;346:520.
11. Nässberger L, Jonsson H, Sjöholm AG, Sturfelt G. Circulating anti-elastase in systemic lupus erythematosus. Lancet 1989;1:509.
12. Koderisch J, Andrassy K, Ramussen N, et al. False-positive anti-neutrophil cytoplasmic antibodies in HIV infection. Lancet 1990;335:1227-8.
13. Davenport A, Grant PJ. False-positive autoantibodies in HIV infection. Lancet 1990;336:317-8.
14. Cohen JW, Goldschmeding R, Elema JD, et al. Association of autoantibodies to myeloperoxidase with different forms of vasculitis. Arthritis Rheum 1990;33:1264-72.

NEUTROPHIL NICOTINAMIDE ADENINE DINUCLEOTIDE PHOSPHATE (NADPH)OXIDASE

Defective neutrophil neutrophil nicotinamide adenine dinucleotide phosphate (NADPH) oxidase results in the development of chronic granulomatous disease (CGD).[1] The microbicidal activity of neutrophils depends to a large extent on the integrity of the NADPH oxidase system, which when activated generates superoxide and other activated oxygen species.[2] Patients with CGD suffer from recurrent severe infections with catalase-producing organisms. The incidence of CGD is about 1 in 1 million, and is inherited by various modes with approximately 60% of patients having X-linked inheritance, 40% having autosomal recessive inheritance and about 1% having autosomal dominant inheritance.[3] The neutrophil oxidase system is composed of membrane-associated catalytic components and soluble cytosolic catalytic or regulatory components. One of the membrane components, cytochrome b_{558}, is a heterodimer with subunits of 91 and 22 kd. The X-linked form of CGD is associated in most cases with an absence of the cytochrome b and a defect in the gene encoding its 91 kd subunit.[4] Recently two cytosolic oxidase components (proteins of 47 and 67 kd) have been defined; the absence of one or the other of these cytosolic components is found in patients with autosomal recessive forms of CGD.[5] For review of classification of CGD, see 6. Laboratory diagnosis is based on the demonstration of an absence or greatly diminished superoxide production. This is classically determined by nitroblue tetrazolium (NBT) dye reduction test.[7] Measurement of superoxide production in response to soluble stimulus PMA (in continuous O_2^- assay) and in response to opsonized zymosan (examined in end point assay) in conjunction with the NBT test provides a valuable tool for CGD classification as well as detecting the carrier state in the X-linked CGD families.[6] If antibodies to the different components of the oxidase system were available, CGD neutrophils could be analyzed for the presence or absence of the different components by immunoblot analysis or by flow cytometric studies.

REFERENCES:

1. Tauber AI, Bornegaard N, Simons E, Wright J. Chronic granulomatous disease: a syndrome of phagocyte oxidase deficiencies. Medicine (Baltimore) 1983;62:286-309.
2. Lehrer RI, Ganz T, Selsted ME, et al. Neutrophils and host defense. Ann Intern Med 1988;109:127-42.
3. Gallin JI, Malech HL. Update on chronic granulomatous diseases of childhood. JAMA 1990;263:1533-7.
4. Parkos CA, Allen RA, Cochrane CG, Jesaitis AJ. The quaternery structure of the plasma membrane b-type cytochrome of human granulocytes. Biochim Biophys Acta 1988;932:71-83.
5. Volpp BD, Nauseef WM, Clark RA. Two cytosolic neutrophil oxidase components absent in autosomal chronic granulomatous disease. Science 1988;242:1295-7.
6. Curnutte JT. Classification of chronic granulomatous disease. Hematol Oncol Clin North Am 1988;2:241-52.
7. Baehner RL, Nathan DJ. Quantitative nitroblue tetrazolium test in chronic granulomatous disease. N Engl J Med 1968;278:971.

NITROBLUE TETRAZOLIUM (NBT) DYE REDUCTION (PMA-NBT TEST)

This screening test is useful for the diagnosis of chronic granulomatous disease (CGD), a heterogeneous disorder caused by three, or possibly four, different mutations[1-3] which result in predisposition to infection due to defects in the NADPH oxidase system of neutrophils. X-linked CGD, which accounts for two-thirds of CGD cases, is usually, but not always due to the absence of neutrophil cytochrome b. Autosomal recessive CGD, in which the neutrophils contain normal amounts of an apparently normal cytochrome b, may be due to failure of phosphorylation of a protein of the oxidase electron transport chain; this form accounts for about one third of CGD cases.[4] Rare variant forms are also recognized (cf. 2 for review). Well controlled assays for NBT reduction by phorbol-myristate-acetate (PMA)-stimulated neutrophils typically, but not invariably, provide a reliable screening test for CGD. The carrier state of the usual X-linked variety of CGD, which is manifest as mosaicism of dye reduction by granulocytes in the NBT test[1,4-6] should be sought in families of affected patients.[5-7] Flow cytometric analysis is also useful for detecting heterozygotes.[8]

REFERENCES:

1. Segal AW. The molecular and cellular pathology of chronic granulomatous disease. Eur J Clin Invest 1988;18:433-43.
2. Curnutte JT. Classification of chronic granulomatous disease. Hematol Oncol Clin North Am 1988;2:241-52.
3. Ezekowitz RAB, Newburger PE. New perspectives in chronic granulomatous disease. J Clin Immunol 1988;8:419-25.
4. Bolscher BGJM, van Zwieten R, Kramer IM, Weening RS, Verhoeven AJ, Roos D. A phosphoprotein of M_r 47,000, defective in autosomal chronic granulomatous disease, copurifies with one of two soluble components required for NADPH:O_2 oxidoreductase activity in human neutrophils. J Clin Invest 1989;83:757-63.
5. Meerhof LJ, Roos D. Heterogeneity in chronic granulomatous disease detected with an improved nitroblue tetrazolium slide test. J Leukocyte Biol 1986;39:699-711.

6. Johansen KS. Nitroblue tetrazolium slide test: use of the phorbol-myristate-acetate-stimulated NBT-reduction slide test for routine and prenatal detection of chronic granulomatous disease and diagnosis of heterozygous carriers. Acta Pathol Microbiol Immuno Scand 1983;91:349-54.
7. Borregaard N, Cross AR, Herlin T, Jones OT, Segal AW, Valerius NH. A variant form of X-linked chronic granulomatous disease with normal nitroblue tetrazolium slide test and cytochrome *b*. Eur J Clin Invest 1983;13:243-8.
8. Hassan NF, Campbell DE, Douglas SD. Flow cytometric analysis of oxidase activity of neutrophils from chronic granulomatous disease patients. Adv Exp Med Biol 1988;239:73-8.

NUCLEOLAR ANTIBODIES

Antibodies to components of nucleoli are most common in systemic sclerosis sera and include autoantibodies to: nucleolar 7-2 RNA (nucleolar 7-2 ribonucleoprotein) which are present in a very small percent of systemic sclerosis;[1,2] RNA polymerase I in about 4% of systemic sclerosis;[3] the fibrillarin component of U3 RNA in about 8% of systemic sclerosis;[4] and PM-Scl in about 3% of polymyositis-scleroderma overlap syndromes.[5-7] See the individual antibodies for discussion and reference 8 for review of early literature.

REFERENCES:
1. Reddy R, Tan EM, Henning D, Nohga K, Busch H. Detection of a nucleolar 7-2 ribonucleoprotein and a cytoplasmic 8-2 ribonucleoprotein with autoantibodies from patients with scleroderma. J Biol Chem 1983;258:1383-6.
2. Hashimoto C, Steitz JA. Sequential association of nucleolar 7-2 RNA with two different autoantigens. J Biol Chem 1983;258:1379-82.
3. Reimer G, Rose KM, Scheer U, Tan EM. Autoantibody to RNA polymerase I in scleroderma sera. J Clin Invest 1987;79:65-72.
4. Reimer G, Pollard KM, Penning CA, et al. Monoclonal autoantibody from a (New Zealand black x New Zealand white) F_1 mouse and some human scleroderma sera target an M_r34,000 nucleolar protein of the U3 RNP particle. Arthritis Rheum 1987;30:793-800.
5. Reimer G, Penning CA, Tan EM. Molecular characterization of the PM-Scl antigen. Arthritis Rheum 1986;29:S74.
6. Reimer G, Scheer U, Peters J-M, Tan EM. Immunolocalization and partial characterization of a nucleolar autoantigen (PM-Scl) associated with polymyositis/scleroderma overlap syndromes. J Immunol 1986;137:3802-8.
7. Targoff IN, Reichlin M. Nucleolar localization of the PM-Scl antigen. Arthritis Rheum 1985;28:226-30.
8. Bernstein RM, Steigerwald JC, Tan EM. Association of antinuclear and antinucleolar antibodies in progressive systemic sclerosis. Clin Exp Immunol 1982;48:43-51.

OLIGOCLONAL IMMUNOGLOBULINS

The term "oligoclonal immunoglobulins" (OI) refers to discrete populations of immunoglobulin (sometimes referred to as oligoclonal bands) detected by electrophoresis in CSF and *not* accompanied by a corresponding band in serum. Oligoclonal bands (i.e., OI) detected in higher concentration in CSF than in serum are considered abnormal (cf. 1-6 for review). Isoelectric focusing (IEF) is the method of choice for detection of OI.[4-6] OI are present in over 90% of patients with multiple sclerosis;[7] in CSF of patients with cerebrovascular accidents;[8] in a wide variety of infections of the CNS, including bacterial,[9] mycobacterial,[10,11] fungal,[12,13] viral,[14-16] borrelial[17,18] and treponemal[19,20] diseases. OI are also found in CSF of patients with lymphoproliferative and other neoplastic diseases infiltrating the leptomeninges of the CNS,[21,22] as well as in patients with CNS lupus.[23] OI are unusual in vascular dementia.[24] They are not detected in patients with Alzheimer disease, nor in patients with parenchymal or extradural metastases of systemic cancer.[22] OI can be detected in tears[25] and are present in some of the siblings of patients with MS.[26,27] Two-dimensional electrophoresis, by which clonal uniformity and temporal invariance have been demonstrated in MS brain and CSF,[28] promises even greater sensitivity for detection of oligoclonal bands.[28,29] As in the case with antibodies to measles virus in MS, the oligoclonal immunoglobulins in CSF of patients with HTLV-I-associated chronic progressive myelopathy are due only in small part to oligoclonal immunoglobulins with specificity for HTLV-I.[30] *B. burgdorferi*-specific oligoclonal immunoglobulins are common with lymphocytic meningoradiculitis.[31] See also **IgG INDEX, IgM INDEX; IgG(loc), IgM(loc), IgA(loc)** and **IgG SYNTHESIS RATE (IBBB IgG SYNTHESIS RATE).**

REFERENCES:

1. Thompson EJ. Laboratory diagnosis of multiple sclerosis: immunological and biochemical aspects. Br Med Bull 1977;33:28-33.
2. Harrington MG, Kennedy PGE. The clinical use of cerebrospinal fluid studies in demyelinating neurological diseases. Postgrad Med J 1987;63:735-40.
3. Tourtellotte WW, Walsh MJ, Baumhefner RW, Staugaitis SM, Shapsak P. The current status of multiple sclerosis intra-blood-brain-barrier IgG synthesis. In: Scheinberg L, Raine CS, eds. Multiple sclerosis: experimental and clinical aspects. New York: NY Academy of Sciences, 1984;436:52-67.
4. Staugaitis SM, Shapshak P, Tourtellotte WW, Lee MM, Reiber HO. Isoelectric focusing of unconcentrated cerebrospinal fluid: applications to ultrasensitive analysis of oligoclonal immunoglobulin G. Electrophoresis 1985;6:287-91.
5. Laurenzi MA, Link H. Comparison between agarose gel electrophoresis and isoelectric focusing of CSF for demonstration of oligoclonal immunoglobulin bands in neurological disorders. Acta Neurol Scand 1978;58;148-56.
6. Rieder HP, Jegge S. Isoelektrische fokussierung und agar-elektrophorese des liquor cerebrospinalis bei neurologischen patienten. Schweiz med Wschr 1979:109;1411-9.
7. Rocchelli B, Poloni M, Mazzarello P, Delodovici M. Clinical and CSF findings in multiple sclerosis patients with or without IgG oligoclonal bands at isoelectric focusing examination of CSF and serum proteins. Eur Neurol 1983;22:35-42.
8. Tsementzis SA, Chao SW, Hitchcock ER, Gill JS, Beevers DG. Oligoclonal immunoglobulin G in acute subarachnoid hemorrhage and stroke. Neurology 1986;36:395-7.
9. Forsberg P, Frydén A, Link H. Immunoglobulin abnormalities in the cerebrospinal fluid during bacterial meningitis. J Neuroimmunol 1986;12:299-310.
10. Bukasa KS-S, Sindic CJM, Limet JN, Laterre C. Antibody activity of CSF oligoclonal IgG in neurological infectious diseases: an immunoblotting study. Acta Neurol Belg 1988;88:203-20.
11. Kinnman J, Link H, Frydén A. Characterization of antibody activity in oligoclonal immunoglobulin G synthesized within the central nervous system in a patient with tuberculosis meningitis. J Clin Microbiol 1981;13:30-5.
12. Van de Wyngaert FA, Sindic CJM, Rousseau JJ, Fernandes Xavier FG, Brucher JM, Laterre EC. Spinal arachnoiditis due to aspergillus meningitis in a previously healthy patient. J Neurol 1986;233:41-3.
13. Porter KG, Sinnamon DG, Gillies RR. Cryptococcus neoformans specific oligoclonal immunoglobulins in cerebrospinal fluid in cyrtococcal meningitis. Lancet 1977;1:1268.
14. Ceroni M, Piccardo P, Rodgers-Johnson P, et al. Intrathecal synthesis of IgG antibodies to HTLV-I supports an etiological role for HTLV-I in tropical spastic paraparesis. Ann Neurol 1988;23:S188-91.
15. Elovaara I, Seppälä I, Poutiainen E, Suni J, Valle S-L. Intrathecal humoral immunologic response in neurologically symptomatic and asymptomatic patients with human immunodeficiency virus infection. Neurology 1988;38:1451-6.
16. Appleman ME, Marshall DW, Brey RL, et al. Cerebrospinal fluid abnormalities in patients without AIDS who are seropositive for the human immunodeficiency virus. J Infect Dis 1988;158:193-9.
17. Henriksson A, Link H, Cruz M, Stiernstedt G. Immunoglobulin abnormalities in cerebrospinal fluid and blood over the course of lymphocytic meningoradiculitis (Bannwarth's syndrome). Ann Neurol 1986;20:337-45.
18. Kristoferitsch W, Lanschützer H. Oligoklonales immunoglobulin M im liquor cerebrospinalis von patienten mit meningopolyneuritis Garin-Bujadoux-Bannwarth. Wien klin Wochenschr 1986;98:386-8.
19. Strandberg-Pedersen N, Kam-Hansen S, Link H, Mvra M. Specificity of immunoglobulins synthesized within the central nervous system in neurosyphilis. Acta Pathol Microbiol Immunol Scand [C] 1982;90:97-104.
20. Vartdal F, Vandvik B, Michaelsen TE, et al. Neurosyphilis: intrathecal synthesis of oligoclonal antibodies to Treponema pallidum. Ann Neurol 1982;11:35-40.

21. Ernerudh J, Olsson T, Berlin G, von Schenck H. Cerebrospinal fluid immunoglobulins and β2-microglobulin in lymphoproliferative and other neoplastic diseases of the central nervous system. Arch Neurol 1987;44:915-20.
22. Schipper HI, Bardosi A, Jacobi C, Felgenhauer K. Meningeal carcinomatosis: origin of local IgG production in the CSF. Neurology 1988;38:413-6.
23. Ernerudh J, Olsson T, Lindström F, Skogh T. Cerebrospinal fluid immunoglobulin abnormalities in systemic lupus erythematosus. J Neurol Neurosurg Psychiatry 1985;48:807-13.
24. Elovaara I, Seppälä I, Palo J, Sulkava R, Erkinjuntti T. Oligoclonal immunoglobulin bands in cerebrospinal fluid of patients with Alzheimer's disease and vascular dementia. Acta Neurol Scand 1988;77:397-401.
25. Coyle PK, Sibony P, Johnson C. Oligoclonal IgG in tears. Neurology 1987;37:853-6.
26. Xu X-H, McFarlin DE. Oligoclonal bands in CSF: twins with MS. Neurology 1984;34:769-74.
27. Duquette P, Charest L. Cerebrospinal fluid findings in healthy siblings of multiple sclerosis patients. Neurology 1986;36:727-9.
28. Walsh MJ, Tourtellotte WW. Temporal invariance and clonal uniformity of brain and cerebrospinal IgG, IgA, and IgM in multiple sclerosis. J Exp Med 1986:163;41-53.
29. Wiederkehr F, Imfeld H, Vonderschmitt DJ. Two-dimensional gel electrophoresis, isoelectric focusing and agarose gel electrophoresis in the diagnosis of multiple sclerosis. J Clin Chem Clin Biochem 1986;24:1017-21.
30. Link H, Cruz M, Gessain A, et al. Chronic progressive myelopathy associated with HTLV-I: oligoclonal IgG and anti-HTLV-I IgG antibodies in cerebrospinal fluid and serum. Neurology 1989;39:1566-72.
31. Hansen K, Cruz M, Link H. Oligoclonal *Borrelia burgdorferi*-specific IgG antibodies in cerebrospinal fluid in Lyme neuroborreliosis. J Infect Dis 1990;161:1194-202.

ORGANISM-SPECIFIC ANTIBODY INDEX

Organism-specific antibody index (OSAI) is a measurement of the ratio of organism-specific IgG to total IgG in CSF compared to the ratio in serum as shown by the formula below.

$$OSAI = \left[\frac{Organism\text{-}specific\ IgG\ in\ CSF}{Total\ IgG\ in\ CSF} \right] \div \left[\frac{Organism\text{-}specific\ IgG\ in\ Serum}{Total\ IgG\ in\ Serum} \right]$$

An index >1 (i.e., more organism-specific immunoglobulin in CSF than in serum) is strong evidence that intra-blood-brain barrier synthesis of organism-specific IgG is occuring and suggests a CNS infection by the specific organism being evaluated. Organism-specific antibody indices can also be determined for antibodies of the IgM and IgA classes. For example, early and prolonged IBBB synthesis of Japanese encephalitis virus-specific IgM (and total IgM as manifest in an elevated IgM index) occurs in most patients with Japanese encephalitis.[1,2] Increases of *Borrelia burgdorferi* IgM antibody index are seen in neuroborreliosis.[3-5] Increases of herpes simplex virus IgG antibody index are seen in HSV encephalitis,[6] as are increases for *Cysticercus cellulosae* IgG antibody index in cerebral cysticercosis;[7] of HTLV-I IgG antibody index in tropical spastic paraparesis;[8] and for mumps virus IgG antibody index in mumps meningoencephalitis.[9] An elevated OSAI is strong evidence for CNS infections due to a variety of other organisms, including arboviruses,[10] HIV,[11,12] *Treponema pallidum*,[13] *Toxoplasma gondii*,[14] Varicella-zoster virus,[15] and *Burcella spp.*,[16] among others (cf. 17 for discussion of the humoral immune reactions in CNS infections). In some infections (e.g., neuroborreliosis) organism-specific antibodies can be found in CSF even when absent in serum.[18] See also **IgA INDEX, IgG INDEX, IgM INDEX.**

REFERENCES:
1. Ehrenkranz NJ, Zemel ES, Bernstein C, et al. Immunoglobulin M in the cerebrospinal fluid of patients with arbovirus encephalitis and other infections of the central nervous system. Neurology 1974;24:976-80.
2. Burke DS, Nisalak A, Ussery MA, et al. Kinetics of IgM and IgG responses to Japanese encephalitis virus in human serum and cerebrospinal fluid. J Infect Dis 1985;151:1093-9.
3. Felgenhauer K. Differentiation of the humoral immune response in inflammatory diseases of the central nervous system. J Neurol 1982;228:223-37.

4. Henriksson A, Link H, Cruz M, Stiernstedt G. Immunoglobulin abnormalities in cerebrospinal fluid and blood over the course of lymphocytic meningoradiculitis (Bannwarth's syndrome). Ann Neurol 1986;20:337-45.
5. Halperin JJ, Luft BJ, Anand AK, et al. Lyme neuroborreliosis: central nervous system manifestations. Neurology 1989;39:753-9.
6. van Loon AM, van der Logt JTM, Heessen FWA, et al. Diagnosis of herpes simplex virus encephalitis by detection of virus-specific immunoglobulins A and G in serum and cerebrospinal fluid by using an antibody-capture enzyme-linked immunosorbent assay. J Clin Microbiol 1989;27:1983-7.
7. Mohammed IN, Heiner DC, Miller BL, et al. Enzyme-linked immunosorbent assay for the diagnosis of cerebral cysticercosis. J Clin Microbiol 1984;20:775-9.
8. Ceroni M, Piccardo P, Rodgers-Johnson P, et al. Intrathecal synthesis of IgG antibodies to HTLV-I supports an etiological role for HTLV-I in tropical spastic paraparesis. Ann Neurol 1988;23:188-91.
9. Vandvik B, Nilsen RE, Vartdal F, Norrby E. Mumps meningitis: specific and non-specific antibody responses in the central nervous system. Acta Neurol Scand 1982;65:468-87.
10. Peter JB, et al. Arbovirus antibody index: a reliable tool for diagnosis of arbovirus encephalitis, in preparation.
11. Elovaara I, Seppälä I, Poutianinen E, et al. Intrathecal humoral immunologic response in neurologically symptomatic and asymptomatic patients with human immunodeficiency virus infection. Neurology 1988;38:1451-6.
12. Peter JB, McKeown KL, Barka NE, Tourtellotte WW, Singer EJ, Syndulko K. Neopterin and β_2-microglobulin and the assessment of IBBB synthesis of HIV-specific and total IgG. 1990; Submitted.
13. Cerny EH, Hambie EA, Lee F, et al. Adenovirus ELISA for the evaluation of cerebrospinal fluid in patients with suspected neurosyphilis. Am J Clin Pathol 1985;84:505-8.
14. Potasman I, Resnick L, Luft BJ, Remington JS. Intrathecal production of antibodies against *Toxoplasma gondii* in patients with toxoplasmic encephalitis and the acquired immunodeficiency syndrome (AIDS). Ann Intern Med 1988;108:49-51.
15. Martinez-Martin P, Garcia-Saíz A, Rapún JL, Echevarria JM. Intrathecal synthesis of IgG antibodies to varicella-zoster virus in two cases of acute aseptic meningitis syndrome with no cutaneous lesions. J Med Virol 1985;16:201-9.
16. Sanchez-Sousa A, Torres C, Campello MG, et al. Serological diagnosis of neurobrucellosis. J Clin Pathol 1990;43:79-81.
17. Felgenhauer K, Ackermann R, Schliep G. The process dynamics of viral and bacterial diseases of the central nervous system. J Neurol Sci 1980;47:21-34.
18. Stiernstedt GT, Granström M, Hederstedt B, Sköldenberg B. Diagnosis of spirochetal meningitis by enzyme-linked immunosorbent assay and indirect immunofluorescence assay in serum and cerebrospinal fluid. J Clin Microbiol 1985;21:819-25.

OVARY ANTIBODIES

Anti-ovary antibodies (AOA) are found in 15-50% of patients with premature ovarian failure, i.e., cessation of ovarian function after puberty but before age 40 which is associated with high levels of serum gonadotropins and low levels of serum estradiol.[1-3] Patients with premature ovarian failure have an increased frequency of DR3.[4] AOA are anti-steroid cell antibodies (SCA) which also stain testes, placenta and (usually) adrenals.[5,6] SCA reactive with steroid-producing cells are almost always present in patients with Addison disease and ovarian failure (polyendocrine type 1).[5-9] In contrast, antibodies to LH receptors were not found in 14 patients with premature ovarian failure,[10] nor were antibodies to FSH receptor found in a patient with resistant ovary syndrome.[11] Antibodies to FSH receptor were, however, described in the serum of patients with myasthenia gravis (MG) who had hypergonadotropic ovarian failure (12, cf. 13 for review). Another single patient with premature ovarian failure and antibodies to FSH receptor has been mentioned but not published.[14] The significance of a report of a wide variety of anti-ovary (and other) antibodies in infertile couples is dubious.[15] Multiple organ-localized autoimmune diseases develop in nude mice after reconstitution of T cell function by fetal rat thymus graft.[16] Resumption of menses during administration of corticosteroids has been reported in 3 patients with autoimmune ovarian disease (cf. 17 for review). The ovary is now a well documented target for autoantibodies in polyglandular failure, primary ovarian failure, SLE, infertility, autoimmune oophoritis and endometriosis.[14-25] IgG/IgA and IgM anti-ovary antibodies are seen in 70% and 47% of women after repeated attempts at in-vitro fertilization (IVF).[25-27] By IFA, these antibodies are reactive with theca interna and atretic follicles,[28] as might be expected to result from release of proteins altered by repeated trauma of the follicles during IVF. Antibodies to corpora lutea and the hCG-occupied or hCG-unoccupied receptor for LH/hCG are found in primary sterility and endometriosis (50%) and in about 38%of patients with secondary sterility and endometriosis.[25] See also **STEROID CELL ANTIBODIES**.

REFERENCES:
1. Coulam CB. Premature gonadal failure. Fertil Steril 1982;38:645-55.
2. Coulam CB. The prevalence of autoimmune disorders among patients with primary ovarian failure. Am J Reprod Immunol 1983;4:63-6.
3. Coulam CB, Ryan RJ. Prevalence of circulating antibodies directed toward ovaries among women with premature ovarian failure. Am J Reprod Immunol Microbiol 1985;9:23-4.
4. Alper MM, Garner PR. Premature ovarian failure: its relationship to autoimmune disease. Obstet Gynecol 1985;66:27-30.
5. Sotsiou F, Bottazzo GF, Doniach D. Immunofluorescence studies on autoantibodies to steroid-producing cells, and to germline cells in endocrine disease and infertility. Clin Exp Immunol 1980;39:97-111.
6. Ahonen P, Miettinen A, Perheentupa J. Adrenal and steroidal cell antibodies in patients with autoimmune polyglandular disease type I and risk of adrenocortical and ovarian failure. J Clin Endocrinol Metab 1987;64:494-500.
7. Elder M, Maclaren N, Riley W. Gonadal autoantibodies in patients with hypogonadism and/or Addison's disease. J Clin Endocrinol Metab 1981;52:1137-42.
8. Neufeld M, MacLaren NK, Blizzard RM. Two types of autoimmune Addison's disease associated with different polyglandular autoimmune (PGA) syndromes. Medicine 1981;60:355-62.
9. Saenger P, Levine LS, Irvine WJ, et al. Progressive adrenal failure in polyglandular autoimmune disease. J Clin Endocrinol Metab 1982;54:863-8.
10. Austin GE, Coulam CB, Ryan RJ. A search for antibodies to luteinizing hormone receptors in premature ovarian failure. Mayo Clin Proc 1979;54:394-400.
11. Talbert LM, Raj MHG, Hammond MG, Greer T. Endocrine and immunologic studies in a patient with resistant ovary syndrome. Fertil Steril 1984;42:741-4.
12. Chiauzzi V, Cigorraga S, Escobar ME, Rivarola MA, Charreau EH. Inhibition of follicle-stimulating hormone receptor binding by circulating immunoglobulins. J Clin Endocrinol Metab 1982;54:1221-8.
13. Huhtaniemi IT. Gonadotrophin receptors: correlates with normal and pathological functions of the human ovary and testis. J Clin Endocrinol Metab 1983;12:117-31.
14. Trence DL, Morley JE, Handwerger BS. Polyglandular autoimmune syndromes. Am J Med 1984;77:107-16.
15. Case Records of the Massachusetts General Hospital (Case 46-1986). N Engl J Med 1986;315:1336-43.
16. Donat VH, Morenz J. Nachweis humoraler antikörper gegen genitalorganantigene bei sterilen ehepaaren. Zentralbl Gynakol 1983;105:493-50.
17. Taguchi O, Takahashi T, Seto M, Namikawa R, Matsuyama M, Nishizuka Y. Development of multiple organ-localized autoimmune diseases in nude mice after reconstitution of T cell function by rat fetal thymus graft. J Exp Med 1986;164:60-71.
18. Rabinowe SL, Berger MJ, Welch WR, Dluhy RG. Lymphocyte dysfunction in autoimmune oophoritis: resumption of menses with corticosteroids. Am J Med 1986;81:347-50.
19. Wolfe CD, Stirling RW. Premature menopause associated with autoimmune oophoritis: case report. Br J Obstet Gynaecol 1988;95:630-2.
20. Moncayo-Naveda HE, Moncayo R, Benz R, et al. Organ specific antibodies against ovary in patients with systemic lupus erythematosus. Am J Obstet Gynecol 1989;160:1227-9.
21. Mathur S, Peress MR, Williamson HO, et al. Autoimmunity to endometrium and ovary in endometriosis. Clin Exp Immunol 1982;50:259-66.
22. Luborsky JL, Visintin I, Boyers S, et al. Ovarian antibodies detected by immobilized antigen immunoassay in patients with premature ovarian failure. J Clin Endocrinol Metab 1990;70:69-75.

23. Moncayo-Naveda HE, Moncayo R, Benz R, et al. Organ-specific antibodies against ovary in patients with systemic lupus erythematosus. Am J Obstet Gynecol 1989;160:1227-9.
24. Sedmark DD, Hart WR, Tubbs RR. Autoimmune oophoritis: a histopathologic study of involved ovaries with immunologic characterization of the mononuclear cell infiltrate. Int J Gynecol Pathol 1987;6:73-81.
25. Moncayo H, Moncayo R, Benz R, et al. Ovarian failure and autoimmunity. Detection of autoantibodies directed against both the unoccupied luteinizing hormone/human chronic gonadotropin receptor and the hormone-receptor complex of bovine corpus luteum. J Clin Invest 1989;84:1857-65.
26. Moncayo R, Moncayo H, Dapunt O. Immunological risks of IVF [Letter]. Lancet 1990;335:180.
27. Gobert B, Barabarino-Monnier P, Guillet-Rosso F, Bene MC, Faure GC. Ovary antibodies after IVF. Lancet 1990;335:723.
28. Sacco AG, Shivers CA. Localization of tissue antigens in the rabbit ovary, oviduct and uterus by the fluorescent antibody technique. J Reprod Fertil 1973;32:415-9.

PARATHYROID ANTIBODIES

Anti-parathyroid antibodies are said to occur in idiopathic hypoparathyroidism (IHP), and in IHP associated with other endocrinopathies.[1] Others, however, find them only in a minority of IHP patients[2,3] and sometimes in other endocrinopathies in the absence of hypoparathyroidism.[3] The existence of latent hypoparathyroidism is debatable.[4] Complement-dependent, antibody-mediated lysis of parathyroid cells in autoimmune hypoparathyroidism[5] appears to be due to anti-endothelial cell antibodies of IgM isotype.[6]

REFERENCES:
1. Blizzard RM, Chee D, Davis W. The incidence of parathyroid and other antibodies in the sera of patients with idiopathic hypoparathyroidism. Clin Exp Immunol 1966;1:119-28.
2. Irvine WJ, Scarth L. Antibody to the oxyphil cells of the human parathyroid in idiopathic hypoparathyroidism. Clin Exp Immunol 1969;4:505-10.
3. Bottazzo GF, Florin-Christensen A, Pouplard A, Doniach D. Autoantibodies to prolactin-secreting cells of human pituitary. Lancet 1975;1:97-101.
4. Burckhardt P. Idiopathic hypoparathyroidism and autoimmunity. Hormone Res 1982;16:304-7.
5. Brandi ML, Aurbach GD, Fattorossi A, Quarto R, Marx SJ, Fitzpatrick LA. Antibodies cytotoxic to bovine parathyroid cells in autoimmune hypoparathyroidism. Proc Natl Acad Sci USA 1986;83:8366-9.
6. Fattorossi A, Aurbach GD, Sakaguchi K, et al. Anti-endothelial cell antibodies: detection and characterization in sera from patients with autoimmune hypoparathyroidism. Proc Natl Acad Sci USA 1988;85:4015-9.

PARIETAL CELL ANTIBODIES

Found in approximately 2% of normal populations, the frequency of anti-parietal (APCA) antibodies increases with age, as well as in the presence of insulin-dependent diabetes mellitus.[1,2] APCA, which cause reduced production of acid and mucosal atrophy when injected into rats,[3] are found in 50-100% of patients with pernicious anemia (PA) in frequencies which decrease with the duration of the PA (cf. 4 for review). This contrasts with the duration-related increase in frequency of antibodies to intrinsic factor in PA.[5,6] APCA in high titers are reliable predictors of minimal to severe atrophic gastritis,[7] and in the elderly with autoimmune atrophic gastritis APCA are predictive of a 3% per year rate of developing latent PA.[8] The acid-producing H^+/K^+ adenosine triphosphatase (proton pump) of gastric mucosa reacts with and is inhibited by APCA which interact with the α and β subunits of the pump.[9-11] APCA are reported to interfere with carbonic and hydrase secretion.[12] Blocking antibodies to the gastrin receptor are found in some patients with PA.[13] The relative contributions of these antibodies to reduced acid production and mucosal atrophy remain to be quantified. The relationship of anti-parietal cell antibodies to type A gastritis, (characterized by atrophy of the fundal mucosa, achlorhydria, tendency to evolve to latent or overt pernicious anemia and association with autoimmune endocrine disease) is well known.[14,15] Antibodies reactive with parietal cells in patients with pernicious anemia can be detected by IFA,[16] flow cytometry[17] and cytotoxicity.[18] At least some of these antibodies are reactive with the gastrin receptor in the fundal mucosa and may be very important in the pathogenesis of achlorhydria of PA.[13] Other anti-receptor antibodies may lead to excessive c-AMP production by gastric cells.[19] As noted above, approximately 75% of patients with PA have APCA.[20] Approximately 50% of patients with PA have thyroid antibodies and 30% of patients with thyroiditis have anti-parietal cell antibodies.[4,20] In type B (antral), none of these relationships are found, but antibodies to gastrin-producing cells are often detectable.[4] APCA are found in approximately 3% of normal adult caucasoids.[1]

Type B (antral gastritis, the most common form) increases in prevalence with age, typically is present in patients with duodenal ulcer, and is a common precursor of gastric carcinoma than type A gastritis. *Helicobater pylori* is etiologically associated with type A gastritis and is highly associated with duodenal ulcer; clearance of *H. pylori* is associated with decreased rates of ulcer recurrence. The absence of serum antibodies to *H. pylori* is strong evidence against H. pylori-associated gastritis or duodenal ulcer. See also **GASTRIN-PRODUCING CELL ANTIBODIES, GASTRIN RECEPTOR ANTIBODIES** and **GASTRIC CELL c-AMP STIMULATING ANTIBODIES**.

REFERENCES:
1. Hawkins BR, O'Connor KJ, Dawkins RL, Dawkins B, Rodger B. Autoantibodies in an Australian population: I. prevalence and persistence. J Clin Lab Immunol 1979;2:211-5.
2. Riley WJ, Toskes PP, Maclaren NK, Silverstein JH. Predictive value of gastric parietal cell autoantibodies as a marker for gastric and hematologic abnormalities associated with insulin-dependent diabetes. Diabetes 1982;31:1051-5.
3. Inada M, Glass GBJ. Effect of prolonged administration of homologous and heterologous intrinsic factor antibodies on the parietal and peptic cell masses and the secretory function of the rat gastric mucosa. Gastroenterology 1975;69:396-408.
4. Vandelli C, Bottazzo GF, Doniach D, Franceschi F. Autoantibodies to gastrin-producing cells in antral (type B) chronic gastritis. N Engl J Med 1979;300:1406-10.
5. Ungar B, Stocks AE, Martin FIR, Whittingham S, Mackay IR. Intrinsic-factor antibody, parietal-cell antibody, and latent pernicious anemia in diabetes mellitus. Lancet 1968;2:415-7.
6. Ungar B, Whittingham S, Francis CM. Pernicious anemia: incidence and significance of circulating antibodies to intrinsic factor and to parietal cells. Aust Ann Med 1967;16:226-9.
7. Wright R, Whitehead R, Wangel AG, et al. Autoantibodies and microscopic appearance of gastric mucosa. Lancet 1966;1:618-21.
8. Irvine WK. The association of atrophic gastritis and autoimmune thyroid disease. Clin Endocrinol Metab 1975;4:351-77.
9. Karlsson FA, Burman P, Loof L, Mardh S. Major parietal cell antigen in autoimmune gastritis with pernicious anemia is the acid-producing H^+, K^+-adenosine triphosphatase of the stomach. J Clin Invest 1988;81:475-9.
10. Burman P, Mardh S, Norberg L, Karlsson FA. Parietal cell antibodies in pernicious anemia inhibit H^+, K^+adenosine triphosphatase, the proton pump of the stomach. Gastroenterology 1989;96:1434-8.
11. Toh B-H, Gleeson PA, Simpson RJ, et al. The 60-to 90-kDa parietal cell autoantigen associated with autoimmune gastritis is a β subunit of the gastric H^+/K^+ATPase (proton pump). Proc Natl Acad Sci USA 1990;87:6418-22.
12. Bitensky L, Loveridge N, Chayen J, et al. Inhibition of gastrin-responsiveness by parietal cell antibodies. Clin Sci Mol Med 1979;53:15.
13. De Aizpurua HJ, Ungar B, Toh B-H. Autoantibody to the gastrin receptor in pernicious anemia. N Engl J Med 1985;313:479-83.
14. Strickland RG, Bhathal PS, Korman MG, et al. Serum gastrin and the antral mucosa in atrophic gastritis. Br Med J 1971;4:451-3.
15. Strickland RG, Mackay IR. A reappraisal of the nature and significance of chronic atrophic gastritis. Am J Dig Dis 1973;18:426-40.
16. De Aizpurua HJ, Toh B-H, Ungar B. Parietal cell surface reactive autoantibody in pernicious anaemia demonstrated by indirect membrane immunofluorescence. Clin Exp Immunol 1983;52:341-9.
17. De Aizpurua HJ, Ungar B, Toh B-H. Flow microfluorometric analysis of autoantibody reactions with parietal cell surface membranes in pernicious anaemia. Clin Exp Immunol 1983;54:405-10.
18. De Aizpurua HJ, Cosgrove LJ, Ungar B, Toh B-H. Autoantibodies cytotoxic to gastric parietal cells in serum of patients with pernicious anaemia. N Engl J Med 1983;309:625-9.

19. De Lazzari F, Mirakian R, Hammond L, Venturi C, Naccarato R, Bottazzo GF. Gastric cell c-AMP stimulating autoantibodies in duodenal ulcer disease. Gut 1988;29:94-100.
20. Irvine WJ, Davies SH, Teitelbaum S, Delamore IW, Williams AW. The clinical and pathological significance of gastric parietal cell antibody. Ann N Y Acad Sci 1965;124:657-91.

PERIPHERAL NERVE MYELIN and PERIPHERAL NERVE TISSUE ANTIBODIES

These complement-fixing antibodies, which are present in highest concentration at hospital admission of Guillain-Barré syndrome patients, fall to very low levels by day 15-20 (cf. 1 for review). Antibodies to peripheral nerve tissue are found in about 58% of GBS, 3% of patients with polyneuropathy of other origin and 9% of patients without polyneuropathy.[2] The clinical utility of measuring these antibodies is dubious. See also **MYELIN BASIC PROTEIN** and **MYELIN ANTIBODIES.**

REFERENCES:
1. Koski CL, Sanders ME, Swoveland PT, et al. Activation of terminal components of complement in patients with Guillain-Barré syndrome and other demyelinating neuropathies. J Clin Invest 1987;80:1492-7.
2. van Doorn PA, Brand A, Vermeulen M. Clinical significance of antibodies against peripheral nerve tissue in inflammatory polyneuropathy. Neurology 1987;37:1798-1802.

PEPSINOGEN (PG) I and II

The decrease in PG I in serum of patients with pernicious anemia (PA) is a reflection of loss of chief cells in the gastric fundus. PG II, which is produced in the gastric fundus and gastric pylorus, is not affected by the type A gastric (fundic) atrophy typical of PA. PG I levels less than 30 ug/l and PG I/PG II ratios less than 3.0 are found in approximately 92% and 82% of patients with PA respectively.[1] The specificity of PG I levels and PG I/PG II ratios is, however, insufficient to allow diagnosis based on these tests alone, even when serum cobalamin levels are low.[2,3] When combined with an abnormal result for antibodies to intrinsic factor and a low serum level of cobalamin (which together have high sensitivity and specificity for PA),[4] a low serum PG I and a low PG I/PG II ratio are strongly suggestive of PA. A normal result for both serum PG I and serum PG I/PG II ratio are strong evidence against PA. See also **PARIETAL CELL ANTIBODIES** and **INTRINSIC FACTOR ANTIBODIES.**

REFERENCES:
1. Carmel R. Pepsinogens and other serum markers in pernicious anemia. Am J Pathol 1988;90:442-5.
2. Samloff IM, Varis K, Ihamaki T, et al. Relationship among serum pepsinogen I, serum pepsinogen II and gastric mucosal histology. Gastroenterology 1982;83:204-9.
3. Varis K, Samloff IM, Ihamaki T, Siurala M. An appraisal of tests for severe atrophic gastritis in relatives of patients with pernicious anemia. Dig Dis Sci 1979;24:187-91.
4. Lindenbaum J. Status of laboratory testing in the diagnosis of megaloblastic anemia. Blood 1983;61:624-7.

PEPTIDE GROWTH FACTORS

Peptide growth factors (PGFs) include epidermal growth factor (EGF), fibroblast growth factor (FGF), insulin-like growth factors (IGF), platelet-derived growth factor (PDGF). PGFs have been largely characterized for their capacity to stimulate tumor cell proliferation in a wide variety of neoplasms for which they are mitogenic *in vitro* and in which they enhance expression of the characteristics of transformation, including anchorage-independent growth, decreased density-dependent growth inhibition and increased expression of some oncogenes (cf. 1 and 2 for review). Changes in PGFs and their receptors as well as the effects of autoantibodies thereto are increasingly recognized in other diseases and are expected to be very important. See also **PEPTIDE REGULATORY FACTORS, TRANSFORMING GROWTH FACTORS** α & β and individual growth factors.

REFERENCES:
1. Tappy L, Fujita-Yamaguchi Y, LeBon TR, Boden G. Antibodies to insulin-like growth factor I receptors in diabetes and other disorders. Diabetes 1988;37:1708-14.
2. Gansler T, Furlanetto R, Stokes Gramling T, et al. Antibody to type I insulin-like growth factor receptor inhibits growth of Wilms' tumor in culture and in athymic mice. Am J Pathol 1989;135:961-6.

PEPTIDE REGULATORY FACTORS: NON-MALIGNANT DISEASE

Peptide regulatory factors (PRFs) are low molecular weight (less than 80 kd), short- or intermediate-range mediators which bind to high-affinity receptors on the surface of adjacent cells (paracrine effect) or the surface of the cells by which the PRF is secreted (autocrine effect). PRFs affect differentiation and/or proliferation. The term "PRFs" includes cytokines (monokines/lymphokines/interleukins), growth factors, colony-stimulating factors (hematopoietic growth factors) and interferons.[1-14] See also **COLONY-STIMULATING FACTORS, CYTOKINES, INTERFERONS, MACROPHAGE INFLAMMATORY PROTEINS, NEUROPEPTIDES** and **PEPTIDE GROWTH FACTORS.**

REFERENCES:
1. Green AR. Peptide regulatory factors: multifunctional mediators of cellular growth and differentiation. Lancet 1989;1:705-7.
2. Michell RH. Post-receptor signalling pathways. Lancet 1989;1:765-7.
3. Metcalf D. Haemopoietic growth factors 1. Lancet 1989;1:825-7.
4. Metcalf D. Haemopoietic growth factors 2: clinical applications. Lancet 1989;1:885-7.
5. Metcalf D. The molecular control of cell division, differentiation commitment and maturation in haemopoietic cells. Nature 1989;339:27-30.
6. Balkwell FR. Interferons. Lancet 1989;1:1060-3.
7. Tracey KJ, Vlassara H, Cermai A. Peptide regulatory factors. Lancet 1989;1:1122-5.
8. Ross R. Platelet-derived growth factor. Lancet 1989;1:1179-82.
9. Waterfield MD. Epidermal growth factor and related molecules. Lancet 1989;1:1243-6.
10. Slack JMW. Peptide regulatory factors in embyonic development. Lancet 1989;1:1312-5.
11. Hanley MR. Peptide regulatory factors in in the nervous system. Lancet 1989;1:1373-6.
12. Duff GW. Peptide regulatory factors in non-malignant disease. Lancet 1989;1:1432-4.
13. Steel CM. Peptide regulatory factors and malignancy. Lancet 1989;2:30-4.
14. Wolpe SD, Cerami A. Macrophage inflammatory proteins 1 and 2: members of a novel superfamily of cytokines. FASEB J 1989;3:2565-73.

PERFORIN

This granule protein of natural killer cells and cytotoxic T cells[1] is involved in formation of pore-like lesions in target cells which resemble those produced by the terminal components of complement (C6-C9), with which perforin shares highly conserved sequences (cf. 2 for review).

REFERENCES:
1. Shinkai Y, Takio K, Okumura K. Homology of perforin to the ninth component of complement (C9). Nature 1988;334:525-7.
2. Reid KBM, Day AJ. Structure-function relationships of the complement components. Immunol Today 1989;10:177-80.

PERINUCLEAR ANTIBODIES

Antibodies reactive with perinuclear granules of human buccal mucosal cells (so-called perinuclear factors in the older literature) are positive in 40% of patients with IgM RF-negative RA[1] and may be useful for prognosis because they are found in the RF-negative subgroup with a poor prognosis.[2] Anti-perinuclear antibody-positive, rheumatoid factor-negative RA is associated with HLA-DR4 as is RF-positive RA.[3] These antibodies are, however, found in a variety of other rheumatic diseases[4] and are very common in patients with Epstein-Barr virus infection.[5] About 27% of patients with primary biliary cirrhosis have a perinuclear pattern of ANA which is due to antibodies to a ∿210 kd envelope glycoprotein of the nuclear pore.[6] Other perinuclear ANAs are reactive with lamins A, B and C.[7] An exchange of sera to clarify the relationship of these perinuclear antibodies is indicated.

REFERENCES:
1. Sondag-Tschroots IRJM, Aaij C, Smit JW, Feltkamp TEW. The antiperinuclear factor. 1. The diagnostic significance of the antiperinuclear factor for rheumatoid factor. Ann Rheum Dis 1979;38:248-51.
2. Westgeest AAA, Boerbooms AMTh, Jongmans M, et al. Antiperinuclear factor: indicator of more severe disease in seronegative rheumatoid arthritis. J Rheumatol 1987;14:893-7.
3. Boerbooms AMTh, Westgeest AAA, Reekers P, van de Putte LBA. Immunogenetic heterogeneity of seronegative rheumatoid arthritis and the antiperinuclear factor. Ann Rheum Dis 1990;49:15-7.
4. Vivino FB, Maul GG. Histologic and electron microscopic characterization of the antiperinuclear factor antigen. Arthritis Rheum 1990;33:960-9.
5. Westgeest A, van Loon A, van der Logt J, et al. Antiperinuclear factor, a rheumatoid arthritis specific autoantibody: its relation to Epstein-Barr virus. J Rheumatol 1989;16:626-30.
6. Courvalin J, Lassoued K, Bartnik E, et al. The 210-kD nuclear envelope polypeptide recognized by human autoantibodies in primary biliary cirrhosis is the major glycoprotein of the nuclear pore. J Clin Invest 1990;86:279-85.
7. Lassoued K, Guilly MN, Danon F, et al. Antinuclear autoantibodies specific for lamins: characterization and clinical significance. Ann Intern Med 1988;108:829-33.

PHOSPHOLIPID ANTIBODIES

Antibodies to negatively charged phospholipids are found in patients classified as having SLE, because they meet four or more of the ACR criteria.[1] APA are also found in lupus-like disease in which less than four of the criteria are applicable and in "primary anti-phospholipid syndrome when the only serologic abnormalities detectable are anti-nuclear antibodies, usually in low titer, and antibodies to phospholipids".[2,3] Whether a syndrome defined on the basis of a laboratory test is more a matter of imagination than perspicacity is unresolved, as is the contribution of anti-cardiolipin antibodies to the reduction of erythrocyte CR1 expression in SLE patients.[4] See also **CARDIOLIPIN ANTIBODIES.**

REFERENCES:
1. Tan EM, Cohen AS, Fries JT, et al. The 1982 revised criteria for the classification of SLE. Arthritis Rheum 1982;25:1271-7.
2. Harris EN, Gharavi AE, Hughes GRV. Anti-phospholipid antibodies. Clin Rheum Dis 1985;11:591-609.
3. Asherson RA, Khamashta MA, Gil A, et al. Cerebrovascular disease and antiphospholipid antibodies in systemic lupus erythematosus, lupus-like disease, and the primary antiphospholipid syndrome. Am J Med 1989;86:391-9.
4. Hammond A, Rudge AC, Loizou S, et al. Reduced numbers of complement receptor type I on erythrocytes are associated with increased levels of anticardiolipin antibodies. Arthritis Rheum 1989;32:259-64.

PITUITARY ANTIBODIES

Anti-pituitary antibodies are found most frequently in the empty sella syndrome and less frequently in sera of patients with pituitary adenomas, prolactinomas, acromegaly, idiopathic diabetes insipidus[1] and in POEMS (polyneuropathy, organomegaly, endocrinopathy, M protein, and skin changes) syndrome.[2] These antibodies are detected by their reactions with pituitary tissue and/or with mouse or rat cell lines secreting pituitary hormones. Anti-pituitary cell antibodies are also found in IDDM and ACTH deficiency;[3] they may be a marker for unfavorable outcome after pituitary microsurgery for Cushing disease.[4] Antibodies to FSH-secreting and LH-secreting pituitary cells (but not to the hormones themselves) are found in about 48% of children with cryptorchidism and are more frequent in patients with bilateral rather than unilateral cryptorchidism.[5]

REFERENCES:
1. Komatsu M, Kondo T, Yamauchi K, et al. Antipituitary antibodies in patients with the primary empty sella syndrome. J Clin Endocrinol Metab 1988;67:633-8.

2. Reulecke M, Dumas M, Meier C. Specific antibody activity against neuroendocrine tissue in a case of POEMS syndrome with IgG gammopathy. Neurology 1988;38:614-6.
3. Sugiura M, Hashimoto A, Shizawa M, et al. Heterogeneity of anterior pituitary cell antibodies detected in insulin-dependent diabetes mellitus and adrenocorticotropic hormone deficiency. Diabetes Res 1986;3:111-14.
4. Scherbaum WA, Schrell U, Gluck M, et al. Autoantibodies to pituitary corticotropin-producing cells: possible marker for unfavourable outcome after pituitary microsurgery for Cushing's disease. Lancet 1987;1:1394-8.
5. Pouplard-Barthelaix A, Lepinard V, Luxembourger L, et al. Circulating pituitary autoantibodies against cells secreting luteinising and follicle stimulating hormones in children with cryptorchidism [Letter]. Lancet 1984;2:631-2.

PLATELET ANTIBODIES

In general, the correlation of anti-platelet antibodies in serum with platelet-associated immunoglobulins (PAIg) is good.[1] Major doubts about the clinical utility of assays for PAIgG and anti-platelet antibodies are well justified[2] despite positive and negative predictive values of 96% and 92% respectively for PAIg.[3] Only occasionally are antibodies to platelets found in the serum of patients with ITP in the absence of PAIg.[1,4] Immunoblot analysis can be used for detection and characterization of the antigens (e.g., a 98 kd platelet glycoprotein consistent with GPIIIa) involved in neonatal isoimmune thrombocytopenia.[5] See also **PLATELET-ASSOCIATED IMMUNOGLOBULINS (PAIg)**.

REFERENCES:
1. Kelton JG, Moore J, Gauldie J, et al. The development and application of a serum assay for platelet bindable IgG(S-PBIgG). J Lab Clin Med 1981;98:272-9.
2. Harrington WJ. Are platelet-antibody tests worthwhile? [Editorial]. N Engl J Med 1987;316:211-12.
3. Corash L, Rheinschmidt M. Detection of platelet antibodies with a fluorescence activated flow cytometric technique. In: Rose NR, Friendman H, Fahey JL, eds. Manual of clinical laboratory immunology. Washington, DC: American Society for Microbiology, 1986;254-7.
4. Moore SB, Wick MR, Richardson LM. Immune thrombocytopenias: tests for platelet antibodies. Mayo Clin Proc 1984;59:860-3.
5. Lazarchick J, Russell R, Horn B. Maternal platelet antibody levels in neonatal isoimmune thrombocytopenia. Ann Clin Lab Sci 1990;20:200-4.

PLATELET-ACTIVATING FACTOR

Platelet-activating factor (PAF) (1-O-alkyl-2-O-acetyl-sn-glycero-3 phosphocholine) produces platelet activation at $\sim$0.1 nM as well as other diverse actions.[1] Sensitive (0.02-2 pmol), specific RIAs, although requiring lipid extraction,[2] should permit critical evaluation of PAF's role in allergy, anaphylaxis, asthma, graft rejection, ulcer disease and renal disease (cf. 3). PAF is synthesized by cells thought to be important in asthma, including endothelial cells, mast cells, monocytes, eosinophils and neutrophils. PAF is released in increased quantities in the sputum of patients with asthma and chronic lung disease, in nasal secretions and skin after antigen challenge, and in blood after cold challenge in cold-induced urticaria. Inhalation of PAF causes transient bronchospasm, eosinophil influx and increased microvascular permeability in the central and peripheral airways. Intradermal injection of PAF causes wheal and flare followed by an indurated red papule. Severe childhood asthma is associated with deficiency of specific hydrolases which metabolize PAF (cf. 4 and 5 for review).

REFERENCES:
1. Hanahan DJ, Kumar R. Platelet activating factor; chemical and biochemical characteristics. Prog Lipid Res 1987;26:1.
2. Smal MA, Baldo BA, McCaskill A. A specific, sensitive radioimmunoassay for platelet-activating factor (PAF). J Immunol Methods 1990;128:183-8.
3. Braquet P, Mencia-Huerta JM, Chabrier PE, Touqui L, Vargaftig BB. The promise of platelet-activating factor. In: ISI atlas of science: Pharmacology 1987;1:187-98.
4. Braquet P, Touqui L, Shen TY, et al. Perspectives in platelet-activating factor research. Pharmacol Rev 1987:39;97-145.
5. Anonymous. PAF antagonists in asthma [Editorial]. Lancet 1989;1:592-3.

PLATELET-ASSOCIATED IMMUNOGLOBULINS (PAIg)

Flow cytometry with paraformaldehyde-fixed platelets is the method of choice for detection and quantitation of PAIg (IgG and IgM) and antibodies to platelet glycoproteins, because the number of platelets needed is less than most other methods.[1-4] By flow cytometry, PAIgG and PAIgM can also be assessed separately with a 15% increase in diagnostic sensitivity without loss of specificity in immune thrombocytopenic purpura.[2-4] PAIgG levels are generally much higher in ITP than in malignancy or sepsis.[3] Only occasionally does separate testing of serum for anti-platelet antibodies yield positive results when PAIg levels by flow cytometry are normal.[5,6] As with ITP, however, anti-platelet antibodies in serum are sometimes found in thrombotic thrombocytopenic purpura[7] and in heparin-induced thrombocytopenia.[8] Recent reviews on platelet antibodies are available.[9,10] Sensitivity and specificity of approximately 95% each are reported for the diagnosis of immune vs. "non immune" thrombocytopenia.[1,2] Platelet-associated and plasma anti-glycoprotein (GPIIb/IIIa and GPIb) antibodies are found in 75% and 58% respectively of patients with chronic ITP.[11] Despite positive and negative predictive values of 96% and 92% respectively,[1] major doubts about the clinical utility of assays for PAIgG and anti-platelet antibodies have been expressed.[12] Negative results for PAIg, however, are strong evidence against ITP (cf. 13 for recent review). See also **PLATELET ANTIBODIES.**

REFERENCES:
1. Corash L, Rheinschmidt M. Detection of platelet antibodies with a fluorescence activated flow cytometric technique. In: Rose NR, Friedman H, Fahey JL, eds. Manual of clinical laboratory immunology. Washington, DC: American Society for Microbiology, 1986;254-7
2. Rosenfeld CS, Nichols G, Bodensteiner DC. Flow cytometric measurement of antiplatelet antibodies. Am J Clin Pathol 1987;87:518-22.
3. Szal M, Blumberg N. Clinical correlates in patients with elevated platelet-associated immunoglobulins. Ann Clin Lab Sci 1988;18:24-33.
4. Lazarchick J, Genco PV, Hall SA, Ponzio AD, Burdash NM. Detection of platelet antibodies by flow cytometric analysis. Diag Immunol 1984;2:238-41.
5. Moore SB, Wick MR, Richardson LM. Immune thrombocytopenias: tests for platelet antibodies. Mayo Clin Proc 1984;59:860-3.
6. Kelton JG, Moore J, Gauldie J, Neame PB, Hirsh J, Tozman E. The development and evaluation of a serum assay for platelet bindable IgG (S-PBIgG). J Lab Clin Med 1981;98:272-9.
7. Lazarchick J, Graddick SL, Hall SA, Genco PV. Platelet directed antibody in the serum of patients with primary thrombotic thrombocytopenic purpura. Ann Clin Lab Sci 1987;17:339-44.
8. Silberman S, Kovarik P. Heparin-induced thrombocytopenia: use of indirect immunofluorescence. Ann Clin Lab Sci 1987;17:106-10.
9. Karpatkin S. Autoimmune thrombocytopenic purpura. Semin Hematol 1985;22:260-88.
10. Kelton JG, Gibbons S. Autoimmune platelet destruction: idiopathic thrombocytopenic purpura. Semin Thromb Hemost 1982;8:83-104.
11. McMillan R, Tani P, Millard F, Berchtold P, Renshaw L, Woods VL Jr. Platelet-associated and plasma anti-glycoprotein autoantibodies in chronic ITP. Blood 1987;70:1040-5.
12. Harrington WJ. Are platelet-antibody tests worthwhile? [Editorial]. N Engl J Med 1987;316:211-2.
13. Ault KA. Flow cytometric measurement of platelet-associated immunoglobulin. Pathol Immunopathol Res 1988;7:395-408.

PLATELET-DERIVED GROWTH FACTOR

Originally isolated from human platelets, PDGF is synthesized and secreted by a wide variety of cells (including tumor cells, activated vascular endothelial cells and activated macrophages). Platelet-derived growth factor (PDGF), which accounts for much of the capacity of serum to promote growth of fibroblasts and other mesenchymal connective-tissue-forming cells (cf. 1 and 2 for review), is distinct from epidermal growth factor (EGF) which stimulates growth and division of capillary endothelial cells.[3] In addition to its role in normal growth and development, PDGF is probably important in inflammatory, fibroproliferative processes such as myelofibrosis, pulmonary fibrosis and rheumatoid arthritis[4] as well as in atherosclerosis[5] and in some forms of cancer.[4,6]

REFERENCES:
1. Ross R. Platelet-derived growth factor. Lancet 1989;1:1179-82.
2. Waterfield MD. Epidermal growth factor and related molecules. Lancet 1989;1:1243-9.
3. Fisher DA, Salido EC, Barajas L. Epidermal growth factor and the kidney. Annu Rev Physiol 1989;51:67-80.
4. Ross R, Raines EW, Bowen-Pope DF. The biology of platelet-derived growth factor. Cell 1986;46:155-69.
5. Ross R. The pathogenesis of artherosclerosis - an update. N Engl J Med 1986;314:488-500.
6. Betsholtz C, Westermark B, Ek B, Heldin C-H. Coexpression of a PDGF-like factor and PDGF receptors in a human osteosarcoma cell line: implications for autocrine receptor activation. Cell 1984;39:447-57.

PM-Scl (ANTI-PM-1) ANTIBODIES

These antibodies are apparently localized in nucleoli and cytoplasm by IF. They react with a complex of 11 proteins (20-110 kd) and are identified by immunodiffusion in about 8% of patients with features of polymyositis and scleroderma.[1-3]

REFERENCES:
1. Reichlin M, Maddison PJ, Targoff I, et al. Antibodies to a nuclear/nucleolar antigen in patients with polymyositis overlap syndromes. J Clin Immunol 1987;4:40-4.
2. Targoff IN, Reichlin M. Nucleolar localization of the PM-Scl antigen. Arthritis Rheum 1985;28:226-30.
3. Reimer G, Scheer U, Peters JM, Tan EM. Immunolocalization and partial characterization of a nucleolar autoantigen (PM-Scl) associated with polymyositis/scleroderma overlap syndromes. J Immunol 1986;137:3802-8.

POLYETHYLENE GLYCOL (PEG) ASSAY FOR CIC

This assay is useful for the detection, characterization and quantitation of antigens and antibodies in complexes which sediment in PEG.[1] Aggregates of immunoglobulins found in certain paraproteinemias also sediment in PEG. Recent adaptations of the original PEG precipitation method have not improved the borderline clinical utility of this assay.[2,3] Some authorities recommend the C1q binding assay and the conglutinin assay for detection of circulating immune complexes, because these assays "may be helpful for assessing and monitoring of disease activity in conditions such as rheumatoid arthritis and SLE".[4]

REFERENCES:
1. Digeon M, Laver M, Riza J, Bach JF. Detection of circulating immune complexes in human sera by simplified assays with polyethylene glycol. J Immunol Methods 1977;16:165-83.
2. Swierczynska Z, Milgrom F. Comparison of some procedures detecting circulating immune complexes. Immunol Invest 1985;14:485-91.
3. Levinson SS, Goldman JO, Feldkamp CS. Anti-IgG binding test to assay circulating IgG-containing immune complexes from polyethylene glycol precipitates. Clin Chem 1984;30:1502-6.
4. IUIS/WHO Working Group. Laboratory investigations in clinical immunology: methods, pitfalls, and clinical indications: a second IUIS/WHO report. Clin Immunol Immunopathol 1988;49:478-97.

PROCOLLAGEN III AMINOTERMINAL PEPTIDE (PIIINP)

Serum levels of PIIINP are increased in PSS,1 RA2 and coronary artery disease.[3] In alcoholic cirrhosis, primary biliary cirrhosis and chronic active hepatitis, serum levels of PIIINP are much higher than the elevated levels found in the rheumatic diseases.[4,5] Serum levels of PIIINP rise dramatically and serum levels of neopterin and beta 2-microglobulin decrease in patients treated with Praziquantel® for hepatomegaly due to *Schistosoma mansoni* infection.[6,7]

Increased levels of serum PIIINP correlate with degree of hepatic fibrosis in hemophilic patients with chronic non-A, non-B hepatitis,[8] and in alcohol-related chronic liver disease.[9] Serum PIIINP increases as early as one week after growth hormone treatment of short children who will experience acceleration of growth during treatment with recombinant growth hormone.[10] Minor decreases in serum PIIINP are reported in primary fibromyalgia,[11] but the differences are small, as is also true of the increased levels of serum PIIINP reported in asymptomatic children with α_1-antitrypsin deficiency.[12]

REFERENCES:
1. Hørslev-Petersen K, Ammitzbøll T, Engström-Laurent A, et al. Serum and urinary aminoterminal type III procollagen peptide in progressive systemic sclerosis: relationship to sclerodermal involvement, serum hyaluronan and urinary collagen metabolites. J Rheumatol 1988;15:460-7.
2. Hørslev-Petersen K, Bentsen KD, Halberg P, et al. Connective tissue metabolites in serum as markers of disease activity in patients with rheumatoid arthritis. Clin Exp Rheumatol 1988;6:129-34.
3. Bonnet J, Garderes PE, Aumailley M, et al. Serum type III procollagen peptide levels in coronary artery disease (a marker of atherosclerosis). Eur J Clin Invest 1988;18:18-21.
4. Rohde H, Vargas L, Hahn E, Kalbfleisch H, Bruguera M, Timpl R. Radioimmunoassay for type III procollagen peptide and its application to human liver disease. Eur J Clin Invest 1979;9:451-9.
5. van Zanten RAA, van Leeuwen REW, Beukers R, Wilson JHP. Procollagen III peptide levels in alcoholic liver disease and primary biliary cirrhosis. Neth J Med 1988;32:278-84.
6. Zwingenberger K, Harms G, Feldmeier H, Moller O, Steiner A, Bienzle U. Liver involvement in human schistosomiasis mansoni. Regression of immunological and biochemical disease markers after specific treatment. Acta Tropica 1988;45:263-75.
7. Zwingenberger K, Feldmeier H, Nogueira Queiroz JA, et al. Liver involvement in human schistosomiasis mansoni. Assessment by immunological and biochemical markers. Parasitol Res 1988;74:448-55.
8. Miller EJ, Lee CA, Karayiannis P, et al. Non-invasive investigation of liver disease in haemophilic patients. J Clin Pathol 1988;41:1039-43.
9. Gabrielli GB, Faccioli G, Casaril M, et al. Procollagen III peptide and fibronectin in alcohol-related chronic liver disease: correlations with morphological features and biochemical tests. Clin Chim Acta 1989;179:315-22.
10. Tapanainen P, Risteli L, Knip M, Kaar M-L, Risteli J. Serum aminoterminal propeptide of type III procollagen: a potential predictor of the response to growth hormone therapy. J Clin Endocrinol Metab 1988;67:1244-9.
11. Jensen LT, Jacobsen S, Hørsley-Petersen K. Serum procollagen type III aminoterminal peptide in primary fibromyalgia (fibrositis syndrome). Br J Rheum 1988;27:496.
12. Eriksson S, Sveger T. Procollagen type III peptide in asymptomatic children with α_1-antitrypsin deficiency [Letter]. J Pediatr Gastroenterol Nutr 1988;7:938.

PROLIFERATING CELL NUCLEAR ANTIGEN

Anti-proliferating cell nuclear antigen (PCNA) are found in 2-10% of patients with SLE. These antibodies react with PCNA (cyclin) which is the auxiliary protein of DNA polymerase-delta.[1,2] No correlation with distinctive clinical or laboratory features has been noted.[2]

REFERENCES:
1. Bravo R, Frank R, Blundell PA, Macdonald-Bravo H. Cyclin/PCNA is the auxiliary protein of DNA polymerase-δ. Nature 1987;326:515-7.
2. Fritzler MJ, McCarty GA, Ryan JP, Kinsella TD. Clinical features of patients with antibodies directed against proliferating cell nuclear antigen. Arthritis Rheum 1983;26:140-5.

PROPERDIN DEPENDENT NEPHRITIC FACTOR (NF$_{I/III}$)

These IgG autoantibodies are found in patients with membranoproliferative glomerulonephritis (MPGN) types I and III.[1] In contrast to NFII, which rapidly activates C3 *in vitro* and usually decreases only serum C3 *in vivo* in MPGN type II, NF$_{I/III}$ is properdin-dependent and slowly converts C5 and C9 as well as C3 *in vitro*. See also **C3 AND C4 NEPHRITIC FACTOR (NF$_{II}$/C3NEF; C4NeF)** and **COMPLEMENT COMPONENTS.**

REFERENCES:
1. Clardy CW, Forristal J, Strife CF, West CD. A properdin dependent nephritic factor slowly activating C3, C5, and C9 in membranoproliferative glomerulonephritis, types I and III. Clin Immunol Immunopathol 1989;50:333-47.

PROSTAGLANDINS

The cyclooxygenase pathway by which arachidonic acid is converted to prostaglandins and thromboxanes is inhibited by non-steroidal anti-inflammatory drugs. Now that reliable methods for detection of urinary metabolites are available, we can expect that eicosanoid formation *in vivo* in health and disease will be rapidly defined and that methodologic problems and artifactual *ex vivo* formation will be avoided.[1-4] Assays for prostaglandins are not yet of proven clinical utility except for clinical research, including the use of aspirin to prevent pregnancy-induced hypertension (and lower the ratio of serum thromboxane A_2 to prostacyclin) in high risk pregnancies.[5] See also **THROMBOXANE A_2**.

REFERENCES:
1. Zipser RD, Laffi G. Prostaglandins, thromboxanes and leukotrienes in clinical medicine. West J Med 1985;143:485-97.
2. Oates JA, FitzGerald GA, Branch RA, et al. Clinical implications of prostaglandins and thromboxane A_2 formation (First of two parts). N Engl J Med 1988;319:689-98.
3. Oates JA, FitzGerald GA, Branch RA, et al. Clinical implications of prostaglandins and thromboxane A_2 formation (Second of two parts). N Engl J Med 1988;319:761-7.
4. Fuster V, Cohen M, Halperin J. Aspirin in the prevention of coronary disease [Editorial]. N Engl J Med 1989;321:183-5.
5. Schiff E, Peleg E, Goldenberg M, et al. The use of aspirin to prevent pregnancy-induced hypertension and lower the ratio of thromboxane A_2 to prostacyclin in relatively high risk pregnancies. N Engl J Med 1989;321:351-6.

PROTHYMOSIN α ANTIBODIES

These antibodies, which are found in about 18% of SLE and 2% of controls, correlate with anti-dsDNA antibodies but are of no clinical utility.[1] The time may have come for a moratorium on description of other antibodies in SLE in the absence of data on the binding constants and hence the probable clinical relevance of such antibodies. The same applies to monoclonal antibodies which cross-react with a variety of antigens.

REFERENCES:
1. Vlachoyiannopoulos PG, Frillingos S, Tzioufas AG, et al. Circulating antibodies to prothymosin α in systemic lupus erythematosus. Clin Immunol Immunopathol 1989;53:151-60.

PURKINJE CELL (Yo) ANTIBODIES

Yo antibodies, which characteristically stain Purkinje cell cytoplasm in a coarse granular pattern, react with 34-38 and 62-64 kd component(s) of Purkinje cell cytoplasm. They are found in patients with subacute or paraneoplastic cerebellar degeneration (PCD), which is a rare complication of some cancers, including carcinomas of the lung (usually the small cell variety), ovary and breast as well as Hodgkin disease.[1-3] Other antibodies, the reactivity of which is not restricted to Purkinje cytoplasm, are found in some patients with PCD, subacute sensory neuropathy or paraneoplastic encephalomyelitis.[4-9] Patients (especially postmenopausal women) with cerebellar syndromes of recent onset should have prompt testing for antibodies to Purkinje cytoplasm followed by tumor search (especially gynecologic) if Purkinje cell antibodies are detected.[10] Neurologically normal patients with ovarian neoplasms[11] and patients with small cell lung cancer without subacute sensory neuropathy or other paraneoplastic neurologic disorders[9] can have large amounts of these antibodies; decreases in antibody titers after tumor removal need not be followed by increases in titer with recurrence of the tumor.[11] Cloning of a brain protein and identification of a sequence reactive with Ig from serum containing Purkinje cell antibodies could lead to an improved assay.[12] Paraneoplastic syndromes can be divided into those affecting the central nervous system (cerebellar dysfunction[4] and loss of visual acuity)[13,14] and those affecting the peripheral nervous system (Lambert-Eaton myasthenic syndrome[15,16] and sensory neuronopathy).[6,17] For succinct review, see 18. The recently cloned 34 kd cerebellar degeneration-related antigen (CDR34), which is an immunogenic protein containing a tandemly repeated hexapeptide, the mRNA of which is highly expressed in brain neurons (especially Purkinje cells), neuroectodermal cell lines, some epithelial cancer lines and tumor tissue from patients with PCD.[19] Increased IBBB synthesis of anti-Yo antibodies is common in PCD; plasmapheresis decreases serum but not CSF levels of anti-Yo and is typically without clinical benefit.[20] See also **Hu (NEURONAL ANTINUCLEAR) ANTIBODIES, RETINA ANTIBODIES** and **VOLTAGE-GATED-CALCIUM CHANNEL ANTIBODIES.**

REFERENCES:

1. Henson RA, Urich H. Cancer and the nervous system: the neurological manifestations of systemic malignant disease, 1st ed. Oxford: Blackwell Scientific 1982:3-623.
2. Smith JL, Finley JC, Lennon VA. Autoantibodies in paraneoplastic cerebellar degeneration bind to cytoplasmic antigens of Purkinje cells in humans, rats and mice and are of multiple immunoglobulin classes. J Neuroimmunol 1988;18:37-48.
3. Anderson NE, Budde-Steffen C, Wiley RG, et al. A variant of the anti-Purkinje cell antibody in a patient with paraneoplastic cerebellar degeneration. Neurology 1988;38:1018-26.
4. Greenlee JE, Lipton HL. Anticerebellar antibodies in serum and cerebrospinal fluid of a patient with oat cell carcinoma of the lung and paraneoplastic cerebellar degeneration. Ann Neurol 1986;19:82-5.
5. Greenlee JE, Brashear HR, Jaeckle KA, Stroop WG. Anti cerebellar antibodies in sera of patients with paraneoplastic cerebellar degeneration: studies of antibody specificity and response to plasmapheresis. Ann Neurol 1986;20:139.
6. Graus F, Elkon KB, Lloberes P, et .al. Neuronal antinuclear antibody (anti-Hu) in paraneoplastic encephalomyelitis simulating acute polyneuritis. Acta Neurol Scand 1987;75:249-52.
7. Anderson NE, Rosenblum MK, Graus F, et al. Autoantibodies in paraneoplastic syndromes associated with small-cell lung cancer. Neurology 1988;38:1391-98.
8. Grisold W, Drlicek M, Popp W, Jellinger K. Antineuronal antibodies in small cell lung carcinoma - a significance for paraneoplastic syndromes? Acta Neuropathol 1987;75:199-202.
9. Popp W, Drlicek M, Grisold W, Zwick H. Circulating antineuronal antibodies in small cell lung cancer. Lung 1988;166:243-51.
10. Rodriguez M, Truh LI, O'Neill BP, Lennon VA. Autoimmune paraneoplastic cerebellar degeneration: ultrastructural localization of antibody-binding sites in Purkinje cells. Neurology 1988;38:1380-86.
11. Brashear, HR, Greenlee, JE, Jaeckle, KA, Rose, JW. Anticerebellar antibodies in neurologically normal patients with ovarian neoplasms. Neurology 1989;39:1605-9.
12. Dropcho EJ, Chen Y-T, Posner JB, Old LJ. Cloning of a brain protein identified by autoantibodies from a patient with paraneoplastic cerebellar degeneration. Proc Natl Acad Sci USA 1987;84:4552-6.
13. Grunwald GB, Klein R, Simmonds MA, Kornguth SE. Autoimmune basis for visual paraneoplastic syndrome in patients with small-cell lung carcinoma. Lancet 1985;1:658-61.
14. Thirkill CE, FitzGerald P, Sergott RC, et al. Cancer associated retinopathy (CAR syndrome) with antibodies reacting with retinal, optic-nerve, and cancer cells. N Engl J Med 1989;321:1589-94.
15. Sher E, Gotti C, Canal N, et al. Specificity of calcium channel autoantibodies in Lambert-Eaton myasthenic syndrome. Lancet 1989;2:640-3.
16. Dropcho EJ, Stanton C, Oh SJ. Neuronal antinuclear antibodies in a patient with Lambert-Eaton myasthenic syndrome and small cell lung carcinoma. Neurology 1989;39:249-51.
17. Graus F, Elkon KB, Cordon-Cardo C, Posner JB. Sensory neuronopathy and small cell lung cancer: antineuronal antibody that also reacts with the tumor. Am J Med 1986;80:45-52.
18. Kornguth SE. Neuronal proteins and paraneoplastic syndromes [Editorial]. N Engl J Med 1989;321:1607-8.
19. Chen Y-T, Rettig WJ, Yenamandra AK, et al. Cerebellar degeneration-related antigen: a highly conserved neuroectodermal marker mapped to chromosomes X in human and mouse. Proc Natl Acad Sci USA 1990;87:3077-81.

20. Furneaux HF, Reich L, Posner JB. Autoantibody synthesis in the central nervous system of patients with paraneoplastic syndromes. Neurology 1990;40:1085-91.

RA33 ANTIBODIES

These anti-nuclear antibodies, which react with a 33 kd proteinaceous component of HeLa Ohio cells, are found in 36% of RA patients and in about 0.6% (1/170) of normal/disease controls.[1] Anti-RA33 antibodies do not correlate with presence or absence of ANA or with ANA pattern by IFA testing on rat liver, are less frequent in RA than IgM RF (50-70%), and are not affected by the removal of IgM-RF. Confirmation of these important results and detailed correlation with clinical and laboratory variables in RA is awaited.

REFERENCES:

1. Hassfeld W, Steiner G, Hartmuth K, et al. Demonstration of a new antinuclear antibody (anti-RA33) that is highly specific for rheumatoid arthritis. Arthritis Rheum 1989;32:1515-20.

RAJI CELL ASSAY FOR CIC

The Raji cell assay is among the least analytically sensitive assays and is among the least diagnostically specific assays for CIC.[1-3] Especially in SLE, positive results often reflect the presence of anti-lymphocyte antibodies.[4] If C3-binding CIC are to be sought, the anti-C3 immune complex assay is currently the most reliable.[5] Some authorities recommend the C1q binding assay and conglutinin binding assay for detection of circulating immune complexes because these assays "may be helpful for assessing and monitoring of disease activity in conditions such as rheumatoid arthritis and SLE".[3] See also **C1q, CONGLUTININ** and **POLYETHYLENE GLYCOL ASSAYS FOR CIC.**

REFERENCES:

1. McDougal JS, Hubbard M, Strobel PL, McDuffie FC. Comparison of five assays for immune complexes in the rheumatic diseases: performance characteristics of the assays. J Lab Clin Med 1982;100:705-19.
2. Lessard J, Nunnery E, Cecere F, McDuffy S, Pope RM. Relationship between the articular manifestations of rheumatoid arthritis and circulating immune complexes detected by three methods and specific classes of rheumatoid factors. J Rheumatol 1983;10:411-7.
3. Bentwich Z, Beverley PCL, Hammarstrom L, et al. Laboratory investigations in clinical immunology: methods, pitfalls, and clinical indications. Clin Immunol Immunopathol 1988;49:478-97.
4. Anderson CL, Stillman WS. Raji cell assay for immune complexes: evidence for detection of Raji-directed immunoglobulin G antibody in sera from patients with systemic lupus erythematosus. J Clin Invest 1980;66:353-60.
5. Arndt R. Detection of C3-binding circulating immune complexes Raji-, conglutinin- and anti-C3 assays--critical review. Immun Infekt 1984;12:3-11.

RAST TESTING

Testing for allergen-specific IgE is useful when skin testing is unreliable due to generalized dermatitis, or severe dermatographism, or when the patient is unable to discontinue antihistamines (see 1-6 for review). Assays for allergen-specific IgG4 are useful largely in patients undergoing desensitization to hymenoptera.[3] Detection of IgG4 antibodies to foods is of no proven diagnostic value,[2] as is also the case for immune complexes composed of food antigens and IgE and/or IgG.[7] Reagents for assessment of allergic contact dermatitis by epicutaneous patch testing are again available in the U.S.[8]

REFERENCES:

1. Van Arsdel PP Jr, Larson EB. Diagnostic tests for patients with suspected allergic disease. Ann Intern Med 1989;110:304-12.
2. Homburger HA. Diagnosis of allergy: in vitro testing. CRC Crit Rev Lab Sci 1986;23:279-314.
3. Hamilton RG, Adkinson NF Jr. Clinical laboratory methods for the assessment and management of human allergic diseases. Clin Lab Med 1986;6:117-38.

4. Allergy Council on Scientific Affairs. *In vitro* testing for allergy: report II of the allergy panel. JAMA 1987;258:1639-43.
5. Marshall E. Immune system theories on trial. Science 1986;234:1490-2.
6. Grieco MH. Controversial practices in allergy. JAMA 1982;247:3105-11.
7. Sheffer AL, Lieberman PL, Aaronson DW, et al. Measurement of circulating IgG and IgE food-immune complexes. J Allergy Clin Immunol 1988;81:758-60.
8. Fransway AF. Epicutaneous patch testing: current trends and controversial topics. Mayo Clin Proc 1989;64:415-23.

RETINA ANTIBODIES

Antibodies reactive with nuclear components of the retina and with certain tumors (e.g., small cell carcinomas of the lung) are reported in ANA-negative patients with cancer-associated retinopathy (CAR syndrome); passive transfer of serum causes extensive demyelinization of guinea pig optic nerve.[1] Other neuronal ANAs are well defined in subacute sensory neuronopathy,[2] sensory neuropathies,[3,4] and Lambert-Eaton myasthenic syndrome.[5] See also **PURKINJE (Yo) ANTIBODIES, Hu (NEURONAL ANTINUCLEAR) ANTIBODIES and VOLTAGE-GATED CALCIUM CHANNEL ANTIBODIES.**

REFERENCES:
1. Thirkill CE, FitzGerald P, Sergott RC, et al. Cancer associated retinopathy (CAR syndrome) with antibodies reacting with retinal, optic-nerve, and cancer cells. N Engl J Med 1989;321:1589-94.
2. Kimmel DW, O'Neill BP, Lennon VA. Subacute sensory neuronopathy associated with small cell carcinoma: diagnosis aided by autoimmune serology. Mayo Clin Proc 1988;63:29-32.
3. Graus F, Cordon-Cardo C, Posner JB. Neuronal antinuclear antibody in sensory neuronopathy from lung cancer. Neurology 1985;35-538-43.
4. Graus F, Elkon KB, Cordon-Cardo C, Posner JB. Sensory neuronopathy and small cell lung cancer: antineuronal antibody that also reacts with the tumor. Am J Med 1986;80:45-52.
5. Dropcho EJ, Stanton C, Oh SJ. Neuronal antinuclear antibodies in a patient with Lambert-Eaton myasthenic syndrome and small-cell lung carcinoma. Neurology 1989;39:249-51.

RETICULIN ANTIBODIES

Of the 5 different types of ARA,[1,2] R_1-ARA is the most important. IgA-R_1-ARA are highly specific (greater than 98%) for untreated coeliac disease,[3] although sensitivity may be only about 25-30% (3; cf. 4 for review). Combined screening for coeliac disease with IgA-AGA and IgA-R_1-ARA has been recommended (5; but see 6), as has screening with both these antibodies and IgA-AEmA.[4,6]

IgA-ARA, like IgA anti-gliadin and IgA anti-endomysial antibodies, are found in dermatitis herpetiformis (DH) and can be used to monitor compliance with a gluten-free diet which requires an average of 2 years for clearing of DH.[7-9]

REFERENCES:
1. Unsworth DJ, Johnson GD, Haffenden G, Fry L, Holborow EJ. Binding of wheat gliadin *in vitro* to reticulin in normal and dermatitis herpetiformis skin. J Invest Dermatol 1981;76:88-93.
2. Rizzetto M, Doniach D. Types of 'reticulin' antibodies detected in human sera by immunofluorescence. J Clin Pathol 1973;26:841-51.
3. Unsworth DJ, Walker-Smith JA, Holborow EJ. Gliadin and reticulin antibodies in childhood coeliac disease. Lancet 1983;1:874-5.
4. Kumar V, Beutner EH, Chorzelski TP. Antiendomysial antibody - useful serological indicator of dermatitis herpetiformis. Arch Dermatol Res 1987;279:454-8.
5. Dias J, Unsworth DJ, Walker-Smith JA. Antigliadin and antireticulin antibodies in screening for coeliac disease. Lancet 1987;2:157-8.
6. Volta U, Bonazzi C, Pisi E, Salardi S, Cacciari E. Antigliadin and antireticulin antibodies in coeliac disease and at onset of diabetes in children. Lancet 1987;2:1034-5.

7. Kapuscinska A, Zalewski T, Chorzelski TP, et al. Disease specificity and dynamics of changes in IgA class anti-endomysial antibodies in celiac disease. J Pediatr Gastroenterol Nutr 1987;6:529-34.
8. Fry L, Leonard JN. Intestinal humoral immunity in dermatitis herpetiformis. Lancet 1990;336:378-9.
9. Fry L, Riches DJ, Seah PP, Hoffbrand AV. Clearance of skin lesions in dermatitis herpetiformis after gluten withdrawal. Lancet 1973;1:288-91.

RHEUMATOID FACTORS

Autoantibodies of the IgG, IgA or IgM isotype which are reactive with the crystallizable fraction (Fc) of IgG are called rheumatoid factors. Assays for IgM rheumatoid factors employ human IgG coated to latex particles (latex fixation) or rabbit IgG coated to sheep cells (SCAT, sheep cell agglutination titer). The SCAT is less sensitive but more specific for rheumatoid arthritis (RA) than is latex fixation (cf. 1 for review). Other techniques such as nephelometry and ELISA can be used.[2] IgM RFs are found in about 2-10% of apparently healthy caucasoid adults (1,3,4, cf. 5 for review) and in about 50-70% of adults with classical rheumatoid arthritis as defined by accepted criteria.[6,7] Over several years, there is an inverse relation between functional capacity in RA and titer of IgM RF (cf. 8 for review). The best available data indicate that positive titers of IgM RFs in apparently healthy adults are risk factors for development of RA in proportion to the height of the IgM RF titer.[5,8-10] These data suggest that IgM RF maybe an early marker of the pathogenetic process of RA.

IgA rheumatoid factors are particularly common in IgA nephropathy, but like IgM RFs in RA, their role in pathogenesis is unclear.[11] IgA RFs and IgA-containing CIC are said to correlate with cartilage loss and bone erosion in RA,[12] but (sadly) predictive values were not established and hence evidence for clinical utility of these assays is lacking. IgG rheumatoid factors are reported in a variety of conditions, including vasculitis but the clinical utility of assay for IgG RFs is dubious.[13,14]

The genes which epxress the variable regions of RFs are conserved and commonly present in normals;[15] similar conservation is often found in the variable regions of $\varkappa$ light chains of RFs from different patients.[16] Likewise the presence of the gene for a certain constant region of $\varkappa$ light chains yields a relative risk of 2.8 for RA.[17,18] These data on RF genes and the data on susceptibility genes in the MHC suggest that the predisposition to RA is multifactorial and not restricted to a single susceptibility locus in the MHC or elsewhere.

IgG in RA shows markedly reduced glycosylation,[19] which is associated with lower levels of B cell galactosyltransferase.[20] These abnormalities, which are not restricted to RA, are probably epiphenomena with no important role in etiology or pathogenesis.

REFERENCES:
1. Carson DA. Rheumatoid factor. In: Kelley WN, Harris ED Jr, Ruddy S, Sledge CB, eds. Textbook of Rheumatology. Philadelphia: Saunders WB, 1985;2.
2. Scott DL, Dawes PT, Collins M, Stone R. ELISA assays for IgM and IgG rheumatoid factors: their clinical correlations during therapy with slow-acting anti-rheumatic drugs. Clin Rheum 1987;6:358-68.
3. Hawkins BR, O'Connor KJ, Dawkins RL, Dawkins B, Rodger B. Autoantibodies in an Australian population. I. Prevalence and pesistence. J Clin Lab Immunol 1979;2:211-15.
4. Bennett PH, Wood PHN. Population studies of the rheumatic diseases. Excerpta Medica. International Congress Series No. 148, 1968.
5. del Puente A, Knowler WC, Pettitt DJ, Bennett PH. The incidence of rheumatoid arthritis is predicted by rheumatoid factor titer in a longitudinal population study. Arthritis Rheum 1988;31:1239-44.
6. Masi AT, Medsger TA Jr. Epidemiology of the rheumatic diseases. In: McCarty DJ, ed. Arthritis and allied conditions. Philadelphia: Lea & Febiger, 1979.
7. Ropes MW, Bennett GA, Cobb S, Jacox R, Jessar RA. 1958 revision of diagnostic criteria for rheumatoid arthritis. Bull Rheum Dis 1958;9:175-6.
8. McKenna F. Clinical and laboratory assessment of outcome in rheumatoid arthritis. Br J Rheumatol 1988;27:12-20.
9. Aho K, Palosuo T, Raunio V, Puska P, Aromaa A, Salonen JT. When does rheumatoid disease start? Arthritis Rheum 1985;28:485-9.

10. Walker DJ, Pound JD, Griffiths ID, Powell RJ. Rheumatoid factor tests in the diagnosis and prediction of rheumatoid arthritis. Ann Rheum Dis 1986:45;684-90.
11. Jackson S. Immunoglobulin-antiimmunoglobulin interactions and immune complexes in IgA nephropathy. Am J Kidney Dis 1988;12:425-9.
12. Withrington RH, Teitsson I, Valdimarsson H, Seifert MH. Prospective study of early rheumatoid arthritis. II. Association of rheumatoid factor isotypes with fluctuations in disease activity. Ann Rheum Dis 1984;43:679-85.
13. Robbins DL, Feigal DW Jr, Leek JC. Relationship of serum IgG rheumatoid factor to IgM rheumatoid factor and disease activity in rheumatoid arthritis. J Rheum 1986;13:259-62.
14. Procaccia S, Gasparini A, Colucci A, et al. ELISA determined IgM, IgG and IgA rheumatoid factors in rheumatoid arthritis and in other connective tissue diseases. Clin Exp Rheumatol 1987;5:335-42.
15. Carson DA, Chen PP, Kipps TJ, et al. Idiotypic and genetic studies of human rheumatoid factors. Arthritis Rheum 1987;30:1321-5.
16. Silverman GJ, Goldfien RD, Chen P, et al. Idiotypic and subgroup analysis of human monoclonal rheumatoid factors: implications for structural and genetic basis of autoantibodies in humans. J Clin Invest 1988;82:469-75.
17. Moxley G. DNA polymorphism of immunoglobulin kappa confers risk of rheumatoid arthritis. Arthritis Rheum 1989;32:634-7.
18. Moxley G. Immunoglobulin kappa genotype confers risk of rheumatoid arthritis among HLA-DR4 negative individuals. Arthritis Rheum 1989;32:1365-70.
19. Parekh RB, Dwek RA, Sutton BJ, et al. Association of rheumatoid arthritis and primary osteoarthritis with changes in the glycosylation pattern of total serum IgG. Nature 1985;316:452-7.
20. Axford SJ, Mackenzie L, Lydyard PM, et al. Reduced B-cell galactosyltransferase activity in rheumatoid arthritis. Lancet 1987;2:1486-8.

RIBOSOMAL ANTIBODIES

Antibodies to ribosomes and to ribosomal ribonucleoprotein (anti-rRNP) are found in about 5-12% of patients with systemic lupus erythematosus and are quite rare in other rheumatic diseases.[1-6] The clinical significance of antibodies to ribosomes (i.e., to rRNP) is disputed, but some data suggest an association with nephritis (cf. 5 for review). These antibodies are distinct from those reactive with nuclear ribonucleoproteins (nRNP) which differ in physico-chemical properties from rRNP.[6] Antibodies to ribosomes of the chief cells of rat and mouse stomach (the usual substrates for their detection) are very rare in the normal adult caucasoid population.[7] See also **RIBOSOMAL P PROTEIN ANTIBODIES.**

REFERENCES:
1. Homberg J-C, Rizzetto M, Doniach D. Ribosomal antibodies detected by immunofluorescence in systemic lupus erythematosus and other collagenoses. Clin Exp Immunol 1974;17:617-28.
2. Miyachi K, Tan EM. Antibodies reacting with ribosomal ribonucleoprotein in connective tissue diseases. Arthritis Rheum 1979;22:87-93.
3. Koffler D, Miller TE, Lahita RG. Studies on the specificity and clinical correlation of antiribosomal antibodies in systemic lupus erythematosus sera. Arthritis Rheum 1979;22:463-70.
4. Schur PH, Moroz LA, Kunkel HG. Precipitating antibodies to ribosomes in the serum of patients with systemic lupus erythematosus. Immunochemistry 1967;4:447-453.
5. Meroni PL, de Bartolo G, Barcellini W, et al. Anti-ribosomal ribonucleoprotein autoantibodies in systemic lupus erythematosus. J Clin Immunol 1984;4:45-54.
6. Cortés JJ, Mendoza F, Reyes PA. Antibodies to ribosomal ribonucleoprotein, prevalence in systemic rheumatic diseases and partial characterization of the antigen. J Rheumatol 1987;14:727-31.
7. Hawkins BR, O'Connor KJ, Dawkins RL, Dawkins B, Rodger B. Autoantibodies in an Australian population. I. Prevalence and persistence. J Clin Lab Immunol 1979;2:211-15.

RIBOSOMAL P PROTEIN ANTIBODIES

Anti-P antibodies, which were reported in 90% (18/20) of patients with psychosis due to systemic lupus erythematosus (SLE), are also common (12-20%) in non-psychotic patients with SLE.[1] A positive test for anti-P antibodies (a chemically synthesized C-terminal peptide common to PO, P1 and P2 ribosomal phosphoproteins is used as antigen) is not diagnostic of lupus psychosis, because almost 50% of patients with anti-P antibodies have no severe behavioral problems.[1-3] Independent data evaluating the suggestion that an increase in anti-P might predict lupus psychosis[1] have not been published nor have additional studies showing enrichment of anti-P in CSF (cf. 2). Anti-P antibodies were not found in a large group of patients with CNS abnormalities associated with Sjögren syndrome including 32% with focal disease in the presence or absence of cognitive and/or psychiatric dysfunction and in 24% with cognitive and/or psychiatric dysfunction alone.[4] Anti-P antibodies are, however, occasionally found in Sjögren syndrome associated with SLE and CNS complications.[4] Other data suggest that the association of anti-P antibodies with neuropsychiatric disease in SLE was over ascertained,[5] and the clinical utility of these assays for evaluation of neuropsychiatric disease in SLE is in great doubt. However, anti-P antibodies may well be as diagnostically sensitive and specific for the diagnosis of SLE as are anti-Sm antibodies. See also **NEURONAL ANTIBODIES**.

REFERENCES:
1. Bonfa E, Golombek SJ, Kaufman LD, et al. Association between lupus psychosis and anti-ribosomal P protein antibodies. N Engl J Med 1987;317:265-71.
2. Golombek SJ, Graus F, Elkon KB. Autoantibodies in the cerebrospinal fluid of patients with systemic lupus erythematosus. Arthritis Rheum 1986;29:1090-7.
3. Elkon K, Skelly S, Parnassa A, et al. Identification and chemical synthesis of a ribosomal protein antigenic determinant in systemic lupus erythematosus. Proc Natl Acad Sci USA 1986;83:7419-23.
4. Spezialetti R, Bluestein HG, Alexander EL. Frequency of antibodies to human ribosomal P protein (P) and neuronal cells in Sjögren's syndrome (SS) [Abstract]. Singapore: Second International Conference on Systemic Lupus Erythematosus. 1989.
5. van Dam, de Jong J, Nossent H, et al. Diagnostic value of antibodies against ribosomal phosphoproteins [Abstract]. Singapore: Second International Conference on Systemic Lupus Erythematosus. 1989.

RNA POLYMERASE I

Anti-RNA polymerase I antibodies give a speckled or punctuate nucleolar staining pattern[1] and are present in 4% of scleroderma sera. Similar antibodies are said to be found in 100% of individuals with systemic lupus erythematosus or mixed connective tissue disease and in 78% of individuals with rheumatoid arthritis.[2,3] These results however, are not yet confirmed.

REFERENCES:
1. Reimer G, Rose KM, Scheer U, Tan EM. Autoantibody to RNA polymerase I in scleroderma sera. J Clin Invest 1987;79:65-72.
2. Stetler DA, Jacob ST. Phosphorylation of RNA polymerase I augments its interaction with autoantibodies of systemic lupus erythematosus patients. J Biol Chem 1984;259:13629-32.
3. Stetler DA, Rose KM, Wenger ME, et al. Antibodies to distinct polypeptides of RNA polymerase I in sera from patients with rheumatic autoimmune disease. Proc Natl Acad Sci USA 1982;79:7499-7503.

Scl-70 (TOPOISOMERASE I)

Reacting with human topoisomerase I of 100 kd molecular weight as well as its 67 ($\sim$70) kd fragment, these IgG (and IgA)[1] antibodies are best referred to as anti-topoisomerase I antibodies or less aptly as anti-Scl-100.[2] Anti-topoisomerase I antibodies are present in 43% of diffuse scleroderma patients; but 2/3 of patients with these antibodies have diffuse scleroderma.[3] Anti-topoisomerase I antibodies are also found in about 18% of patients with limited scleroderma. These frequencies are expected to change when EIA, a more sensitive technology, is used with purified antigen or with proteins expressed by the topoisomerase I gene which has been cloned.[4-6] Positivity does not predict cardiac or renal involvement or survival.

Anti-Scl-86, an antibody found in proportions of diffuse and limited scleroderma patients similar to anti-Scl-70, probably reacts with the partially degraded form of anti-Scl-100.[7] See also **CENTROMERE ANTIBODIES.**

REFERENCES:
1. Hildebrandt S, Weiner E, Senécal J, et al. The IgG, IgM, and IgA isotypes of anti-topoisomerase I and anticentromere autoantibodies. Arthritis Rheum 1990;33:724-7.
2. Shero JH, Bordwell B, Rothfield NF, Earnshaw WC. High titers of autoantibodies to topoisomerase I (Scl-70) in sera from scleroderma patients. Science 1986;231:737-40.
3. Steen VD, Powell DL, Medsger TA Jr. Clinical correlations and prognosis based on serum autoantibodies in patients with systemic sclerosis. Arthritis Rheum 1988;31:196-203.
4. D'Arpa P, Machlin PS, Ratrie H III, Rothfield NF, Cleveland DW, Earnshaw WC. cDNA cloning of human DNA topoisomerase I: catalytic activity of a 67.7-kda carboxyl-terminal fragment. Proc Natl Acad Sci USA 1988;85:2543-7.
5. Juarez C, Vila JL, Gelpi C, et al. Characterization of the antigen reactive with anti-Scl-70 antibodies and its application in an enzyme-linked immunosorbent assay. Arthritis Rheum 1988;31:108-15.
6. Verheijen R, van den Hoogen F, Beijer R, et al. A recombinant topoisomerase I used for autoantibody detection in sera from patients with systemic sclerosis. Clin Exp Immunol 1990;80:38-43.
7. van Venrooij WJ, Stapel SO, Houben H, et al. Scl-86, a marker antigen for diffuse scleroderma. J Clin Invest 1985;75:1053-60.

SECRETORY IgA (sIgA)

Secretory IgA is a complex of two molecules of IgA produced by plasma cells and covalently linked to a J chain via disulfide bonds to the four heavy chains. This complex is in turn linked to a molecule of secretory component which is a solubilized part of the IgA receptor of mucosal epithelial cells (cf. 1-3 for review). Selective deficiency of sIgA is not well recognized, but low levels of sIgA in urine are found in some individuals with recurrent non-obstructive urinary tract infections (4,5; cf. 6 for review).

REFERENCES:
1. Russell MW, Mestecky J. Induction of the mucosal immune response. Rev Infect Dis 1988;10:S440-6.
2. Mestecky J. Immunologic considerations of IgA and IgA containing immune complexes. Am J Kidney Dis 1988;12:378-83.
3. Lamm ME. The IgA mucosal immune system. Am J Kidney Dis 1988;12:384-7.
4. Fliedner M, Mehis O, Rauterberg EW, Ritz E. Urinary sIgA in children with UTI. J Pediatr 1986;109:416-21.
5. Riedasch G, Heck P, Rauterberg E, Ritz E. Does low urinary sIgA predispose to urinary tract infection? Kidney Int 1983;23:759-63.
6. Anonymous. Secretory IgA in recurrent urinary tract infections in childhood [Editorial]. Lancet 1988;2:433-4.

SENSITIVITY, SPECIFICITY, PREDICTIVE VALUES AND EFFICIENCY

Tests of very high sensitivity [positivity in disease or p(T/D)] can be used to exclude the relevant disease (cf. 1 and 2 for review). For example, a negative anti-nuclear antibody (ANA) in a non-immunosuppressed patient with a normal immune system is strong evidence against the diagnosis of systemic lupus erythematosus (SLE) if the cutoff point of the ANA assay has been set that essentially all untreated patients with SLE are ANA-positive and that the fewest possible individuals without SLE are ANA-positive. Tests of very high specificity [negativity in health, i.e., p(T/D) as well as negativity in other unrelated diseases] are used as confirmatory tests. For example, a positive test for acetylcholine receptor antibodies is strong evidence for the diagnosis of myasthenia gravis or of a subclinical early or latent MG as can occur, albeit rarely in patients with Graves disease, SLE or thymoma.[2] Likewise positive tests for thyroid-stimulating immunoglobulins are essentially confirmatory of Graves disease, be it of the classical or euthyroid variety. The most useful information about the performance of laboratory tests devolves from their positive and negative predictive values (PVs) which relate the results (+ or −) to the prevalence of the relevant disease(s) in the population being studied. PVs of tests are necessarily approximations and are best based on data derived from tests for which the cutoff point was assigned after inspection of the receiver (or relative) operating characteristic curve for the test being evaluated (cf. 1-7 for review). In all cases, special attention must be given to potential problems arising from unrepresentative spectrum of patients and from possible bias in associating the test result with the disease.[8]

REFERENCES:
1. Dawkins RL, Peter JB. Laboratory tests in clinical immunology: a critique. Am J Med 1980;68:3-5.
2. Dawkins RL. Sensitivity and specificity of autoantibody testing. In: Rose NR, Mackay IR, eds. The autoimmune diseases. Sydney: Academic Press, 1985;669-93.
3. Griner PF, Mayewski RJ, Mushlin AI, Greenland P. Selection and interpretation of diagnostic tests and procedures: principles and application. Ann Intern Med 1981;94:553-600.
4. Beck JR, Shultz EK. The use of relative operating characteristic (ROC) curves in test performance evaluation. Arch Pathol Lab Med 1986;110:13-20.
5. Nierenberg AA, Feinstein AR. How to evaluate a diagnostic marker test. JAMA 1988;259:1699-702.
6. Linnet K. A review on the methodology for assessing diagnostic tests. Clin Chem 1988;347:1379-86.
7. Anderson RE, Hill RB, Key CR. The sensitivity and specificity of clinical diagnostics during five decades. JAMA 1989;261:1610-7.
8. Ransohoff DF, Feinstein AR. Problems of spectrum and bias in evaluating the efficacy of diagnostic tests. N Engl J Med 1978;299:926-30.

SEVERE COMBINED IMMUNE DEFICIENCY

Severe combined immune deficiency (SCID), a group of genetically determined diseases characterized by abnormal T and B cell functions, includes X-linked lymphopenic SCID (Swiss type agammaglobulinemia) and adenosine deaminase deficiency, which together account for 40-50% of SCID. Among the remaining patients, abnormalities of T lymphocyte function include defects of signal transduction[1] and defects of antigen recognition and proliferative responses (due to failure to express IL-1R[2] or CD3[3] or failure to produce IL-2/IL-2 R[4,5]).

In some patients with severe combined immune deficiency of humans and mice, B cells as well as T cells and NK cells are present, but the genes for T cell receptors and immunoglobulins are maintained in their germline configurations, i.e., the genes have not been rearranged (recombined via recombinases) to produce the diversity of T cell receptors and immunoglobulins characteristic of a normal immune system. Abnormalities of gene(s) of the long-sought-after recombinase enzyme system are expected to be found in one or more immune deficiencies, including SCID. RAG-1 (recombination-activating gene-1) is activated only in T and B cells that have recombinase activity.[6] SCID[7] and $bg/nu/xid$[8] mice are very useful for study of the biology of autoimmunity,[9] bone marrow[10-12] and leukemia.[13]

REFERENCES:
1. Chatila T, Wong R, Young M, et al. An immunodeficiency characterized by defective signal transduction in T lymphocytes. N Engl J Med 1989;320:696-702.
2. Chu ET, Rosenwasser LJ, Dinarello CA, et al. Immunodeficiency with defective T-cell response to interleukin 1. Proc Natl Acad Sci USA 1984;81:4945-9.
3. Doi S, Saiki O, Tanaka T, et al. Cellular and genetic analyses of IL-2 production and IL-2 receptor expression in a patient with familial T-cell-dominant immunodeficiency. Clin Immunol Immunopathol 1988;46:24-36.
4. Alarcon B, Regueiro JR, Arnaiz-Villena A, Terhorst C. Familial defect in the surface expression of the T-cell receptor-CD3 complex. N Engl J Med 1988;319:1203-8.
5. Weinberg K, Parkman R. Severe combined immunodeficiency due to a specific defect in the production of interleukin-2. N Engl J Med 1990;322:1718-23.
6. Schatz DG, Oettinger MA, Baltimore D. The V(D)J recombination activating gene, RAG-1. Cell 1989;59:1035-48.
7. Bosma GC, Custer RP, Bosma MJ. A severe combined immunodeficiency mutation in the mouse. Nature 1983;301:527-30.

8. Andriole GL, Mulé JJ, Hansen CT, et al. Evidence that lymphokine-activated killer cells and natural killer cells are distinct based on an analysis of congenitally immunodeficient mice. J Immunol 1985;135:2911-3.
9. Krams SM, Dorshkind K, Gershwin ME. Generation of biliary lesions after transfer of human lymphocytes into severe combined immunodeficient (SCID) mice. J Exp Med 1989;170:1919-30.
10. Mosier DE, Gulizia RJ, Baird SM, Wilson DB. Transfer of a functional human immune system to mice with severe combined immunodeficiency. Nature 1988;335:256-9.
11. McCune JM, Namikawa R, Kaneshima H, et al. The SCID-hu mouse: murine model for the analysis of human hematolymphoid differentiation and function. Science 1988;241:1632-9.
12. Kamel-Reid S, Dick JE. Engraftment of immune-deficient mice with human hematopoietic stem cells. Science 1988;242:1706-9.
13. Kamel-Reid S, Letarte M, Sirard C, et al. A model of human acute lymphoblastic leukemia in immune-deficient SCID mice. Science 1989;246:1597-1600.

SINGLE DOMAIN ANTIBODIES

Single domain antibodies (dAbs) cloned from the variable regions of heavy chains can bind antigens with good affinity even in the absence of light chains.[1-3] Speed of production (days/weeks for dAbs versus weeks/months for mAbs) and the small size of dAbs are special advantages (cf. 4-6). This new technology for producing antigen-specific VH domains will be as scientifically useful as that of monoclonal antibody production by hybridomas.

REFERENCES:
1. Ward ES, Güssow D, Griffiths AD, et al. Binding activities of a repertoire of single immunoglobulin variables domains secreted from *Escherichia coli*. Nature 1989;341:544-6.
2. Orlandi R, Güssow DH, Jones PT, Winter G. Cloning immunoglobulin variable domains for expression by the polymerase chain reaction. Proc Natl Acad Sci USA 1989;86:3833-7.
3. Huse WD, Sastry L, Iverson SA, et al. Generation of a large combinatorial library of the immunoglobulin repertoire in Phage lambda. Science 1989;246:1275-81.
4. Austin P. Will dAbs challenge mAbs? Nature 1989;341:484-5.
5. Dick HM. Single domain antibodies. A simpler and possibly better alternative to monoclonal antibodies in diagnosis and treatment. Br Med J 1990;300:959-60.
6. Anonymous. Single domain antibodies [Editorial]. Lancet 1990;2:1370-1.

SKIN ANTIBODIES

INTER-EPITHELIAL ANTIBODIES, which typically bind via desmosomal components to the surface of cells throughout the epidermis, are found by direct immunofluorescence in skin of approximately 80% of patients with pemphigus vulgaris (PV) and pemphigus foliaceus (PF), and by indirect immunofluorescence in serum of about 90% of patients with these diseases. Why the fluorescence patterns are usually similar, but the blisters in PV (lower epidermis) and PF (upper epidermis) differ in location is unknown. The inter-epithelial antibodies in PV react to higher titers with monkey esophagus, whereas in PF the antibodies react to higher titers with guinea pig esophagus. Rises or falls of titer may indicate impending relapse or effective control of disease respectively (1, cf. 2 for review). These antibodies are of high sensitivity but lower specificity. In endemic pemphigus foliaceus (fogo selvagem), IgG4 inter-epithelial autoantibodies, which are found in 100% of patients,[3] react with desmoglein I and may thereby interrupt keratocyte adhesion; passive transfer into neonatal mice by Fab' suggests that complement activation and surface cross-linking are not crucial to keratinocyte detachment.[4]

DERMAL-EPIDERMAL [EPIDERMAL BASEMENT MEMBRANE ZONE (BMZ)] ANTIBODIES, which bind via hemidesmosomal components to the BMZ, are found by direct fluorescence in skin of approximately 90% of patients with bullous pemphigoid (BP), 90% of cicatricial pemphigoid (and Brunsting-Perry variant), and approximately 100% of epidermolysis bullosa acquisita. Antibodies to epidermal BMZ are found by indirect immunofluorescence in serum of approximately 70%, 10% and 25% frequency in these diseases, respectively. Similar antibodies to epithelial BMZ are detected by direct immunofluorescence in 30-50% of herpes gestationis (C3 at BMZ in 100%) and by indirect immunofluorescence in serum of approximately 20% of herpes gestationis. Immunoblotting, a more sensitive method, allows detection of serum antibodies to hemidesmosomal components of the BMZ in approximately 90% of patients with herpes gestationis.[5] See also **HERPES GESTATIONIS ANTIBODIES**.

REFERENCES:
1. Jablonska S, Chrozelski TP, Beutner EH. Uses of immunofluorescence tests of skin and sera. Arch Dermatol 1975;111:371-81.
2. Stanley JR. Pemphigus and pemphigoid as paradigms of organ-specific, autoantibody-mediated diseases. J Clin Invest 1989;83:1443-8.
3. Squiquera HL, Diaz LA, Sampaio AP, et al. Serological abnormalities in patients with endemic pemphigus foliaceus (fogo selvagem), their relatives and normal donors from endemic and non-endemic areas of Brazil. J Invest Dermatol 1988;91:189-91.
4. Rock B, Labib RS, Diaz LA. Monovalent Fab' immunoglobulin fragments from endemic pemphigus foliaceus autoantibodies reproduce the human disease in neonatal balb/c mice. J Clin Invest 1990;85:296-9.
5. Morrison LH, Labib RS, Zone JJ, Diaz LA, Anhalt GJ. Herpes gestationis autoantibodies recognize a 180-kD human epidermal antigen. J Clin Invest 1988;81:2023-6.

Sm (ANTI-*Sm*ith) ANTIBODIES

These antibodies, which are specific for systemic lupus erythematosus, react with the B'/B and D polypeptides which are shared by U1, U2, and U4/6 snRNP (small nuclear ribonucleoproteins) particles which have an essential role in splicing pre-mRNA (cf.1-4 for review). Anti-Sm antibodies do not correlate with any particular feature of SLE.[5] These antibodies are detected by EIA in about 29% of SLE patients compared with about 17% detected by indirect hemagglutination/double diffusion.[6] In contrast to anti-dsDNA antibodies which tend to fluctuate in parallel with disease activity,[7] anti-Sm antibodies do not vary greatly with time,[8] although there is some disagreement on this.[9] The *Sm*ith antigen is composed of 5 small nuclear RNAs (U1, U2, U4, U5 and U6) and is associated with 11 or more polypeptides (including 70 kd, A, A', B'/B'', C, D, E, F and G). Some data suggest anti-Sm antibodies may be a result of, rather than a cause of flares of SLE.[10] EIA is now the method of choice for detection and quantitation of anti-Sm antibodies.[6] Recent cloning of a full-length polypeptide identical with, or closely related to polypeptide B promises great clinical utility for assays for these antibodies.[11] See also **U1 snRNP ANTIBODIES, SMALL NUCLEAR RIBONUCLEOPROTEIN (snRNP) ANTIBODIES** and **U2 snRNP**.

REFERENCES:
1. Conner GE, Nelson D, Wisniewolski R, et al. Protein antigens of the RNA-protein complexes detected by anti-Sm and anti-RNP antibodies found in serum of patients with systemic lupus erythematosus and related disorders. J Exp Med 1982;156:1475-85.
2. Hardin JA. The lupus autoantigens and the pathogenesis of systemic lupus erythematosus. Arthritis Rheum 1986;29:457-60.
3. Tan EM, Chan EKL, Sullivan KF, Rubin RL. Antinuclear antibodies (ANAs): diagnostically specific immune markers and clues toward the understanding of systemic autoimmunity. Clin Immunol Immunopathol 1988;47:121-41.
4. Sperling R. Autoantibodies against nuclear ribonucleoprotein (RNP) complexes. Isr J Med Sci 1988;24:358-62.
5. Field M, Williams DG, Charles P, Maini RN. Specificity of anti-Sm antibodies by ELISA for systemic lupus erythematosus: increased sensitivity of detection using purified peptide antigens. Ann Rheum Dis 1988;47:820-5.
6. Tsay GJ, Chan EKL, Peebles CL, Pollard KM, Tan EM. An immunoassay differentiating sera with antibodies to Sm alone, antibodies to Sm/RNP complex, and antibodies to RNP alone. Arthritis Rheum 1987;30:389-96.
7. Swaak AJG, Aarden LA, Statius van Eps LW, Feltkamp TEW. Anti-dsDNA and complement profiles as prognostic guides in systemic lupus erythematosus. Arthritis Rheum 1979;22:226-35.
8. McCarty GA, Rice JR, Bembe ML, Pisetsky DS. Independent expression of autoantibodies in systemic lupus erythematosus. J Rheumatol 1982;9:691-5.

9. Barada FA Jr, Andrews BS, Davis JS IV, Taylor RP. Antibodies to Sm in patients with systemic lupus erythematosus. Correlation of Sm antibody titers with disease activity and other laboratory parameters. Arthritis Rheum 1981;24:1236-44.

10. ter Borg EJ, Horst G, Hummel E, Jaarsma D, Limburg PC, Kallenberg CGM. Sequential development of antibodies to specific Sm polypeptides in a patient with systemic lupus erythematosus: evidence for independent regulation of anti-double-stranded DNA and anti-Sm antibody production. Arthritis Rheum 1988;31:1563-7.

11. Ohosone Y, Mimori T, Griffith A, et al. Molecular cloning of cDNA encoding Sm autoantigen: derivation of a cDNA for a B polypeptide of the U series of small nuclear ribonucleoprotein particles. Proc Natl Acad Sci USA 1989;86:4249-53.

SMALL NUCLEAR RIBONUCLEOPARTICLE (snRNP) ANTIBODIES

Particles responsible for mRNA processing (spliceosomes) are composed of small nuclear ribonucleoparticles (snRNPs), including U1, U2 and U4-U6 which are well characterized. The snRNP-associated proteins [B' (28 kd), B (27 kd), D (16 kd), D' (15.5 kd), E (12 kd), F (11 kd) and G (91 kd)] are found in all snRNPs, whereas the 70 kd, A (34 kd) and C (22 kd) proteins are unique to U1 snRNPs and A' (33 kd) and B'' (28.5 kd) are unique to U2 snRNPs. Antibodies reactive with 68 kd, A and C are found in mixed connective tissue disease (MCTD) and anti-Sm antibodies are reactive with B, B' and D (cf. 1-5 for review). The E, F and G polypeptides of U1 snRNP are only rarely targets for antibodies in autoimmune diseases. The structure of snRNPs helps explain why anti-U1 RNP antibodies can be found alone, whereas anti-Sm antibodies are typically accompanied by antibodies to U1 snRNP.[1] High titers of antibodies to U1 snRNP (previously referred to as anti-U1 RNP antibodies) are a hallmark of mixed connective tissue disease (cf. 1-4 for review). In lower titers, anti-U1 sRNP antibodies are common in SLE, often in association with anti-Sm antibodies which are pathognomonic of SLE.[1-5] EIAs using chemically purified snRNP polypeptides or recombinant proteins as antigens are very promising.[6] Relationship of the known distribution of Sm antigens in tissues[7] to the clinical manifestations of SLE is not known. Anti-Sm sera are also reactive with snRNP-associated protein termed "N" which has a tissue specificity corresponding to the calcitonin gene-related peptide distribution (cf. 8). See also **Sm ANTIBODIES, U1 snRNP ANTIBODIES** and **U2 RNP ANTIBODIES.**

REFERENCES:

1. Hardin JA. The lupus autoantigens and the pathogenesis of systemic lupus erythematosus. Arthritis Rheum 1986;29:457-60.

2. Tan EM, Chan EKL, Sullivan KF, Rubin RL. Antinuclear antibodies (ANAs): diagnostically specific immune markers and clues toward the understanding of systemic autoimmunity. Clin Immunol Immunopathol 1988;47:121-41.

3. Craft J, Mimori T, Olsen TL, Hardin JA. The U2 small nuclear ribonucleoprotein particle as an autoantigen. Analysis with sera from patients with overlap syndromes. J Clin Invest 1988;81:1716-24.

4. Sperling R. Autoantibodies against nuclear ribonucleoprotein (RNP) complexes. Isr J Med Sci 1988;24:358-62.

5. Ohosone Y, Mimori T, Griffith A, et al. Molecular cloning of cDNA encoding Sm autoantigen: derivation of a cDNA for a B polypeptide of the U series of small nuclear ribonucleoprotein particles. Proc Natl Acad Sci USA 1989;86:4249-53.

6. Takeda Y, Wang GS, Wang RJ, et al. Enzyme-linked immunosorbent assay using isolated (U) small nuclear ribonucleoprotein polypeptides as antigens to investigate the clinical significance of autoantibodies to these polypeptides. Clin Immunol Immunopathol 1989;50:213-30.

7. McAllister G, Amara SG, Lerner MR. Tissue-specific expression and cDNA cloning of small nuclear ribonucleoprotein-associated polypeptide N. Proc Natl Acad Sci USA 1989;85:5296-300.

8. Li Sen, Klein ES, Russo AF, et al. Isolation of cDNA clones encoding small nuclear ribonucleoparticle-associated proteins with different tissue specificities. Proc Natl Acad Sci USA 1989;86:9778-82.

SMOOTH MUSCLE ANTIBODIES

Smooth muscle antibodies (SMA) are found in approximately 3% of normal adult caucasoids.[1] High titers (greater than or equal to 1:160) of SMA of anti-actin specificity (i.e., a broad reactivity on muscular and non-muscular cells including polygonal, pericellular and canalicular patterns on rat liver) are found in approximately 97% of patients with autoimmune chronic active hepatitis.[2] SMA are found less frequently in uveitis,[3] drug-induced hepatitis,[4] alopecia,[5] alcoholic liver disease,[6] primary pulmonary hypertension[7] and transiently in acute hepatitis and other viral infections, including infectious mononucleosis. The anti-actin variety of SMA are particularly associated with autoimmune liver disease,[8] whereas SMA directed to intermediate filaments can be present in virus-induced liver disease.[9] In general, IFA patterns of SMA are not readily or reliably translated into reactivities with specific proteins;[10] this may account for many conflicting reports. The presence of SMA is not predictive of the development of liver disease[11] and is not helpful for prognosis in patients with autoimmune chronic active hepatitis.[12] In general, the absence of SMA and ANA argues for non-autoimmune forms of chronic hepatitis. See also **MITOCHONDRIAL ANTIBODIES, SOLUBLE LIVER ANTIGEN, LIVER-SPECIFIC MEMBRANE LIPOPROTEIN** and **LIVER MEMBRANE ANTIGEN.**

REFERENCES:

1. Hawkins BR, O'Connor KJ, Dawkins RL, Dawkins B, Rodger B. Antoantibodies in an Australian population. I. Prevalence and persistence. J Clin Lab Immunol 1979;2:211-15.
2. Lidman K, Biberfeld G, Fagraeus A, et al. Anti-actin specificity of human smooth muscle antibodies in chronic active hepatitis. Clin Exp Immunol 1976;24:266-72.
3. Murray P. Serum autoantibodies and uveitis. Br J Opthalmol 1986;70:266-8.
4. Homberg J-C, Abuaf N, Helmy-Khalil S, et al. Drug-induced hepatitis associated with anticytoplasmic organelle autoantibodies. Hepatology 1985;5:722-7.
5. Zauli D, Veronesi S, Fusconi M, et al. Non-organ-specific autoimmunity in alopecia. Dermatologica 1985;171:12-15.
6. Cunningham AL, Mackay IR, Frazer IH, et al. Antibody to G-actin in different categories of alcoholic liver disease: quantification by an ELISA and significance for alcoholic cirrhosis. Clin Immunol Immunopathol 1985;34:158-64.
7. Asherson RA, Harris EN, Bernstein RM, Mackworth-Young CGT, Hughes GRV. Immunological studies in "primary" idiopathic pulmonary hypertension. Eur J Rheumatol Inflamm 1984;7:75-9.
8. Kurki P, Miettinen A, Salaspuro M, et al. Cytoskeleton antibodies in chronic active hepatitis, primary biliary cirrhosis, and alcoholic liver disease. Hepatology 1983;3:297.
9. Bretherton L, Brown C, Pedersen JS, et al. ELISA assay for IgG autoantibody to G actin: comparison of chronic active hepatitis and acute viral hepatitis. Clin Exp Immunol 1983;51:611.
10. Fusconi M, Cassani F, Zauli D, et al. Anti-actin antibodies: a new test for an old problem. J Immunol Methods 1990;130:1-8.
11. Jorde R, Skogen B, Rekvig OP. A re-examination of patients with previously detected autoantibodies to smooth muscle. Acta Med Scand 1987;222:471-5.
12. Hirschmann E, Dold UW. Detection of tissue antibodies and long-term prognosis in liver diseases--a catamnestic matched-pair study. Leber Magen Darm 1988;18:84-94.

SOLUBLE LIVER ANTIGEN ANTIBODIES

These antibodies, which react with liver but not kidney and which are not detectable by IFA assay, are found by RIA in a subgroup of chronic active hepatitis (CAH) patients characterized by negative ANA and negative anti-LKM as well as low prevalences of antibodies to smooth muscle, mitochondria and liver membrane antigens.[1-4] Anti-SLA are probably identical to anti-LP2 antibodies which are found in about 45% of patients with cryptogenic CAH.[4] Anti-soluble liver antigen antibodies probably recognize the same subgroup(s) of autoimmune CAH patients described as having anti-LP (liver/pancreas-specific) antibodies.[2,5] For review of the immunology of liver disease, see references 6 and 7.

REFERENCES:

1. Manns M, Gerken G, Kyriatsoulis A, Staritz M, Meyer zum Büschenfelde K-H. Characterisation of a new subgroup of autoimmune chronic active hepatitis by autoantibodies against a soluble liver antigen. Lancet 1987;1:292-7.

2. Stechemesser E, Strienz J, Berg PA. Serological definition of new subgroup of patients with autoimmune chronic active hepatitis. Lancet 1987;1:683.

3. Meliconi R, Facchini A, Parracino O, et al. Antibodies to a liver cytoplasmic protein complex (LP2) in acute and chronic liver disease. IRCS J Med Sci 1986;14:55.

4. Meliconi R, Facchini A, Miglio F, Gasbarrini G. Antibodies to liver cytoplasmic protein complex in chronic hepatic disease. Lancet 1987;1:683-4.

5. Berg PA. Klinik und immunologie der autoimmunen chronisch aktiven hepatitis und der primär-biliären zirrhose. Immun Infekt 1982;10:3-14.

6. Meyer zum Buschenfelde K-H. Immunologie der lebererkrankungen. Schweiz Med Wochenschr 1987;117:1065-75.

7. Manns MP, Nakamura RM. Autoimmune liver diseases. Clin Lab Med 1988;8:281-301.

SPERM ANTIBODIES

There is growing evidence that anti-sperm antibodies play a role in infertility,[1,2] although infertility due to antibodies is probably not an absolute condition[3,4] and not all antibodies directed toward spermatozoa interfere with sperm function and thus fertilization.[5] It is now well established that both men and women can make antibodies against human spermatozoa,[6] and IgG anti-sperm antibodies are known to inhibit *in vitro* fertilization.[7] Vasectomy is a known cause of production of anti-sperm antibodies.[8] In vasovasostomized men, a combination of IgA anti-sperm antibodies on all sperm and a strong immune response (titer in serum $\geq$ 256) is associated with a conception rate of zero.[9]

Anti-sperm antibodies have traditionally been measured by a variety of agglutination and immobilization techniques.[10] New procedures are based on rosette formation between viable sperm and erythrocytes or plastic beads coated with anti-serum to human immunoglobulins. These include the indirect mixed antiglobulin reaction (MAR)[11,12] and the immunobead test[13-16] which detect various types of antibodies bound to the sperm. These tests, which have virtually replaced the agglutination and immobilization assays, allow measurement of class-specific antibody (IgG, IgM or IgA) as well as the site of attachment of antibodies to sperm (i.e., head, tail). Antibodies can be measured in serum or as an antigen-antibody complex on the surface of donor sperm; direct assessment of anti-sperm antibodies on the sperm surface is preferred.[17] Enzyme immunoassays (EIAs) using various sperm antigens have been useful to some investigators[18-23] but not to others.[24,25] They promise to be more useful when more is known about sperm antigens and their importance in immunological-based infertility. More studies are needed of the interrelationships among semen characteristics, anti-sperm antibodies, and cervical mucus penetration assays in infertile couples.[26] A new monoclonal antibody-based, complement-dependent sperm immobilization assay should help define the epitope structures reactive with anti-sperm antibodies and may well be very useful clinically.[27] IgA and IgG anti-sperm antibodies react with the same populations of sperm;[28] anti-sperm antibodies include those reactive with galactosyltransferase.[29]

REFERENCES:

1. Bronson R, Cooper G, Rosenfeld D. Sperm antibodies: their role in infertility. Fertil Steril 1984;42:171-83.

2. Tung K. Immunologic basis of male infertility [Editorial]. Lab Invest 1987;57:1-4.

3. Rumke P, Renckens CNM, Bezemer PD, Amstel N. Prognosis of fertility in women with unexplained infertility and sperm agglutinins in the serum. Fertil Steril 1984;42:561.

4. Shulman S. Sperm antigens and autoantibodies: effects on fertility. Am J Reprod Immunol Microbiol 1986;10:82.

5. Alexander NJ. Treatment for antisperm antibodies: voodoo or victory? Fertil Steril 1990;53:602-3.

6. Shulman S. Infertility as caused by sperm antibodies. Gynecol Obstet Invest 1986;22:113-27.

7. Clarke GN, Hyne RV, du Plessis Y, Johnston WIH. Sperm antibodies and human in vitro fertilization. Fertil Steril 1988;49:1018-25.

8. Hussey HH. Vasectomy--a note of concern: reprise [Editorial]. JAMA 1981;245:2333.

9. Meinertz H, Linnet L, Fogh-Andersen P, Hjort T. Antisperm antibodies and fertility after vasovasostomy: a follow-up study of 216 men. Fertil Steril 1990;54:315-21.

10. Shulman S. Sperm antibodies and human infertility. Clin Immunol Newsletter 1982;3:167-73.

11. Hinting A, Vermeulen L, Comhaire F. The indirect mixed antiglobulin reaction test using a commercially available kit for the detection of antisperm antibodies in serum. Fertil Steril 1988;49:1039-44.

12. Meinertz H, Hjort T. Detection of autoimmunity to sperm: mixed antiglobulin reaction (MAR) test or sperm agglutination? A study on 537 men from infertile couples. Fertil Steril 1986;46:86-91.

13. Carson SA, Reiher J, Scommegna A, Prins GS. Antibody binding patterns in infertile males and females as detected by immunobead test, gel-agglutination test, and sperm immobilization test. Fertil Steril 1988;49:487-92.

14. Pattinson HA, Mortimer D. Prevalence of sperm surface antibodies in the male partners of infertile couples as determined by immunobead screening. Fertil Steril 1987;48:466-9.

15. Clarke GN. An improved immunobead test procedure for detecting sperm antibodies in serum. Am J Reprod Immunol Microbiol 1987;13:1-3.

16. Shulman S, Pretorius E, Keane T. Antibodies to spermatozoa: XI. The use of immunobeads for the detection of sperm antibodies in serum. Am J Reprod Immunol Microbiol 1985;9:62-6.

17. Hellstrom WJG, Overstreet JW, Samuels SJ, Lewis EL. The relationship of circulating antisperm antibodies to sperm surface antibodies in infertile men. J Urol 1988;140:1039-44.

18. Berry AJ, Roberts D, Peter JB. An enzyme-linked immunosorption assay for serum antisperm antibodies (IgG, IgM, and IgA) [Abstract]. Am J Clin Pathol 1986;85:390.

19. Alexander NJ, Bearwood D. An immunosorption assay for antibodies to spermatozoa: comparison with agglutination and immobilization tests. Fertil Steril 1984;41:270-6.

20. Lynch DM, Leali BA, Howe SE. A comparison of sperm agglutination and immobilization assays with a quantitative ELISA for anti-sperm antibody in serum. Fertil Steril 1986;46:285-92.

21. Witkin SS, David SS. Effect of sperm antibodies on pregnancy outcome in a subfertile population. Am J Obstet Gynecol 1988;158:59-62.

22. Rousseaux-Prevost R, De Almeida M, Arrar L, et al. Antibodies to sperm basic nuclear proteins detected in infertile patients by dot-immunobinding assay and by enzyme-linked immunosorbent assay. Am J Reprod Immunol Microbiol 1989;20:17-20.

23. Windt M-L, Bouic PJD, Menkveld R, Kruger TF. Use of specific monoclonal antibodies to secretory IgA for the detection of spermatozoal antibodies in serum and seminal plasma by enzyme-linked immunosorbent assay. Am J Reprod Immunol Microbiol 1989;20:9-12.

24. Saji F, Negoro T, Ohashi K, Tanizawa O, Kato M. Clinical evaluation of the enzyme-linked immunosorbent assay (ELISA) kit for antisperm antibodies. Fertil Steril 1988;50:644-7.

25. Clarke GN. Lack of correlation between the immunobead test and the enzyme-linked immunosorbent assay for sperm antibody detection. Am J Reprod Immunol Microbiol 1988;18:44-6.

26. Menge AC, Beitner O. Interrelationships among semen characteristics, antisperm antibodies, and cervical mucus penetration assays in infertile human couples. Fertil Steril 1989;51:486-92.

27. Tsuji Y, Clausen H, Nudelman E, Kaizu T, Hakomori S-I, Isojima S. Human sperm carbohydrate antigens defined by an antisperm human monoclonal antibody derived from an infertile woman bearing antisperm antibodies in her serum. J Exp Med 1988;168:343-56.

28. Haas GG, D'Cruz OJ, DeBault LE. Assessment of fluorescence-activated cell sorting of whether sperm-associated immunoglobulin (Ig)G and IgA occur on the same sperm population. Fertil Steril 1990;54:127-32.

29. Humphreys-Beher MG, Garrison PW, Blackwell RE. Detection of antigalac-tosyltransferase antibodies in plasma from patients with antisperm antibodies. Fertil Steril 1990;54:133-7.

SS-A/Ro ANTIBODIES

Antibodies to SS-A/Ro antigen (a 60 kd polypeptide complexed with Ro RNAs [including hY1, hY3, hY4 and hY5]) are detected by immunodiffusion in about 60% of Sjögren syndrome (SS) and in about 35% of SLE (probably denoting a subgroup with photosensitivity, rheumatoid factor and active or latent SS).[1] Anti-SS-A antibodies are detected by EIA in over 96% of patients with primary SS and in the vast majority of patients with SS secondary to RA or SLE.[2] The dual terminology (SS-A/Ro), like that of SS-B/La reflects the names given by two research groups.[3,4] Levels of anti-SS-A antibodies are much higher in primary than in secondary (RA or SLE) SS.

As with other ANAs, antibodies to SS-A/Ro and SS-B/La are best detected using a composite of cryostat sections of solid tissue and acetone-fixed cell lines of human tissue.[5,6] The presence of anti-SS-A/Ro antibodies increases to about 1:20 the risk of a woman with lupus having an infant with congenital heart block.[7] These maternal antibodies may actually cause the development of some cases of congenital heart block.[8] Transplacental passage of maternal anti-SS-A antibodies is a serologic marker for neonatal LE. The mothers of infants with neonatal LE may be asymptomatic, have symptoms only of sicca syndrome or thyroiditis, or have SLE.[9] Antibodies to SS-A/Ro are found in C2 and C4 deficiency states,[10] in vasculitis with SS[11,12] and in high prevalence in subacute cutaneous lupus.[13]

Antibodies to SS-A/Ro are present in low amounts in only a few (less than 1%) normal individuals.[14,15] The method of choice for quantitation of these antibodies is EIA.[15,16] So-called ANA-negative SLE (a small percentage [2-5%] of lupus patients) is typified by subacute cutaneous lupus, positive IgM-RF and anti-SS-A antibodies.[17] Genes of the $C\beta2$ constant region of the TCR and of the HLA class II region may regulate production of anti-SS-A/Ro antibodies.[18]

About 50% of patients with SS as well as those with SLE react with both the 60 kd and 52 kd components of the SS-A (Ro) particle[19] which is composed of at least these proteins and RNA. About 40% of SS react only with the 52 kd protein, and about 20% of SLE react only with the 60 kd component.[19] Antibodies to both the 52 kd SS-A/Ro protein and the 48 kd SS-B/La protein are common in mothers of patients with neonatal LE and complete heart block and are also abundant in fetal cardiac tissue of 18-24 weeks gestation (20; cf. 21 for review). The stable structural association of Ro/RNP with the La polypeptide probably explains why antibodies to Ro and La occur together so commonly.[22]

Remarkable conservation of SSA/Ro-like molecules (most likely human calreticulin) suggests that its calcium-binding function is of fundamental biological significance.[23]

REFERENCES:

1. Tan EM, Chan EKL, Sullivan KF, Rubin RL. Antinuclear antibodies (ANAs): diagnostically specific immune markers and clues toward the understanding of systemic autoimmunity. Clin Immunol Immunopathol 1988;47:121-41.
2. Harley JB, Alexander EL, Bias WB, et al. Anti-Ro (SS-A) and anti-La (SS-B) in patients with Sjögren's syndrome. Arthritis Rheum 1986;29:196-206.
3. Alspaugh MA, Talal N, Tan EM. Differentiation and characterization of autoantibodies and their antigens in Sjögren's syndrome. Arthritis Rheum 1976;19:216-22.
4. Mattioli M, Reichlin M. Heterogeneity of RNA protein antigens reactive with sera of patients with systemic lupus erythematosus. Description of a cytoplasmic nonribosomal antigen. Arthritis Rheum 1974;17:421-9.
5. Harmon CE, Deng J-S, Peebles CL, Tan EM. The importance of tissue substrate in the SS-A/Ro antigen-antibody system. Arthritis Rheum 1984;27:166-73.
6. Quality Control Records of Specialty Laboratories, Inc.
7. Ramsey-Goldman R, Hom D, Deng J-S, et al. Anti-SS-A antibodies and fetal outcome in maternal systemic lupus erythematosus. Arthritis Rheum 1986;29:1269-73.
8. Taylor PV, Scott JS, Gerlis LM, Esscher E, Scott O. Maternal antibodies against fetal cardiac antigens in congenital complete heart block. N Engl J Med 1986;315:667-72.
9. Lane AT, Watson RM. Neonatal lupus erythematosus. AJDC 1984;138:663-6.
10. Provost TT, Arnett FC, Reichlin M. Homozygous C2 deficiency, lupus erythematosus, and anti-Ro(SS-A) antibodies. Arthritis Rheum 1983;26:1279-82.
11. Alexander EL, Arnett FC, Provost TT, Stevens MB. Sjögren's syndrome: association of anti-Ro(SS-A) antibodies with vasculitis, hematologic abnormalities, and serologic hyperreactivity. Ann Intern Med 1983;98:155-9.
12. Hochberg MC, Boyd RE, Ahearn JM, et al. Systemic lupus erythematosus: a review of clinico-laboratory features and immunogenetic markers in 150 patients with emphasis on demographic subsets. Medicine 1985;64:285-95.
13. Tsokos GC, Pillemer SR, Klippel JH. Rheumatic disease syndromes associated with antibodies to the Ro(SS-A) ribonuclear protein. Arthritis Rheum 1987;16:237-44.

14. Fritzler MJ, Pauls JD, Kinsella TD, Bowen TJ. Antinuclear, anticytoplasmic, and Sjögren's syndrome antigen A (SS-A/Ro) antibodies in female blood donors. Clin Immunol Immunopathol 1985;36:120-8.
15. Gaither KK, Fox OF, Yamagata H, Mamula MJ, Reichlin M, Harley JB. Implications of anti-Ro/Sjögren's syndrome A antigen autoantibody in normal sera for autoimmunity. J Clin Invest 1987;79:841-6.
16. Yamagata H, Harley JB, Reichlin M. Molecular properties of the Ro/SSA antigen and enzyme-linked immunosorbent assay for quantitation of antibody. J Clin Invest 1984;74:625-33.
17. Maddison PJ, Provost TT, Reichlin M. Serological findings in patients with "ANA-negative" systemic lupus erythematosus. Medicine 1981;60:87-94.
18. Frank MB, McArthur R, Harley JB, Fujisaku A. Anti-Ro(SSA) autoantibodies are associated with T cell receptor β genes in systemic lupus erythematosus patients. J Clin Invest 1990;85:33-9.
19. Ben-Chetrit E, Fox RI, Tan EM. Dissociation of immune responses to the SS-A (Ro) 52-kd and 60-kd polypeptides in systemic lupus erythematosus and Sjögren's syndrome. Arthritis Rheum 1990;33:349-55.
20. Buyon JP, Ben-Chetrit E, Karp S, et al. Acquired congenital heart block. Pattern of maternal antibody response to biochemically defined antigens of the SSA-Ro-SSB/La system in neonatal lupus. J Clin Invest 1989;84:627-34.
21. Buyon JP, Winchester R. Congenital complete heart block. A human model for passively acquired autoimmune injury. Arthritis Rheum 1990;33:609-14.
22. Boire G, Craft J. Human Ro ribonucleoprotein particles: characterization of native structure and stable association with the La polypeptide. J Clin Invest 1990;85:1182-90.
23. McCauliffe DP, Zappi E, Lieu T, et al. A human Ro/SS-A autoantigen is the homologue of calreticuln and is highly homologous with onchocercal RAL-1 antigen and an aplysia "memory molecule". J Clin Invest 1990;86:332-5.

SS-B/La ANTIBODIES

Antibodies to SS-B/La antigen [a 48 kd nucleoplasmic phosphoprotein complexed to some, but not all Ro small RNA (Ro hY1-hY5), which are RNA polymerase III transcripts[1,2]] are detected by EIA in patients with primary Sjögren syndrome (SS) and in most patients with Sjögren syndrome secondary to RA or SLE.[3] Hence, there is little diagnostic value of anti-SS-B/La antibodies for primary SS, except that the presence of anti-SS-B can suggest early primary SS even when systemic rheumatoid complaints are not accompanied by sicca symptoms.[4,5] These antibodies are found only rarely in SS secondary to rheumatic arthritis, progressive systemic sclerosis and primary biliary cirrhosis. The prevalences as assessed by the less sensitive immunodiffusion technique are, of course, much smaller. Antibodies to both SS-A and SS-B are now best detected by EIA.[3,6] Anti-SS-B/La positive patients (who are always anti-SS-A/Ro positive) in general have a later age of onset of SLE and a low frequency of nephritis.[7] An immunodominant epitope (amino acid 88-101) of SS-B/La protein has striking sequence similarity to a retroviral gag polyprotein.[8] Striking similarities and immunologic cross-reactivities are also seen with part of the 70 kd protein of U1 snRNP and retroviral p30^{gag} and with an epitope on DNA topoisomerase I to a different region of p30^{gag}.[9,10]

REFERENCES:
1. Chan EKL, Tan EM. The small nuclear ribonucleoprotein in SS-B/La binds RNA with a conserved protease-resistant domain of 28 kilodaltons. Mol Cell Biol 1987;7:2588:91.
2. Mamula MJ, Silverman ED, Laxer RM, et al. Human monoclonal anti-La antibodies. The La protein resides on a subset of Ro particles. J Immunol 1989;143:2923-8.
3. Harley JB, Alexander EL, Bias WB, et al. Anti-Ro SS-A and anti-La (SS-B) in patients with Sjögren's syndrome. Arthritis Rheum 1986;29:196-206.
4. Martinez-Lavin M, Vaughan JH, Tan EM. Autoantibodies and the spectrum of Sjögren's syndrome. Ann Intern Med 1979;91:185-90.
5. Tan EM. Autoantibodies to nuclear antigens (ANA): their immunobiology and medicine. Adv Immunol 1982;33:167-240.
6. St. Clair EW, Pisetsky DS, Reich CF, Chambers JC, Keene JD. Quantitative immunoassay of anti-La antibodies using purified recombinant La antigen. Arthritis Rheum 1988;31:506-14.

7. Maddison PJ, Isenberg DA, Goulding NJ, Leddy J, Skinner RP. Anti La(SSB) identifies a distinctive subgroup of systemic lupus erythematosus. Br J Rheumatol 1988;27:27-31.
8. Kohsaka H, Yamamoto K, Fujii H, et al. Fine epitope mapping of the human SS-B/La protein. Identification of a distinct autoepitope homologous to a viral gag polyprotein. J Clin Invest 1990;85:1566-74.
9. Query CC, Keene JD. A human autoimmune protein associated with U1 RNA contains a region of homology that is cross-reactive with retroviral p30^{gag} antigen. Cell 1987;51:211-20.
10. Maul GG, Jimenez SA, Riggs E, Ziemnicka-Kotula D. Determination of an epitope of the diffuse systemic sclerosis marker antigen DNA topoisomerase I: sequence similarity with retroviral p30^{gag} protein suggests a possible cause for autoimmunity in systemic sclerosis. Proc Natl Acad Sci USA 1989;86:8492-6.

STEROID CELL ANTIBODIES

Anti-steroid cell antibodies (SCA) react with cytoplasmic antigens of steroid-producing cells in testes and ovary (testicular Leydig cells and their ovarian equivalent; thecal cells in antral follicles and in corpus luteum) as well as placenta and (usually, but not invariably) adrenal cortex. These IgG antibodies are uniformly present in Addisonian patients with ovarian failure or associated hypoparathyroidism.[1-3]

SCA accompanied by antibodies reactive with all 3 layers of adrenal cortex are also found in 51% of Addison disease with clinical thyroid disease, type I diabetes mellitus or pernicious anemia. However, SCA are present in only 22% of autoimmune adrenalitis without other clinically apparent endocrine disorders.[1]

Only those steroid cell antibodies confirmed positive on human gonads, and found together with adrenal antibodies, are associated with polyendocrine autoimmunity type I (also known as autoimmune polyendocrinopathy-candidosis-ectodermal dystrophy) and ovarian failure in adults (or in children with hypoparathyroidism).[2] Note, however, that 20% of polyendocrine patients without Addison disease or ovarian failure have SCA. In general, there is no evidence that SCA found in these patients are specific for only one gonadal tissue.[2,3] See also **OVARY ANTIBODIES**.

REFERENCES:
1. Sotsiou F, Bottazzo GF, Doniach D. Immunofluorescence studies on autoantibodies to steroid-producing cells, and to germline cells in endocrine disease and infertility. Clin Exp Immunol 1980;39:97-111.
2. Elder M, Maclaren N, Riley W. Gonadal autoantibodies in patients with hypogonadism and/or Addison's disease. J Clin Endocrinol Metab 1981;52:1137-42.
3. Ahonen P, Mietinen A, Perheentupa J. Adrenal and steroidal cell antibodies in patients with autoimmune polyglandular disease type I and risk of adrenocortical and ovarian failure. J Clin Endocrinol Metab 1987;64:494-500.

STREPTOKINASE ACTIVITY

About 96% of patients treated with streptokinase (SK) have large amounts of neutralizing activity (presumably mediated by antibodies) in their serum.[1] No data are available on the relationship of the SK-neutralizing activity to SK-associated complications, such as anaphylactic reactions,[2,3] symptomless proteinuria, hematuria and granular casts few hours after treatment,[4] and delayed hypersensitivity reactions characterized by arthralgia, fever, hematuria, proteinuria, rash and diffuse vasculitis sometimes accompanied by azotemia.[4] Appropriate management of patients with recurrent myocardial infarction who were previously treated with streptokinase (with or without previous demonstration of anti-streptokinase activity) is under discussion.[5] In acute post-streptococcal (*Strep. pyogenes*) glomerulonephritis,[6,7] serum contains antibodies to SK and to potential pathogenic immunogens, including nephritis-strain-associated protein (NSAP, a variant SK enzyme which binds to glomerular basement membrane),[8] and endostreptosin (ESS, an intracellular precursor of NSAP).[9]

REFERENCES:
1. Jalihal S, Morris GK. Antistreptokinase titres after intravenous streptokinase. Lancet 1990;1:184-5.

2. Dykewicz MS, McGrath KG, Davison R, et al. Identification of patients at risk for anaphylaxis due to streptokinase. Arch Intern Med 1986;146:305-7.

3. McGrath KG, Patterson R. Anaphylactic reactivity to streptokinase. JAMA 1984;252:1314-7.

4. Argent N, Adams PC, Callan MFC, et al. Proteinuria and thrombolytic agents [Letters]. Lancet 1990;1:106-7.

5. Sinclair DG, Lynch M, Littler WA, et al. Antistreptokinase titres after intravenous streptokinase [Letters]. Lancet 1990;1:534.

6. Ohkuni H, Friedman J, van de Rijn I, et al. Immunological studies of post-streptococcal sequelae: serological studies with an intracellular protein associated with nephritogenic streptococci. Clin Exp Immunol 1983;54:185-93.

7. Domnisoru L, Ionescu M, Donea E, et al. The dynamics of antistreptokinase and serum complement in poststreptococcal glomerulonephritis. Med Interne 1975;27:359-64.

8. Johnston KH, Zabriskie JB. Purification and partial characterization of the nephritis strain-associated protein from Streptococcus pyogenes, group A. J Exp Med 1986;163:697-712.

9. Cronin W, Deol H, Azadegan A, Lange K. Endostreptosin: isolation of the probable immunogen of acute post-streptococcal glomerulonephritis. Clin Exp Immunol 1989;76:198-203.

STRIATIONAL ANTIBODIES

Present in 80-100% of patients with myasthenia gravis (MG) with thymoma, anti-striational antibodies (AStrA) are found in less than 18% of patients with MG without thymoma.[1-3] The absence of AStrA argues against a thymoma in a patient with MG.[4] Elevated values of AStrA (predominantly IgM) are found in 25% of patients with rheumatoid arthritis treated with penicillamine.[1,5] Striational antibodies are also useful when monitoring immunosuppressive therapy, e.g., by the EIA method[1,3] for detection of autoimmune complications of bone marrow transplantation, including graft-versus-host disease (1, 5; cf. 6 for discussion of GVH disease). The measurement of AStrA and acetylcholine receptor antibodies is useful for predicting risk of MG in patients with thymoma[1,7] and for predicting recurrence of thymoma.[1]

REFERENCES:

1. Cikes N, Momoi MY, Williams CL, et al. Striational autoantibodies: quantitative detection by enzyme immunoassay in myasthenia gravis, thymoma, and recipients of d-penicillamine or allogeneic bone marrow. Mayo Clin Proc 1988;63:474-81.

2. Carrano JA, Zilko PJ, Dawkins RL. Autoantibodies induced by d-penicillamine. In: Dawkins RL, Christiansen FT, Zilko PJ, eds. Immunogenetics in rheumatology, musculoskeletal disease and d-penicillamine. Amsterdam: Excerpta Medica, 1982:362-7.

3. Carrano JA, Swanson NR, Dawkins RL. An enzyme-linked immunosorbent assay for antistriational antibodies associated with myasthenia gravis and thymoma: comparison with indirect immunofluorescence. J Immunol Methods 1983;59:301-14.

4. Keesey J, Bein M, Mink J, et al. Detection of thymoma in myasthenia gravis. Neurology 1980;30:233-9.

5. Dighiero G, Intrator L, Cordonnier C, et al. High levels of anti-cytoskeleton autoantibodies are frequently associated with chronic GVHD. Br J Haematol 1987;67:301-5.

6. Anonymous. Transfusions and graft-versus-host disease [Editorial]. Lancet 1989;1:529-30.

7. Cuénoud S, Feltkamp TEW, Fulpius BW, Oosterhuis HJGH. Antibodies to acetylcholine receptor in patients with thymoma but without myasthenia gravis. Neurology 1980;30:201-3.

SUBSTANCE P

Substance P, the local release of which might correlate with joint inflammation,[1,2] is known to stimulate production of IL-1, IL-6 and TNF-α by monocytes[3] as well as production of prostaglandins by synovial cells.[4] These observations could be relevant to the lack of synovitis in paralyzed limbs of patients with RA (cf. 1). See also **NEUROPEPTIDES.**

REFERENCES:
1. Levine JD, Collier DH, Basbaum AI, et al. Hypothesis: the nervous system may contribute to the pathophysiology of rheumatoid arthritis. J Rheumatol 1985;12:406-11.
2. Levine JD, Goetzl EJ, Basbaum AI. Contribution of the nervous system to the pathophysiology of rheumatoid arthritis and other polyarthritides. Rheum Dis Clin North Am 1987;13:369-83.
3. Lotz M, Vaughan JH, Carson DA. Effect of neuropeptides on production of inflammatory cytokines by human monocytes. Science 1988;241:1218-21.
4. Lotz M, Carson DA, Vaughan JH. Substance P activation of rheumatoid synoviocytes: neural pathway in pathogenesis of arthritis. Science 1987;235:893-5.

SYMPATHETIC NERVOUS SYSTEM ANTIBODIES

Complement-fixing anti-sympathetic ganglia (CF-SG) antibodies and complement-fixing anti-adrenal medullary (CF-ADM) antibodies found in some at risk, prediabetic and insulin-dependent diabetic patients are associated with decreased catecholamine response to posture.[1,2]

REFERENCES:
1. Rabinowe SL, Brown FM, Watts M, et al. Anti-sympathetic ganglia antibodies and postural blood pressure in IDDM subjects of varying duration and patients at high risk of developing IDDM. Diabetes Care 1989;12:1-6.
2. Brown FM, Brink SJ, Freeman R, Rabinowe SL. Anti-sympathetic nervous system autoantibodies. Diabetes 1989;38:938-41.

THREONYL-TRANSFER RNA SYNTHETASE (PL-7) ANTIBODIES

This antibody to threonyl-tRNA synthetase protein is apparently highly specific for myositis. As assayed, it was found in approximately 4% (4/109) of patients with polymyositis/dermatomyositis.[1-5]

REFERENCES:
1. Mathews MB, Reichlin M, Hughes GRV, Bernstein RM. Anti-threonyl-tRNA synthetase, a second myositis-related autoantibody. J Exp Med 1984;160:420-34.
2. Targoff IN, Arnett FC. Clinical manifestations in patients with antibody to PL-12 antigen (alanyl-tRNA synthetase). Am J Med 1990;88:241-51.
3. Targoff IN, Arnett FC, Reichlin M. Antibody to threonyl-transfer RNA synthetase in myositis sera. Arthritis Rheum 1988;31:515-24.
4. Fudman EJ, Schnitzer TJ. Clinical and biochemical characteristics of autoantibody systems in polymyositis and dermatomyositis. Arthritis Rheum 1986;15:255-60.
5. Dang CV, Tan EM, Traugh JA. Myositis autoantibody reactivity and catalytic function of threonyl-tRNA synthetase. FASEB J 1988;2:2376-9.

THROMBOXANE A$_2$

Measurement of 2,3-dinor-thromboxane B$_2$ (an index of endogenous synthesis of thromboxane A$_2$) and 2,3-dinor-6-keto-prostaglandin F1α (an index of endogenous synthesis of prostaglandins) is expected to prove clinically useful in the near future,[1-3] including research on the relationship of vasoactive prostaglandins (thromboxane A$_2$ and prostacyclin) to some varieties of pregnancy-induced hypertension.[4]

REFERENCES:
1. Zipser RD, Laffi G. Prostaglandins, thromboxanes and leukotrienes in clinical medicine. West J Med 1985;143:485-97.
2. Oates JA, FitzGerald GA, Branch RA, et al. Clinical implications of prostaglandin and thromboxane A$_2$ formation (First of two parts). N Engl J Med 1988;319:689-98.

3. Oates JA, FitzGerald GA, Branch RA, et al. Clinical implications of prostaglandin and thromboxane A_2 formation (Second of two parts). N Engl J Med 1988;319:761-7.
4. Schiff E, Peleg E, Goldenberg M, et al. The use of aspirin to prevent pregnancy-induced hypertension and lower the ratio of thromboxane A2 to prostacyclin in relatively high risk pregnancies. N Engl J Med 1989;321:351-6.

THYROID ANTIBODIES

Combined testing for antibodies to thyroglobulin (anti-Tg) and antibodies to thyroid microsome antigens (anti-TM) will detect almost all goitrous thyroiditis (Hashimoto disease), atrophic thyroiditis (myxedema) and about 70-90% of Graves disease.[1,2] Anti-thyroid microsome antibodies are found in about 6-7% of normal adult caucasoids[3] and their prevalence increases with age.[3] These antibodies are persistent over a period of at least 6 years in 57% of adults.[4] By the 6th decade, 15% of females are positive for anti-TM antibodies, which even in asymptomatic individuals can be predictive of hypothyroidism.[4] Early diagnosis by fine needle aspiration is expected to increase the number of patients with Hashimoto disease who are negative for antibodies to thyroid microsomes and thyroglobulin.[1,5] The presence of these antibodies does not exclude thyroid cancer. The association of thyroid disease and thyroid antibodies with adrenal antibodies and parietal cell antibodies is well established in children and adults with[6] and without insulin-dependent diabetes mellitus.[7] The major thyroid microsome antigen is now identified as thyroid peroxidase (cf. 8 for review). When high or low results for total and free thyroid hormones do not fit the clinical findings, the presence of autoantibodies to thyroid hormones or iodothyronine should be sought.[9] Testing for anti-TM antibodies is thought to be a cost-effective screening method for postpartum thyroid dysfunction.[10] Patients with Graves disease, who have neither anti-Tg nor anti-TM antibodies before and during treatment, are more likely to have relapse of hyperthyroidism than those who have both antibodies.[11] See also **THYROID-STIMULATING IMMUNOGLOBULINS**.

REFERENCES:
1. Anonymous. Autoimmune thyroid disease and thyroid antibodies [Editorial]. Lancet 1988;1:1261-2.
2. Peter JB. Thyroid autoimmunity: in search of antibodies. Diagnostic Medicine 1981:4(5):19-25.
3. Hawkins BR, O'Connor KJ, Dawkins RL, Dawkins B, Rodger B. Autoantibodies in an Australian population. I. Prevalence and persistence. J Clin Lab Immunol 1979;2:211-5.
4. Hawkins BR, Cheah PS, Dawkins RL, et al. Diagnostic significance of thyroid microsomal antibodies in randomly selected population. Lancet 1980;2:1057-9.
5. Baker JR Jr, Saunders NB, Wartofsky L, Tseng YL, Burman KD. Seronegative Hashimoto thyroiditis with thyroid autoantibody production localized to the thyroid. Ann Intern Med 1988;108:26-30.
6. Riley WJ, Maclaren NK, Lezotte DC, Spillar RP, Rosenbloom AL. Thyroid autoimmunity in insulin-dependent diabetes mellitus: the case for routine screening. J Pediatr 1981;98:350-4.
7. Bright GM, Blizzard RM, Kaiser DL, Clarke WL. Organ-specific autoantibodies in children with common endocrine diseases. J Pediatr 1982;100:8-14.
8. Mariotti S, Anelli S, Ruf J, et al. Comparison of serum thyroid microsomal and thyroid peroxidase autoantibodies in thyroid diseases. J Clin Endocrinol Metab 1987;65:987-93.
9. Sakata S, Nakamura S, Miura K. Autoantibodies against thyroid hormones or iodothyronine. Ann Intern Med 1985;103:579-89.
10. Hayslip CC, Fein HG, O'Donnell VM, et al. The value of serum antimicrosomal antibody testing in screening for symptomatic postpartum thyroid dysfunction. Am J Obstet Gynecol 1988;159:203-9.
11. Takaichi Y, Tamai H, Honda K, et al. The significance of antithyroglobulin and antithyroidal microsomal antibodies in patients with hyperthyroidism due to Graves' disease treated with antithyroidal drugs. J Clin Endocrinol Metab 1989;68:1097-1100.

THYROID GROWTH-PROMOTING IMMUNOGLOBULINS

Immunoglobulins thought to promote thyroid growth when assayed in the presence of TSH are found in serum of patients with goitrous Graves' disease, goitrous Hashimoto's thyroiditis, simple and endemic goiter and toxic adenomas.[1-5] The mechanism, which is apparently independent of adenyl cyclase stimulation, is not known, and there is no direct evidence of an antibody acting on a growth factor receptor (cf. 6 for review).

REFERENCES:
1. Zakarija M, Jin S, McKenzie JM. Evidence supporting the identity in Graves' disease of thyroid-stimulating antibody and thyroid growth-promoting immunoglobulin G as assayed in FRTL5 cells. J Clin Invest 1988;81:879-84.
2. Ealey PA, Mitchell SD, Rowless PM, Marshall NJ. An improved metaphase index assay for detecting thyroid growth stimulators using FRTL-5 thyroid cells cultured on a microtiter plate. J Immunol Methods 1988;111:117-23.
3. Drexhage HA, Bottazzo GF, Doniach D. Thyroid growth stimulating and blocking immunoglobulins. In: Chayen J, Bitensky L, eds. Cytochemical bioassays, techniques and clinical applications. New York: Marcel Dekker, 1983:153-72.
4. Dumont JE, Roger PP, Ludgate M. Assays for thyroid growth immunoglobulins and their clinical implications: methods, concepts and misconceptions. Endocrinol Rev 1987;8:448-52.
5. Wilders-Truschnig MM, Drexhage HA, Leb G, et al. Chromatographically purified immunoglobulin G of endemic and sporadic goiter patients stimulates FRTL5 cell growth in a mitotic arrest assay. J Clin Endocrinol Metab 1990;70:444-52.
6. Zakarija M, McKenzie JM. Do thyroid growth-promoting immunoglobulins exist? [Editorial] J Clin Endocrinol Metab 1990;70:308-10.

THYROID-STIMULATING IMMUNOGLOBULINS

Thyroid-stimulating immunoglobulins (TSI), a variety of thyroid receptor antibodies (TRAb), are identified by their capacity to increase adenyl cyclase activity in the Fisher rat thyroid line (FRTL-5). Elevated TSI are found in over 90% of patients with Graves disease (cf. 1 for review). TSI and thyroid growth-promoting immunoglobulin G (TGI) are probably identical.[2] The assay for TSI is more sensitive and specific for Graves disease than is the assay for thyrotropin-binding inhibitory immunoglobulin (TBII).[1] High levels of TBII may be predictive of recurrent disease.[3] Patients who remain positive for TBII after anti-thyroid drug treatment tend to relapse within six months but no relation to long-term relapse was found.[4] HLA-DR3 is not predictive of relapse but the presence of the HLA-DR4 is associated with remission and with absence of TBII.[4] Monitoring TSI is a good guide for duration of anti-thyroid treatment.[5] TBII and TSI are useful during pregnancy for prediction of thyroid dysfunction in infants born of mothers with a history of Graves disease; in infants of mothers who had thyroidectomy for Graves disease; in infants of mothers who have autoimmune thyroiditis.[6] Several assays describing eye muscle-reactive antibodies in thyroid-associated ophthalmopathy were recently described, but the sensitivity and specificity are too low to provide worthwhile clinical information.[7-9] TSI are occasionally found in patients with concomitant Graves disease and metastatic thyroid carcinoma.[10] TSI in the presence or absence of TBII can be detected in the serum of some patients with subclinical Graves disease before the onset of the overt hyperthyroidism.[11] Thyroid-stimulating activity in sera of normal pregnant women is due at least in part to increase levels of hCG;[12] this is not a problem, however, in the usual assay for TSI which uses purified IgG.

REFERENCES:
1. Morris JC III, Hay ID, Nelson RE, Jiang N-S. Clinical utility of thyrotropin-receptor antibody assays: comparison of radioreceptor and bioassay methods. Mayo Clin Proc 1988;63:707-17.
2. Zakarija M, Jin S, McKenzie M. Evidence supporting the identity in Graves' disease of thyroid-stimulating antibody and thyroid growth-promoting immunoglobulin G as assayed in FRTL5 cells. J Clin Invest 1988;81:879-84.
3. Wilson R, McKillop JH, Pearson DWM, Cuthbert GF, Thomson JA. Relapse of Graves' disease after medical therapy: predictive value of thyroidal technetium-99m uptake and serum thyroid stimulating hormone receptor antibody levels. J Nucl Med 1985;26:1024-8.
4. de Bruin TWA, Bolk JH, Bussemaker JK, et al. Graves' disease: immunological and immunogenetic indicators of relapse. Br Med J 1988;296:1292-5.
5. Edan G, Massart C, Hody B, et al. Optimum duration of antithyroid drug treatment determined by assay of thyroid stimulating antibody in patients with Graves' disease. Br Med J 1989;298:359-61.
6. Matsuura N, Konishi J, Fujieda K, et al. TSH-receptor antibodies in mothers with Graves' disease and outcome in their offspring. Lancet 1988;1:14-7.
7. Kendall-Taylor P, Atkinson S, Holcombe M. A specific IgG in Graves' ophthalmopathy and its relation to retro-orbital and thyroid autoimmunity. Br Med J 1984;288:1183-6.

8. Ahmann A, Baker JR Jr, Weetman AP, Wartofsky L, Nutman TB, Burman KD. Antibodies to porcine eye muscle in patients with Graves' ophthalmopathy: identification of serum immunoglobulins directed against unique determinant by immunoblotting and enzyme-linked immunosorbent assay. J Clin Endocrinol Metab 1987;64:454-60.
9. Hiromatsu Y, Fukazawa H, Guinard F, Salvi M, How J, Wall JR. A thyroid cytotoxic antibody that cross-reacts with an eye muscle cell surface antigen may be the cause of thyroid-associated ophthalmopathy. J Clin Endocrinol Metab 1988;67:565-70.
10. Filetti S, Belfiore A, Amir SM, et al. The role of thyroid-stimulating antibodies of Graves' disease in differentiated thyroid cancer. N Engl J Med 1988;318:753-9.
11. Kasagi K, Tamai J, Morita T, et al. Role of thyrotripin receptor antibodies in the development of hyperthyroidism: follow-up studies in nine patients with Graves' disease. J Clin Endocrinol Metab 1989;68:1189-94.
12. Yoshikawa N, Nishikawa M, Horimoto M, et al. Thyroid-stimulating activity in sera of normal pregnant women. J Clin Endocrinol Metab 1989;69:891-5.

TRANSFORMING GROWTH FACTORS α AND β (TGF-α AND TGF-β)

TGF-α, an epithelial growth factor which is angiogenic *in vivo*, is overexpressed as mRNA and protein in lesional psoriatic epidermis.[1] TGF-β1, an inhibitor of epithelial cell growth, is the same in normal, uninvolved and lesional psoriatic epidermis.[1] Whether the documented decrease in protein kinase C (PKC) in chronic psoriatic lesions[2] releases the epidermal growth factor receptor with resultant increased proliferation and TGF-α expression in psoriatic lesions is unknown.

TGF-β (cf. 3 for review), which appears to counteract certain effects of IL-1, IL-6 and TNF, is increased in RA synovial fluid.[4] TGF-β has immunosuppressive actions,[5] suppresses collagenase production by synoviocytes[6] and stimulates synthesis of extracellular matrix.[7] Baseline production of TGF-β, numbers of TGF-β receptors and binding characteristics by fibroblasts cell lines are normal in scleroderma.[8] TGF-β is probably in the fibrosis found in various chronic diseases.[9,10] Antibodies to TGF-β1 inhibit production of extracellular matrix and histological abnormalities of experimental mesangial proliferative glomerulonephritis induced by antibodies reactive with Thy-1.1 epitope and glomerular mesangial cells.[11] Assays for TGFs are not clinically useful at this time.

REFERENCES:
1. Elder JT, Fisher GJ, Lindquist PB, et al. Overexpression of transforming growth factor α in psoriatic epidermis. Science 1988;243:811-14.
2. Horn F, Marks F, Fisher GJ, et al. Decreased protein kinase C activity in psoriatic versus normal epidermis. J Invest Dermator 1987;88:220-2.
3. Roberts AB, Sporn MB. Transforming growth factor β. Adv Cancer Res 1988;51:107-45.
4. Fava R, Olsen N, Keski-Oja J, et al. Active and latent forms of transforming growth factor β activity in syovial effusions. J Exp Med 1989;169:291-6.
5. Wahl SM, Hunt DA, Wong HL, et al. Transforming growth factor-β is a proliferation. J Immunol 1988;140:3026-32.
6. Edwards DR, Murphy G, Reynolds JJ, et al. Transforming growth factor beta modulates the expression of collagenase and metalloproteinase inhibitor. EMBO J 1987;6:1899-904.
7. Ignotz RA, Massagué J. Transforming growth factor-beta stimulates the expression of fibronectin and collagen and their incorporation into the extracellular matrix. J Biol Chem 1986;261:4337-45.
8. Needleman BW, Choi J, Burrows-Mezu A, Fontana JA. Secretion and binding of transforming growth factor β by scleroderma and normal dermal fibroblasts. Arthritis Rheum 1990;33:650-6.
9. Czaja MJ, Weiner FR, Flanders KC, et al. In vitro and in vivo association of transforming growth factor-beta 1 with hepatic fibrosis. J Cell Biol 1989;108:2477-82.
10. MacKay K, Striker LJ, Stauffer JW, et al. Transforming growth factor-β. Murine glomerular receptors and responses of isolated glomerular cells. J Clin Invest 1989;83:1160-7.
11. Border WA, Okua S, Languino LR, et al. Suppression of experimental glomerulonephritis by antiserum against transforming growth factor β1. Nature 1990;346:371-4.

TRANSGENIC ANIMALS

Animals, typically mice, containing new or altered genes (transgenes) as a result of their introduction into the germ line (usually into fertilized ova) are known as transgenic animals[1,2] Transgenics are useful for studying cancer;[2-5] the functional silencing of self-reactive B cells;[6,7] T cell tolerance[8] and autoimmunity[9-12] including IDDM (cf. 13 and 14 for review); immunologically mediated hepatocellular injury in HBV infections;[15] venous, but not arterial thromboses;[16] and neural development and cardiac function.[17]

REFERENCES:
1. Westphal H. Transgenic mammals and biotechnology. FASEB J 1989;3:117-20.
2. Pattengale PK, Stewart TA, Leder A, et al. Animal models of human disease. Pathology and molecular biology of spontaneous neoplasms occurring in transgenic mice carrying and expressing activated cellular oncogenes. Am J Pathol 1989;135:39-61.
3. Heisterkamp N, Jenster G, ten Hoeve J, et al. Acute leukemia in *bcr/abl* transgenic mice. Nature 1990;344:251-3.
4. Muller WJ, Sinn E, Pattengale PK, et al. Single-step induction of mammary adenocarcinoma in transgenic mice bearing the activated *c-neu* oncogene. Cell 1988;54:105-15.
5. Knowles BB, McCarrick J, Fox N. Osteosarcomas in transgenic mice expressing an α-amylase-SV40 T-antigen hybrid gene. Am J Pathol 1990;137:259-62.
6. Nossal GJV. Immunologic tolerance: collaboration between antigen and lymphokines. Science 1989;245:147-53.
7. Arnold B, Messerle M, Jatsch L, et al. Transgenic mice expressing a soluble foreign H-2 class I antigen are tolerant to allogeneic fragments presented by self class I but not to the whole membrane-bound alloantigen. Proc Natl Acad Sci USA 1990;87:1762-6.
8. Arnold B, Goodnow C, Hengartner H, Hämmerling G. The coming of transgenic mice: tolerance and immune reactivity. Immunol Today 1990;11:69-72.
9. Hanahan D. Transgenic mice as probes into complex systems. Science 1989;246:1265-75.
10. Murphy KM, Weaver CT, Elish M, et al. Peripheral tolerance to allogeneic class II histocompatibility antigens expressed in transgenic mice: evidence against a clonal-deletion mechanism. Proc Natl Acad Sci USA 1989;86:10034-8.
11. Zinkernagel RM, Cooper S, Chambers J, et al. Virus-induced autoantibody response to a transgenic viral antigen. Nature 1990;345:68-71.
12. Böhme J, Schuhbaur B, Kanagawa O, et al. MHC-linked protection from diabetes dissociated from clonal deletion of T cells. Science 1990;249:293-5.
13. Parham P. A diversity of diabetes [Editorial]. Nature 1990;345:662-4.
14. Lipes MA, Eisenbarth GS. Transgenic mouse models of type I diabetes. Diabetes 1990;39:879-84.
15. Moriyama T, Guilhot S, Klopchin K, et al. Immunobiology and pathogenesis of hepatocellular injury in hepatitis B virus transgenic mice. Science 1990;248:361-4.
16. Erickson LA, Fici GJ, Lund JE, et al. Development of venous occlusions in mice transgenic for the plasminogen activator inhibitor-1 gene. Nature 1990;346:74-6.
17. Yee S-P, Mock D, Maltby V, et al. Cardiac and neurological abnormalities in v-fps transgenic mice. Proc Natl Acad Sci USA 1989;86:5873-7.

TUBULAR BASEMENT MEMBRANE ANTIBODIES

Anti-tubular basement membrane (TBM) antibodies are found in some patients after kidney transplantation, after treatment with certain drugs and without apparent reason.[1-4] In patients with tubulointerstitial nephritis, TBM antibodies are rarely detected in the absence of other antibodies.[5,6] In some patients with Goodpasture syndrome, anti-TBM are as prominent as anti-GBM autoantibodies. See also **GLOMERULAR BASEMENT MEMBRANE ANTIBODIES.**

REFERENCES:
1. Rotellar C, Noel LH, Droz D, Kreis H, Berger J. Role of antibodies directed against tubular basement membranes in human renal transplantation. Am J Kidney Diseases 1986;7:157-61.
2. Brentjens JR, Noble B, Andres GA. Immunologically mediated lesions of kidney tubules and interstitium in laboratory animals and in man. Springer Semin Immunopathol 1982;5:357-78.
3. Brentjens JR, Matsuo S, Fukatsu A, et al. Immunologic studies in two patients with antitubular basement membrane nephritis. Am J Med 1989;86:603-8.

4. Cameron JS. Allergic interstitial nephritis: clinical features and pathogenesis. Q J Med (New Series) 1988:66:97-115.
5. Bergstein J, Litman N. Interstitial nephritis with anti-tubular-basement-membrane antibody. N Engl J Med 1975;292:875-8.
6. Fliger FD, Wieslander J, Brentjens JR, Andres GA, Butkowski RJ. Identification of a target antigen in human anti-tubular basement membrane nephritis. Kidney Intl 1987;31:800-7.

TUMOR NECROSIS FACTOR-ALPHA (TNF-α CACHECTIN) and TNF-β (LYMPHOTOXIN)

TNF-α, which probably causes cachexia and anemia in a number of conditions,[1-3] is increased after endotoxin administration.[4] Serum TNF-α is said to be increased in some patients with cancer[5-10] and in parasitic infections.[11] High levels of serum TNF in meningococcal meningitis are associated with extremely high (greater than 90%) mortality.[12] Increases of CSF TNF[13] as well as IL-1 and endotoxin[14,15] are found in gram-negative enteric bacterial meningitis. TNF is not increased in aseptic meningitis.[13] Like IL-1, TNF-α is produced in excess in fulminant hepatic failure,[16] is increased in the serum of children with severe infectious purpura[17] and is increased in bronchopulmonary secretions of patients with the adult respiratory distress syndrome.[18,19] TNF is also increased in plasma in tuberculoid leprosy[20] and (with IL-6 and IFN-γ) is commonly elevated in complicated malaria.[21] TNF-α, but not TNF-β is found in approximately 50% of RA joint fluid.[22] TNF-α, TNF-β, IL-1α and IL-1β stimulate production of hyaluronic acids (HA) by synovial fibroblasts[23] (see HYALURON for discussion of HA in RA). TNF (as well as IFN-γ and IL-1) have powerful effects on bone cell proliferation, prostaglandin production, alkaline phosphatase activity, osteocalcin release and B cell function (cf. 24 for review). TNF-α alters red cell kinetics and causes anemia.[25] TNF-α and TNF-β, like IL-1 and IFN-γ, cause early increases in endothelial cell adhesiveness for lymphocytes which is probably important in control of lymphocyte traffic to areas of inflammation (cf. 26 for review). So far, the structures of three cytokines (IL-1β, IL-2 and TNF-α) are known; each has a distinct structural motif which provides no insight into the overlapping biological roles of these molecules.[27] The mechanism of action of TNF-α is unknown, but TNF-specific receptors are required.[28] TNF-α (but not TNF-β) and IFN-α (but not IFN-γ) are increased in synovial fluid of patients with seropositive RA.[22,29] Both TNF-α and IL-1 stimulate resorption and inhibit synthesis of proteoglycan in explants of cartilage.[30] TNF-α is increased in spinal fluid in bacterial, but not viral meningitis.[31] Serum TNF is increased in some patients with Kawasaki disease[32] (see also 33). The secretory products of mononuclear phagocytes, including IL-1 and TNF, were recently reviewed.[34,35] Recently developed assays can distinguish between TNF-α and β, but clinical utility of this differentiation is not yet clear. The importance of membrane-bound TNF is not yet known. Sensitive, reproducible bioassays and immunoassays for TNF are available;[36] bioassay for TNF shows greatly increased serum levels in cachectic patients with severe chronic heart failure.[37] RNA of TNF-α is increased in peripheral blood mononuclear cells of patients with periarteritis nodosa and Wegener granulomatosis.[33] Plasma TNF-α is elevated after endotoxin administration and in septic shock where levels correlate with severity of illness.[28] Like TNF-α, plasma IL-1β is elevated after endotoxin administration and in septic shock, but the elevations are associated with different clinical outcomes and are probably regulated independently.[38] In addition to activated macrophages, TNF is produced by mast cells stimulated with IgE and antigen.[39] A recently defined TNF receptor is probably typical of a family of receptors, including nerve growth factor receptor.[40] Soluble forms of the TNF receptor (referred to sometimes as TNF-α inhibitor) are expected to be important in homeostasis and as disease markers.[41] Granulocytes, which are usually thought of as terminally differentiated, non-secretory cells, can synthesize and secrete TNF-α.[42]

REFERENCES:
1. Oliff A. The role of tumor necrosis factor (cachectin) in cachexia. Cell 1988;54:141-2.
2. Sherry B, Cerami A. Cachectin/tumor necrosis factor exerts endocrine, paracrine, and autocrine control of inflammatory responses. J Cell Biol 1988;107:1269-77.
3. Moldawer LL, Marano MA, Wei H, et al. Cachectin/tumor necrosis factor-α alters red blood cell kinetics and induces anemia in vivo. FASEB J 1989;3:1637-43.
4. Michie HR, Manogue KR, Spriggs DR, et al. Detection of circulating tumor necrosis factor after endotoxin administration. N Engl J Med 1988;318:1481-6.

5. Balkwill F, Osborne R, Burke F, et al. Evidence for tumor necrosis factor/cachectin production in cancer. Lancet 1987;2:1229-32.
6. Selby PJ, Hobbs S, Viner C, Jackson E, Smith IE, McElwain TJ. Endogenous tumor necrosis factor in cancer patients [Letter]. Lancet 1988;1:483.
7. Petersen CM, Moller BK. Immunological reactivity and bioactivity of tumor necrosis factor [Letter]. Lancet 1988;1:934-5.
8. Duncombe AS, Gottlieb DJ, Bianchi A, Brenner MK. Bioactivity and immunoreactivity of tumor necrosis factor in cancer patients [Letter]. Lancet 1988;1:248.
9. Cordingley FT, Bianchi A, Hoffbrand AV, et al. Tumor necrosis factor as an autocrine tumor growth factor for chronic B-cell malignancies. Lancet 1988;1:969-71.
10. Duncombe AS, Brenner MK. Is circulating tumor necrosis factor bioactive? [Letter]. N Engl J Med 1988;319:1227.
11. Scuderi P, Lam KS, Ryan KJ, et al. Raised serum levels of tumor necrosis factor in parasitic infections. Lancet 1986;2:1364-5.
12. Waage A, Halstensen A, Espevik T. Association between tumor necrosis factor in serum and fatal outcome in patients with meningococcal disease. Lancet 1987;1:355-7.
13. Mustafa MM, Ramilo O, Saez-Llorens X, et al. Role of tumor necrosis factor alpha (cachectin) in experimental and clinical bacterial meningitis. Pediatr Dis J 1989;8:907-8.
14. Arditi M, Ables L, Yogev R. Cerebrospinal fluid endotoxin levels in children with *H. influenzae* meningitis before and after administration of intravenous ceftriaxone. J Infect Dis 1989;160:1005-11.
15. McCracken GH Jr, Mustafa MM, Ramilo O, et al. Cerebrospinal fluid interleukin 1-beta and tumor necrosis factor concentrations and outcome from neonatal gram-negative enteric bacillary meningitis. Pediatr Infect Dis J 1989;8:155-9.
16. Muto Y, Nouri-Aria KT, Meager A, Alexander GJM, Eddleston ALWF, Williams R. Enhanced tumor necrosis factor and interleukin-1 in fulminant hepatic failure. Lancet 1988;2:72-4.
17. Girardin E, Grau GE, Dayer J-M, Roux-Lombard P, The J5 Study Group, Lambert P-H. Tumor necrosis factor and interleukin-1 in the serum of children with severe infectious purpura. N Engl J Med 1988;319:397-400.
18. Millar AB, Foley NM, Singer M, et al. Tumour necrosis factor in bronchopulmonary secretions of patients with adult respiratory distress syndrome. Lancet 1989;2:712-4.
19. Roberts DJ, Davies JM, Evans CC, et al. Tumour necrosis factor and adult respiratory distress syndrome [Letter]. Lancet 1989;2:1043-4.
20. Silva CL, Foss NT. Tumor necrosis factor in leprosy patients. J Infect Dis 1989;159:787-90.
21. Kern P, Hemmer CJ, van Damme J, et al. Elevated tumor necrosis factor alpha and interleukin-6 serum levels as markers for complicated *Plasmodium falciparum* malaria. Am J Med 1989;87:139-43.
22. Saxne T, Palladino MA Jr, HeinegTrd D, et al. Detection of tumor necrosis factor α but not tumor necrosis factor β in rheumatoid arthritis synovial fluid and serum. Arthritis Rheum 1988;31:1041-5.
23. Butler DM, Vitti GF, Leizer T, Hamilton JA. Stimulation of the hyaluronic acid levels of human synovial fibroblasts by recombinant human tumor necrosis factor α, tumor necrosis factor β (lymphotoxin), interleukin-1α, and interleukin-1β. Arthritis Rheum 1988;31:1281-9.
24. Gowen M, MacDonald BR, Russell GG. Actions of recombinant human γ-interferon and tumor necrosis factor α on the proliferation and osteoblastic characteristics of human trabecular bone cells in vitro. Arthritis Rheum 1988;31:1500-7.
25. Moldawer LL, Marano MA, Wei H, et al. Cachectin/tumor necrosis factor-α alters red blood cells kinetics and induces anemia in vivo. FASEB J 1989;3:1637-43.
26. Cavender DE, Edelbaum D, Ziff M. Endothelial cell activation induced by tumor necrosis factor and lymphotoxin. Am J Pathol 1989;134:551-60.
27. Jones EY, Stuart DI, Walker NPC. Structure of tumor necrosis factor. Nature 1989;338:225-8.
28. Watanabe N, Neda H, Ohtusuka Y, et al. Signalling pathway of tumor necrosis factor in normal and tumor cells. Cancer Immunol Immunother 1989;28:157-63.
29. Hopkins SJ, Meager A. Cytokines in synovial fluid: II. The presence of tumor necrosis factor and interferon. Clin Exp Immunol 1988;73:88-92.

30. Saklatvala J. Tumor necrosis factor α stimulates resorption and inhibits synthesis of proteoglycan in cartilage. Nature 1986;322:547-9.
31. Leist TP, Frei K, Kam-Hansen S, Zinkernagel RM, Fontana A. Tumor necrosis factor α in cerebrospinal fluid during bacterial, but not viral, meningitis: evaluation in murine model infections and in patients. J Exp Med 1988;167:1743-8.
32. Furukawa S, Matsubara T, Jujoh K, et al. Peripheral blood monocyte/macrophages and serum tumor necrosis factor in Kawasaki disease. Clin Immunol Immunopathol 1988;48:247-51.
33. Deguchi Y, Shibata N, Kishimoto S. Enhanced transcription of TNF in systemic vasculitis [Letter]. Lancet 1989;2:745-6.
34. Nathan CF. Secretory products of macrophages. J Clin Invest 1987;79:319-26.
35. Tracy KJ, Vlassara H, Cerami A. Cachectin/tumor necrosis factor. Lancet 1989;1:1122-6.
36. Meager A, Leung H, Woolley J. Assays for tumor necrosis factor and related cytokines. J Immunol Methods 1989;116:1-17.
37. Levine B, Kalman J, Mayer L, et al. Elevated circulating levels of tumor necrosis factor in severe heart failure. N Engl J Med 1990;323:236-41.
38. Cannon JG, Tompkins RG, Gelfand JA, et al. Circulating interleukin-1 and tumor necrosis factor in septic shock and experimental endotoxin fever. J Infect Dis 1990;161:79-84.
39. Gordon JR, Galli SJ. Mast cells as a source of both performed and immunologically inducible TNF-α/cachectin. Nature 1990;346:274-6.
40. Smith CA, Davis T, Anderson D, et al. A receptor for tumor necrosis factor defines an unusual family of cellular and viral proteins. Science 1990;248:1019-23.
41. Seckinger P, Zhang J, Hauptmann B, Dayer J. Characterization of a tumor necrosis factor α (TNF-α) inhibitor: evidence of immunological cross-reactivity with the TNF receptor. Proc Natl Acad Sci USA 1990;87:5188-92.
42. Dubravec DB, Spriggs DR, Mannick JA, Rodrick ML. Circulating human peripheral blood granulocytes synthesize and secrete tumor necrosis factor α. Proc Natl Acad Sci USA 1990;87:6758-61.

TWO-DIMENSIONAL ELECTROPHORESIS (2 DE)

Two-dimensional electrophoresis (1; cf. 2 for review of early work) combined with ultrasensitive silver stains,[3,4] computer-assisted densitometry[4] and quality control procedures[5] are useful for detection of abnormalities in body fluids (especially CSF) not readily demonstrated by other techniques. Quantitative abnormalities are well documented in multiple sclerosis, inflammatory encephalitides, SSPE, Huntington and Parkinson diseases, schizophrenia and others (6,7; cf. 8 for review). The qualitative abnormalities found in Creutzfeldt-Jakob disease are the most clinically useful abnormalities yet detected by 2 DE (9; cf. 10 for recent review). See also **OLIGOCLONAL IMMUNOGLOBULINS.**

REFERENCES:
1. O'Farrell PH. High resolution two-dimensional electrophoresis of proteins. J Biol Chem 1975;250:4007-21.
2. Goldman D, Merril CR, Ebert MH. Two-dimensional gel electrophoresis of cerebrospinal fluid proteins. Clin Chem 1980;26:1317-22.
3. Merril CR, Switzer RC, Van Keuren ML. Trace polypeptides in cellular extracts and human body fluids detected by two-dimensional electrophoresis and a highly sensitive silver stain. Proc Natl Acad Sci USA 1979;76:4335-9.
4. Merril CR, Harrington MG. "Ultrasensitive" silver stains: their use exemplified in the study of normal human cerebrospinal fluid proteins separated by two-dimensional electrophoresis. Clin Chem 1984;30:1938-42.
5. Daufeldt JA, Harrison HH. Quality control and technical outcome of ISO-DALT two-dimensional electrophoresis in a clinical laboratory setting. Clin Chem 1984;30:1972-80.
6. Harrington MG, Merril CR, Torrey EF. Differences in cerebrospinal fluid proteins between patients with schizophrenia and normal persons. Clin Chem 1985;31:722-6.
7. Walsh MJ, Tourtellotte WW, Roman J, Dreyer W. Immunoglobulin G,A, and M: clonal restriction in multiple sclerosis cerebrospinal fluid and serum--analysis by two-dimensional electrophoresis. Clin Immunol Immunopathol 1985;35:313-27.

8. Harrington MG, Merril CR, Goldman D, Xu X-H, McFarlin DE. Two dimensional electrophoresis of cerebrospinal fluid proteins in multiple sclerosis and various neurological diseases. Electrophoresis 1984;5:236-45.
9. Harrington MG, Merril CR, Asher DM, Gajdusek DC. Abnormal proteins in the cerebrospinal fluid of patients with Creutzfeldt-Jakob Disease. N Engl J Med 1986;;315:279-83.
10. Harrington MG, Merril CR. Cerebrospinal fluid analysis in diseases of the nervous system. J Chromatogr 1988;429:345-58.

U1 snRNP (U1 RNP) ANTIBODIES

These antibodies, which were previously known as anti-RNP (anti-ribonucleoparticle), antibodies or anti-nRNP (anti-nuclear RNP), are found in high titer in patients with mixed connective tissue disease (MCTD) and are common in low titer in SLE for which anti-Sm antibodies are a specific marker (cf. 1-3 for review). The anti-U1sn RNP antibodies in MCTD react with the 70 kd polypeptide of the U1 RNP particle.[4-6] For discussion of the composition of snRNP particles and antibodies reactive with polypeptides of snRNP, see **SMALL NUCLEAR RIBONUCLEOPARTICLE (snRNP) ANTIBODIES.**

REFERENCES:
1. Hardin JA. The lupus autoantigens and the pathogenesis of systemic lupus erythematosus. Arthritis Rheum 1986;29:457-60.
2. Tan EM, Chan EKL, Sullivan KF, Rubin RL. Antinuclear antibodies (ANAs): diagnostically specific immune markers and clues toward the understanding of systemic autoimmunity. Clin Immunol Immunopathol 1988;47:121-41.
3. Sperling R. Autoantibodies against nuclear ribonucleoprotein (RNP) complexes. Isr J Med Sci 1988;24:358-62.
4. Conner GE, Nelson D, Wisniewolski R, Lahita RG, Blobel G, Kunkel HG. Protein antigens of the RNA-protein complexes detected by anti-Sm and anti-RNP antibodies found in serum of patients with systemic lupus erythematosus and related disorders. J Exp Med 1982;156:1475-85.
5. Habets WJ, de Rooij DJ, Hoet MH, van de Putte LB, van Venrooij WJ. Quantitation of anti-RNP and anti-Sm antibodies in MCTD and SLE patients by immunoblotting. Clin Exp Immunol 1985;59:457-66.
6. Pettersson I, Wang G, Smith EI, et al. The use of immunoblotting and immunoprecipitation of (U) small nuclear ribonucleoproteins in the analysis of sera of patients with mixed connective tissue disease and systemic lupus erythematosus. Arthritis Rheum 1986;29:986-95.

U2 snRNP ANTIBODIES

The U2 snRNP (small nuclear ribonucleoparticles) consist of U2sn RNA and eight associated polypeptides. Two of the polypeptides, A' and B'', are unique to U2 snRNP and six (B', B, D, E, F and G) are shared with U1 and other snRNP (cf. 1-3 for review). U2-specific sera which react with B'', with or without A', are commonly found in overlap syndromes with features of myositis[4] and are often accompanied by antibodies to U1 snRNP polypeptides (70 kd, A and C). Previously known as anti-RNP or anti-nRNP, anti-U1 snRNP antibodies reactive with the 70 kd polypeptide at high titers are characteristic of mixed connective tissue disease.[4-6] Anti-Sm antibodies react with the B'/B and D polypeptides which are shared by U1, U2, U4-6 snRNP.[4-6] See also **U1 snRNP ANTIBODIES** and **Sm ANTIBODIES.**

REFERENCES:
1. Hardin JA. The lupus autoantigens and the pathogenesis of systemic lupus erythematosus. Arthritis Rheum 1986;29:457-60.
2. Tan EM, Chan EKL, Sullivan KF, Rubin RL. Antinuclear antibodies (ANAs): diagnostically specific immune markers and clues toward the understanding of systemic autoimmunity. Clin Immunol Immunopathol 1988;47:121-41.
3. Sperling R. Autoantibodies against nuclear ribonucleoprotein (RNP) complexes. Isr J Med Sci 1988;24:358-62.

4. Craft JC, Mimori T, Olsen TL, Hardin JA. The U2 small nuclear ribonucleoprotein particle as an autoantigen: analysis with sera from patients with overlap syndromes. J Clin Invest 1988;81:1716-24.
5. Conner GE, Nelson D, Wisniewolski R, Lahita RG, Blobel G, Kunkel HG. Protein antigens of the RNA-protein complexes detected by anti-Sm and anti-RNP antibodies found in serum of patients with systemic lupus erythematosus and related disorders. J Exp Med 1982;156:1475-85.
6. Habets WJ, de Rooij DJ, Hoet MH, van de Putte LB, van Venrooij WJ. Quantitation of anti-RNP and anti-Sm antibodies in MCTD and SLE patients by immunoblotting. Clin Exp Immunol 1985;59:457-66.

UBIQUITIN ANTIBODIES (AUA)

Found in 79% of patients with SLE, AUA are expected to improve the sensitivity of the laboratory diagnosis of systemic lupus when found in combination with anti-dsDNA antibodies.[1] These observations were not reproducible in our own Laboratories, and technical problems are suspected. The role of ubiquitin in the formation of cytoplasmic non-membrane-bound inclusions, including the intraneuronal neurofibrillary tangles of Alzheimer disease and Mallory bodies (alcoholic hyaline bodies of alcoholic hepatitis and micronodular cirrhosis) is as yet unknown (cf. 2 and 3 for review). See also **DOUBLE STRANDED DNA ANTIBODIES** and **HEAT SHOCK PROTEIN ANTIBODIES**.

REFERENCES:
1. Muller S, Briand J-P, Van Regenmortel MHV. Presence of antibodies to ubiquitin during the autoimmune response associated with systemic lupus erythematosus. Proc Natl Acad Sci USA 1988;85:8176-80.
2. Gallo J-M, Anderton BH. Ubiquitous variations in nerves. Nature 1989;337:687-8.
3. Manetto V, Abdul-Karim FW, Perry G, Tabaton M, Autilio Gambetti L, Gambetti P. Selective presence of ubiquitin in intracellular inclusions. Am J Pathol 1989;134:505-13.

VIRUS RECEPTORS

Virus-specific receptors are often, but not invariably characterized by a specific function and are sometimes present only on certain cells. Such receptors include the CD4 molecule (HIV), ICAM-1 (polio and rhinoviruses), the C3d receptor (EBV), and the EGF receptor (vaccinia) among others (see 1 for review). That the extent of cell differentiation is also important for productive infection is best exemplified by the susceptibility of embryo cells to infection. As our knowledge of virus-specific receptors and the other bases for viral tropism expand, important clues to the genesis of organ-specific autoimmunity can be expected.

REFERENCES:
1. Mims CA. The pathogenetic basis of viral tropism. Am J Pathol 1989;135:447-55.

VISCOSITY

Measurement of plasma viscosity, like that of ESR, is useful for monitoring chronic inflammation.[1,2] However, plasma viscosity results, unlike ESR results, are independent of gender and are less dependent on age in that adult values for plasma viscosity are reached by age 3 years. Some increase is seen in the elderly. Calibration and quality control of plasma viscosity measurements are straight forward. The reference range is narrow and unaffected by anemia or gender; CVs are low. Because storage for several days does not affect result, plasma viscosity is much preferred to ESR (cf. 3 for review). Plasma viscosity is particularly useful for detecting and monitoring hyperviscosity syndromes in myeloma and macroglobulinemia[4] and in autoimmune disease.[5] Increased plasmaviscosity and hyperfibrinogenemia may play a role in unstable angina.[6] Plasma viscosity measurements are vastly under utilized. See also **ERYTHROCYTE SEDIMENTATION RATE.**

REFERENCES:
1. Bull BS, Chien S, Dormandy JA, et al. Laboratory techniques: guidelines on selection of laboratory tests for monitoring the acute phase response. J Clin Pathol 1988;41:1203-12.
2. Boroviczeny KG, Dintenfass L, Fukada E, et al. Recommendation for a selected method for the measurement of plasma viscosity. J Clin Pathol 1984;37:1147-52.

3. Brahn E, Scoville CD. Biochemical markers of disease activity. Baillieres Clin Rheumatol 1988;2:153-83.
4. Crawford J, Cox EB, Cohen HJ. Evaluation of hyperviscosity in monoclonal gammopathies. Am J Med 1985;79:13-22.
5. Levinson SS, Perry M, Goldman J, Nathan LE. Erroneous results with routine laboratory testing for immunoglobulins due to interference from circulating immune complexes in a case of hyperviscosity syndrome associated with autoimmune disease. Clin Chem 1988;34:784-7.
6. Leschke M, Blanke H, Stellwaag M, Motz W, Strauer BE. Hyperfibrinogenaemia and pathological plasma viscosity. Pathogenetic factors in unstable angina pectoris? Dtsch Med Wochenschr 1988;113:1175-81.

VOLTAGE-GATED CALCIUM CHANNEL ANTIBODIES

The Lambert-Eaton myasthenic syndrome (LES) is a form of myasthenia often associated with small cell lung cancer. In some 50% of cases, there is IgG-mediated reduction in presynaptic voltage-gated (voltage-operated) calcium channels.[1,2] These results, however, have not always been confirmed.[3] VGCCA are found on the surface of small cell lung cancers (SCC). With a promising new immunoassay based on a 27-amino acid toxin (ω-conotoxin) which binds to neuronal VGCCs, diagnostic sensitivity of these antibodies is 90-92% for patients with LES in the presence or absence of small cell lung carcinoma and is about 42% for patients with small cell carcinoma without LES.[4] Other data indicate a diagnostic sensitivity for VGCCA of 76% in patients with LES and primary lung cancer (small cancer, squamous or adenocarcinoma), 30% in those with LES and other cancers or no detectable cancer and 10% in patients with SCC without LES.[5] About 40% of patients with LES are clinically free of cancer when first evaluated (cf. 5), but cancers become clinically apparent up to 46 months after diagnosis of LES.[6] See also **Hu (NEURONAL ANTINUCLEAR) ANTIBODIES** and **PURKINJE (Yo) CELL ANTIBODIES.**

REFERENCES:
1. Lang B, Newsom-Davis J, Peers C, Prior C, Wray DW. The effect of myasthenic syndrome antibody on presynaptic calcium channels in the mouse. J Physiol 1987;390:257-70.
2. Chester KA, Lang B, Gill J, Vincent A, Newsom-Davis J. Lambert-Eaton syndrome antibodies: reaction with membranes from a small cell lung cancer xenograft. J Neuroimmunol 1988;18:97-104.
3. Kim YI, Sanders DB, Johns TR, Phillips LH, Smith RE. Lambert-Eaton myasthenic syndrome: the lack of short-term in vitro effects of serum factors on neuromuscular transmission. J Neurol Sci 1988;87:1-13.
4. Sher E, Gotti C, Cahal N, et al. Specificity of calcium channel autoantibodies in Lambert-Eaton myasthenic syndrome. Lancet 1989;2:640-3.
5. Lennon VA, Lambert EH. Autoantibodies bind solubilized calcium channel-ω-conotoxin complexes from small cell lung carcinoma: a diagnostic aid for Lambert-Eaton myasthenic syndrome. Mayo Clin Proc 1989;64:1498-1504.
6. Sher E, Comola M, Nemni R, et al. Calcium channel autoantibody and non-small-cell lung cancer in patients with Lambert-Eaton syndrome. Lancet 1990;335:413.

Yo ANTIBODIES see PURKINJE CELL (Yo) ANTIBODIES

LIST OF ABBREVIATIONS

Ab	=	Antibody
Ab Index	=	Antibody Index

$$\left(\frac{\text{Specific IgG in CSF}}{\text{Total IgG in CSF}}\right) \div \left(\frac{\text{Specific IgG in Serum}}{\text{Total IgG in Serum}}\right)$$

ABIF	=	Avidin-biotin immunofluorescence
ACIF	=	Anticomplement Immunofluorescence
AE	=	Agarose Electrophoresis
Ag	=	Antigen
B	=	Biochemical Assay
bcr	=	Breakpoint cluster region
CAE	=	Cellulose Acetate Electrophoresis
CD	=	Cluster of Differentiation
cDNA	=	Complementary DNA
CF	=	Complement Fixation
CIA	=	Chemiluminescence Assays
CIE	=	Counterimmunoelectrophoresis
CoA	=	Coagglutination
CSF	=	Cerebrospinal Fluid
DA	=	Direct Agglutination
DFA	=	Direct Fluorescent Antibody
DIF	=	Direct Immunofluorescence
DOT BLOT	=	DNA Dot-blot Hybridization
EIA	=	Enzyme Immunoassay
ELISA	=	Enzyme-linked Immunosorbent Assay
EMIT	=	Enzyme-multiplied Immunoassay
EP	=	Electrophoresis
F	=	Fluorimetry
FA	=	Fluorescent Antibody
FC	=	Flow Cytometry
FLO	=	Flocculation
FPIA	=	Fluorescence Polarization Immunoassay
H	=	Hemolytic Assay
HA	=	Hemagglutination
HAI or HI	=	Hemagglutination Inhibition
HPLC	=	High Pressure Liquid Chromatography
ICA	=	Immunocytochemical Assay
ID	=	Immunodiffusion (Double Diffusion)
IEF	=	Isoelectricfocusing
IEP	=	Immunoelectrophoresis
IF	=	Immunofluorescence
IFA	=	Indirect Fluorescent Antibody
IFE	=	Immunofixation Electrophoresis
IFix	=	Immunofixation
IHA	=	Indirect Hemagglutination
Inh EIA	=	Inhibition Enzyme Immunoassay
IP	=	Immunoperoxidase
IRMA	=	Immunoradiometric Assay
kd	=	Kilodalton
LM	=	Light Microscopy
LMC	=	Lymphocyte Microcytotoxicity
LA	=	Latex Agglutination

LIST OF ABBREVIATIONS (continued)

MAb	=	Monoclonal Antibody
MAC	=	IgM Antibody Capture
MAC-ELISA	=	IgM Antibody Capture ELISA
MEIA	=	Microparticle Enzyme Immunoassay
Micro-IF	=	Micro-Immunofluorescence
mRNA	=	Messenger RNA
NB	=	Northern Blot (RNA hybridization)
NEPH	=	Nephelometry
Nt	=	Neutralization
PCR	=	Polymerase Chain Reaction
PEG	=	Polyethylene Glycol
PEP	=	Protein Electrophoresis
PSA	=	Paired Samples Advised (acute and convalescent)
RAST	=	Radioallergosorbent Test
REA	=	Radiative Energy Attenuation
RFU	=	Relative Fluorescent Units
RIA	=	Radioimmunoassay
RID	=	Radial Immunodiffusion
RIP	=	Radioimmunoprecipitation
RIPA	=	Radioimmunoprecipitation Assay
rRNA	=	Ribosomal RNA
S	=	Spectrophotometry, Ultraviolet or Visible
SB	=	Southern Blot (DNA hybridization)
SD	=	Standard Deviation(s)
SF	=	Synovial Fluid
snRNP	=	Small nuclear ribonucleoproteins
TA	=	Tube Agglutination
TCA	=	Tissue Culture Assay
TDE(2DE)	=	Two-dimensional Electrophoresis
WB	=	Western Blot (immunoblot)

METHODOLOGY GUIDE

1. SEPARATION ANALYSES
   EP   Electrophoresis
   FC   Flow Cytometry

2. SOLUBLE ANTIGEN-ANTIBODY REACTION ASSAYS
   ID or DD   Immunodiffusion or Double Diffusion
   RID   Radial Immunodiffusion
   CIE   Counterimmunoelectrophoresis
   IEP   Immunoelectrophoresis
   IFIX   Immunofixation

3. PARTICULATE ANTIGEN-ANTIBODY REACTION ASSAYS
   DA   Direct Agglutination
   HA   Hemagglutination
   LA   Latex Agglutination (Latex Particle Agglutination)
   CoA   Coagglutination
   HI or HAI   Hemagglutination Inhibition
   NEPH   Nephelometry

4. RBC LYTIC ASSAYS FOR DETECTING ANTIGEN-ANTIBODY REACTIONS
   CF   Complement Fixation
   Nt   Neutralization

5. IMMUNOHISTOCHEMICAL ASSAYS
   FA   Fluorescent Antibody
   DFA   Direct Fluorescent Antibody
   IFA   Indirect Fluorescent Antibody
   ACIF   Anticomplement Immunofluorescence
   ABIF   Avidin-biotin Immunofluorescence
   Micro-IF   Micro-immunofluorescence
   IP   Immunoperoxidase
   ICA   Immunocytochemical Assay

6. IMMUNOASSAY PROCEDURES
   RIA   Radioimmunoassay
   IRMA   Immunoradiometric Assay
   RAST   Radioallergosorbent Test
   FPIA   Fluorescence Polarization Immunoassay
   CIA   Chemiluminescence Assays
   EIA   Enzyme Immunoassay
   EMIT   Enzyme-multiplied Immunoassay
   ELISA   Enzyme-linked Immunosorbent Assay
   MAC   IgM Antibody Capture
   MEIA   Microparticle Enzyme Immunoassay
   RIPA   Radioimmunoprecipitation Assay

7. TECHNIQUES IN MOLECULAR BIOLOGY
   DOT BLOT   DNA Dot-Blot Hybridization
   PCR   Polymerase Chain Reaction
   SB   Southern Blot
   NB   Northern Blot
   WB   Immunoblot/Western Blot

SEPARATION ANALYSES

Electrophoresis (EP) is a technique for separation of ionic molecules (principally proteins) by the differential migration through a gel according to the size and ionic charge of the molecules in an electrical field. Smaller molecules with a more negative charge will travel faster and further through the gel toward the anode of an electrophoretic cell when high voltage is applied. Similar molecules will group on the gel. They may be visualized by staining and quantitated, in relative terms, using densitometers which continuously monitor the photometric density of the resulting stain.

Flow cytometry (FC) is an emerging technique which holds great promise for the separation, classification and quantitation of blood cells and antibodies which affect blood cells. Complex computerized instruments are used to pass a monocellular stream of cells, platelets or other microscopic particulate elements through a beam of laser light. The cells are categorized first by size and then computer analyzed to sort the mixture of cellular elements into cell type by size. In addition, monoclonal antibodies to specific cell surface markers are conjugated to fluorescent dyes and each cell displaying appropriate fluorescent light emission is counted. Tabulation of counted data in conjunction with size analysis enables determination of relative percentages of each specific cellular subset for which monoclonal antibody conjugates are utilized, even when the size of the cell is identical to other subset species.

SOLUBLE ANTIGEN-ANTIBODY REACTION ASSAYS

Immunodiffusion (ID), also called Double diffusion (DD) or the Ouchterlony technique, is the classical procedure used to detect the presence of antibodies and determine their specificity by visualization of "lines of identity" (precipitin lines). These precipitin lines (precipitated antigen-antibody complexes) form where the binding concentrations of antigen and antibody are equivalent. Patient serum diffuses from one well through the gel and reacts with a known specific antigen (or antibody) which diffuses through the gel from a second well. DD is strictly qualitative, although the density of the precipitin line and the distance of the line from the sample well may give some indication of the antibody concentration.

Radial immunodiffusion (RID) is a quantitative variation of the Ouchterlony technique (immunodiffusion) in which the agar gel contains evenly distributed antigen (or antibody) and its counterpart from the test sample diffuses into the gel from a single well resulting in a circular precipitin line around the sample well. The diameter of the precipitin ring is proportional to the concentration of the antibody (or antigen) present in the test sample. By comparing the diameter of the test specimen precipitin ring to known standards, a relatively insensitive estimation of the concentration of specific antibody or antigen can be achieved.

Counterimmunoelectrophoresis (CIE) is a procedure in which oppositely charged antigen and antibody are propelled toward each other by an electrical field. This reduces the time necessary for visualization of the antigen-antibody reaction from 18-24 hours in ID to less than one hour and also substantially increases the sensitivity of the analysis. CIE has the capability of detecting concentrations of antigen/antibody 10 times smaller than the lowest concentrations measurable by DD or ID.

Immunoelectrophoresis (IEP) is a two-step procedure which first involves the electrophoretic separation of proteins, followed by the linear diffusion of antibodies into the electrophoretic gel from a trough which extends through the length of the gel adjacent to the electrophoretic path. The antigen-antibody reactions produce precipitin arcs at positions where equivalence occurs. Although quantitation is subjective, an experienced eye can determine not only the presence of the antigen but, through visual comparison to normal control sera, may discriminate relative increases or decreases of antigen by gauging the length and density of the precipitin arcs at positions established for specific antigens using known standards.

Immunofixation (IFIX) is a powerful enhancement of immunoelectrophoresis in which a series of post-electrophoretic gel slabs are layered with cellulose-acetate gels saturated with specific antibodies. The resulting antigen-antibody complexes fixed on the second gel may then be stained, allowing sensitive and specific qualitative visual identification of paraproteins by electrophoretic position.

PARTICULATE ANTIGEN-ANTIBODY REACTION ASSAYS

Direct agglutination (DA) is a general term for techniques which use the agglutination (macroscopic clumping) of particulate reagents as an indicator of the presence of an antigen-antibody reaction. Examples (HA, LA and CoA) follow.

Hemagglutination (HA) is a technique for detecting specific antibodies which, when present, will cause antigen-coated reagent erythrocytes to agglutinate. Crude quantitation of the antibodies can be achieved by performing a serial dilution of the patient serum and noting the highest dilution (titer) at which agglutination is still present.

Latex agglutination (LA), also known as latex particle agglutination, for detection of antibodies is identical to HA in principle, but the substitution of smaller, antigen-coated latex particles for erythrocytes results in improved sensitivity and reagent longevity. Alternatively, antibodies can be absorbed to the latex particles (under appropriate ionic and pH conditions) by binding to the Fc region of antibodies, leaving the Fab region free to interact with antigens present in the applied specimens. This phenomenon has made LA a popular technique for detecting antigens as well.

Coagglutination (CoA) is similar to the LA technique for detecting antigen (described above). Protein A, a uniformly distributed cell wall component of *Staphylococcus aureus*, is able to bind to the Fc region of most IgG isotype antibodies leaving the Fab region free to interact with antigens present in the applied specimens. The visible agglutination of the *S. aureus* particles indicates the antigen-antibody reaction.

Hemagglutination inhibition (HI), also abbreviated HAI, is a variation of the HA technique. Some viral antigens, when coated on erythrocytes, spontaneously cause agglutination in the absence of antibody. In these situations, the specific antigen-antibody reaction actually prevents the agglutination of reagent RBCs. HAI cannot differentiate between isotypes of specific antibodies (IgG, IgA or IgM) although positive HAI analysis of specimens treated with *Staphylococcus aureus* Protein A (discussed above under CoA) to remove the IgG isotype antibodies has been used to imply the presence of specific IgM antibodies to the specific viral antigen. The crude quantitation of the specific antibodies is possible using serial dilution (titer).

Nephelometry (NEPH) is used to quantitate antigen by analyzing increases in turbidity, as measured by increasing scatter of laser light. The interaction of specific antibodies in the reagent with the antigen from the sample results in the formation of antigen-antibody complexes which are rendered insoluble by the presence of precipitating reagents. Most modern nephelometers compare the rate of formation of antigen-antibody complexes (determined by computer analysis of laser light scatter data) to that of known antigenic standards in order to measure precisely the protein antigens (some of which are actually immunoglobulins) present in moderate concentrations.

RBC LYTIC ASSAYS FOR DETECTING ANTIGEN-ANTIBODY REACTIONS

Complement fixation (CF) is an exacting, complex yet sensitive procedure that detects the presence of a specific antigen-antibody reaction by causing the *in vitro* activation of complement via the classical pathway. If complement is not fixed, lysis of the pre-antibody-coated reagent erythrocytes occurs. Again, crude quantitation of antibodies is possible by determining the highest dilution (titer) at which lysis does not occur. The differentiation of specific antibody isotype is not possible.

Neutralization (Nt) is similar to complement fixation but is applicable only in certain pathogenic situations where the antibody being measured is directed against a hemolysin (a bacterial toxin capable of directly lysing erythrocytes). In these situations, the hemolysin and reagent erythrocytes are added, and if the antibody to the hemolysin is present, the lysis of RBCs will not occur. As in CF, crude quantitation is afforded by serial dilution which may be quantitatively compared to established standard material dilutions.

IMMUNOHISTOCHEMICAL ASSAYS

Fluorescent antibody (FA) assay is a general term for procedures which utilize the visual detection of fluorescent dyes coupled (conjugated) to antibodies which react with the antigen when present using fluorescent microscopy. FA allows a competent technologist to identify visually the site of the antigen-antibody reaction thereby rendering significant specificity. Variations are further explained below (DFA, IFA, ACIF, ABIF and Micro-IF).

Direct fluorescent antibody (DFA) is the straightforward detection of antigens using fluorescently labeled antigen-specific antibody. Because detection of the antigen in a substrate of patient sample (cellular smear, fluid or patient-inoculated culture medium) is the goal, DFA is seldom quantitative.

Indirect fluorescent antibody (IFA) is the detection of antibodies to specific antigenic material in the substrate using fluorescent microscopy. Using fluorescently conjugated antibodies which are specific for a particular isotype of antibody, it is possible to distinguish IgG, IgA and IgM isotypes of specific antibodies using IFA. This sensitive technique is highly specific in well-trained hands and recent developments in the establishment of internationally recognized standard materials have led to accurate quantitation of antibody concentrations through endpoint titration (the highest serial dilution of specimen at which specific fluorescence remains) and through measuring visual intensity of fluorescence compared to known reference standard material.

Anticomplement immunofluorescence (ACIF) is a technique used to make certain indirect fluorescent antibody techniques more specific and sensitive. Here the fluorescent dye is conjugated to antibody directed at complement and then added to a complement-fixing complex of antigen and patient antibody.

Avidin-biotin immunofluorescence (ABIF) holds promise for more sensitive and specific amplification of indirect fluorescent antibody procedures. Antibody to the patient's specific antibodies is labeled with biotin, a compound capable of specifically binding avidin in high concentrations. Fluorescently labeled avidin is then added and fluorescent microscopy is used to detect the presence of the complexes.

Micro-immunofluorescence (Micro-IF) is really multiple IFA. Several different substrates are arranged in specific locations on a single microscope slide well allowing a rapid, simultaneous IFA on each substrate.

Immunoperoxidase (IP) assays are analogous to IFA in that antibody presence is identified on antigenic substrates visually. However, in the indirect IP instead of fluorescent dye-antibody conjugates, enzyme-antibody conjugates (principally peroxidase enzymes) are reacted with their corresponding substrates to produce a product which can be seen with a light microscope, eliminating the requirement for costly fluorescent microscopic equipment.

Immunocytochemical asssay (ICA) involves the computerized assessment of microscopic fields following DFA, IFA or indirect or direct IP analysis of biopsy tissue from the patient. In addition to improved specificity with the removal of operator subjectivity, the quantifiability of results through computer data analysis of color, intensity and concentration has only begun to be realized.

IMMUNOASSAY PROCEDURES

Radioimmunoassay (RIA) uses fixed-dose, low-level, radioactive-isotope-labeled antigen ("tracer") to compete with unlabeled antigen from the patient specimen for a fixed number of antibody binding sites. Traditional RIA is done with specific antibodies in liquid solution. Solid-phase RIA involves the use of antibody bound to solid support (e.g., tubes, glass beads or plastic fins). The amount of antigen in the specimen is determined by comparing the bound radioactivity with a standard curve.

Immunoradiometric assay (IRMA) uses low-level radioactively labeled specific antibody to quantitate low concentration compounds. In IRMA, a first antibody is presented on solid-phase (coated on tubes or beads). After binding the antigen present in the sample, a second radioactively labeled antibody is added. Radioactivity remaining after washing the solid phase is proportional to the concentration of antigen present in the sample and is quantitated by comparison to a standard curve.

Radioallergosorbent test (RAST) is the name given to an *in vitro* technique which detects the presence of IgE (and IgG) antibodies to allergens, proteins which may give rise to hypersensitivity reactions seen in allergies. Allergens are coated on a complex carbohydrate matrix called a sorbent. Antibodies specific for the allergen being tested bind to the allergen and, if

151

present, are detected by a low-level radioactively labeled antibody to either human IgE or IgG, depending upon the isotype being tested.

Fluorescence polarization immunoassay (FPIA) is a technique which takes advantage of the increased polarization (non-random propagation of emission) of fluorescent light emissions when a fluorescently labeled antigen is bound by reagent antibody. The higher the concentration of unlabeled patient antigen present in the test mixture, the less bound fluorescent antigen is present and, consequently, the lower the polarization of the fluorescent light emission. Standard calibration yields quantitative results.

Chemiluminescence assays (CIA), including a subcategory using bioluminescence (biologically derived chemiluminescence agents), use the generation of light from oxidative chemical reactions as an indicator of the quantity of unbound luminescently labeled antigen. This allows quantitation of unlabeled antigen from patient specimens in a variety of homogeneous (single phase) or heterogeneous (multiple phase) immunoassay techniques.

Enzyme immunoassay (EIA) is the general term for an expanding technical arsenal of testing which allows a full range of quantitative analyses for both antigen and antibodies. These tests use color-changed products of enzyme-substrate interaction (or inhibition) to measure the antigen-antibody reaction. Examples of EIA procedures (EMIT, ELISA, MAC, MEIA) follow.

Enzyme multiplied immunoassay technique (EMIT) is a homogeneous (single phase) EIA procedure in which the antigen being measured competes for a limited number of antibody binding sites with enzyme labeled antigen. The reagent antibody has the ability to block enzymatic activity when bound with the reagent enzyme-antigen complex preventing its formation of product in the presence of substrate. The free antigen-enzyme complexes resulting from competition with measured antigen in the sample forms color-change products proportional to the concentration of antigen present in the specimen.

Enzyme-linked immunosorbent assay (ELISA) is a sensitive, heterogenous (multiple phase) analytical technique for quantitation of antigen or antibody in which enzyme-labeled antibody or antigen is bound to a solid support (e.g., tubes, beads, microtiter plate wells, plastic tines or fins). After addition of patient specimen and substrate, antigen, antibody or complex are detected by a color change indicating the presence of the product of an enzyme-substrate reaction. Direct ELISA is a technique for measuring antigen using competition for antibody binding sites between enzyme-labeled antigen and patient antigen. Indirect ELISA, or enzyme immunometric assay, measures antibody concentrations using bound antigen to interact with specimen antibodies. Enzyme-labeled reagent antibodies can be isotype-specific (i.e., capable of determining the presence of IgG, IgA, IgM or IgE classes which react with the antigen of interest). The specificity of indirect ELISA assays for IgM isotypes in some infectious diseases is limited by false-positive results due to IgM rheumatoid factor in the presence of IgG-specific antibodies.

IgM antibody capture ELISA (MAC ELISA) has been developed to impart significant improvement in assay specificity to indirect ELISA procedures for IgM isotype antibodies. Solid-phase support (usually microtiter plate wells) are coated with anti-human IgM antibodies capable of binding all IgM isotype antibodies present in the specimen. Reagent antigen is then added, followed by enzyme-labeled antigen-specific antibodies. If IgM antibodies specific for the antigen in question are present, the "sandwich" complex will result in enzymatic color-change proportional to the concentration of IgM-specific antibody present. This technique appears to be the method of choice in many highly specific and more sensitive assays for IgM infectious disease antibodies.

Microparticle enzyme immunoassay (MEIA) is a technique in which the solid-phase support consists of very small microparticles in liquid suspension. Specific reagent antibodies are covalently bound to the microparticles. Antigen, if present, is then "sandwiched" between bound antibodies and antigen-specific, enzyme-labeled antibodies. Antigen-antibody complexes are detected and quantitated by analysis of fluorescence from the enzyme-substrate interaction.

Radioimmunoprecipitation assay (RIPA) is the term used to describe the qualitative assay used as a confirmatory procedure for some antibodies to viral antigens. Viral-infected cell cultures are radioactively labeled and lysed to yield radiolabeled antigen fragments. Specific antibodies, if present, will bind these antigen fragments and the resulting antigen-antibody complexes are precipitated using protein A, boiled to free the immune complexes which are then separated by electrophoresis. The pattern of antigenic moieties to which antibodies are present may then be detected using autoradiography (the exposure of sensitive X-ray film by the radioactive emissions of the bound, labeled antigens). Comparison to labeled molecular weight standards electrophoresed in the same run allows determination of the molecular weight "bands" of antigen to which antibodies are present.

TECHNIQUES IN MOLECULAR BIOLOGY

DNA "dot-blot" hybridization (DOT-BLOT) is a rapid technique used to detect the presence of a specific DNA in a specimen. Dots, or spots of the DNA containing sample are placed onto a nitrocellulose membrane and fixed. This membrane is then hybridized to a radioactively labeled DNA segment of known sequence, specific for the pathogenic DNA being tested. If the pathogenic DNA is present in the specimen, complementary DNA sequences present on the membrane will hybridize, or anneal, producing a double-stranded DNA segment with the radioactive label incorporated into the molecule. The presence of radioactivity is detected by autoradiography.

Polymerase chain reaction (PCR) is a highly efficient method to amplify low levels of specific DNA sequences in a sample to reach the threshold of detection. Two short DNA "primers", oligonucleotides (small portions of a single DNA strand) specific for the pathogenic DNA sought whose sequence flanks that section of DNA to be amplified, are used. Repeated cycles of DNA denaturation (separation of the double DNA strands), primer annealing (recombination of the double-stranded structure) and extension of the primed DNA sequence (by the enzyme DNA polymerase in the presence of added purine and pyrimidine bases) are performed. Each cycle doubles the amount of specific DNA sequence present and results in an exponential accumulation of the DNA fragment being amplified. The reaction products are hybridized to a radioactively labeled DNA segment complementary to a short sequence of the amplified DNA. Following electrophoresis, the radiolabeled product of specific size is detected by autoradiography.

Southern blot (SB) describes the technique first developed by the Scottish molecular biologist Edward M. Southern which now bears his name. Specimen DNA is denatured, treated with restriction enzymes to result in DNA fragments and then the single-stranded DNA fragments are separated by electrophoresis. The electrophoretically separated fragments are then blotted to a nitrocellulose membrane, retaining their electrophoretic position, and hybridized with radiolabeled single-stranded DNA fragments with sequences complementary to those being sought. The resulting double-stranded DNA bearing the radiolabel is then, if present, detected by autoradiography.

Northern blot (NB) uses techniques similar to the Southern blot described above. Messenger-RNA from the specimen is separated by electrophoresis and blotted to a specially modified paper support to result in covalent fixing of the mRNA in the electrophoretic positions. Radiolabeled single-stranded DNA fragments complementary to the specific mRNA being sought are then hybridized to the bound mRNA. If the specific mRNA is present, the radioactivity is detected by autoradiography. The derivation of this technique from the Southern blot used for DNA detection has led to the common usage of the term "Northern blot" for the detection of specific mRNA.

Immunoblot, commonly referred to as "Western blot" (WB) because of the similarity to the procedures described above, is used to detect antibodies to specific epitopes of electrophoretically separated subspecies of antigens. Electrophoresis of antigenic material yields separation of the antigenic components by molecular weight. Blotting of the separated antigen to nitrocellulose, retaining the electrophoretic position, and reacting it with patient specimen will result in the binding of specific antibodies, if present, to each antigenic "band". Electrophoresis of known molecular weight standards allows for the determination of the molecular weight of each antigenic band to which antibodies may be produced. These antibodies are then detected using EIA reactions which characterize antibody specificity. This technique is often used to confirm the specificity of antibodies which are detected by ELISA screening procedures.

NOTES

NOTES

NOTES

Tear Off Here

BUSINESS REPLY MAIL

FIRST-CLASS PERMIT NO 62282 LOS ANGELES, CA 90009

POSTAGE WILL BE PAID BY ADDRESSEE

Specialty Laboratories, Inc.

PO Box 92722
Los Angeles, California 90009-9920

Name _____

Title _____ Dept. _____

Specialty _____

Institution _____

Street _____

City _____ State _____ Zip Code _____

Check for Complimentary Items.

☐ Use and Interpretation of Tests in Clinical Immunology, 7th Ed., 1990.

☐ Use and Interpretation of Tests in Medical Microbiology, 2nd Ed., 1990.

☐ Please provide _____ additional copy(ies) of booklet(s) marked.

☐ Please provide _____ copy(ies) of fee schedule.

☐ Three-ring binder(s) for fee schedule.

Send _____ additional copies to:

Name _____ Title _____

Institution _____ Dept. _____

Street _____

City _____ State _____ Zip Code _____

GB1190